Current Topics in Pathology

Ergebnisse der Pathologie

53

Edited by

H.-W. Altmann, Würzburg · K. Benirschke, Hanover · A. Bohle, Tübingen
K. M. Brinkhous, Chapel Hill · P. Cohrs, Hannover · H. Cottier, Bern
M. Eder, München · P. Gedigk, Bonn · W. Giese, Münster · Chr. Hedinger, Zürich
S. Iijima, Hiroshima · W. H. Kirsten, Chicago · I. Klatzo, Bethesda
K. Lennert, Kiel · H. Meessen, Düsseldorf · W. Sandritter, Freiburg
G. Seifert, Hamburg · H. C. Stoerk, New York · H. U. Zollinger, Basel

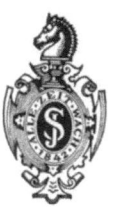

Springer-Verlag Berlin Heidelberg GmbH 1970

This work is subject to copyright. All rights are reserved, whether the whole or part of the material is concerned, specifically those of translation, reprinting, re-use of illustrations, broadcasting, reproduction by photocopying machine or similar means, and storage in data banks.

Under § 54 of the German Copyright Law where copies are made for other than private use, a fee is payable to the publisher, the amount of the fee to be determined by agreement with the publisher.

ISBN 978-3-662-30515-7   ISBN 978-3-662-30514-0 (eBook)
DOI 10.1007/978-3-662-30514-0

© by Springer-Verlag Berlin Heidelberg 1970
Originally published by Springer-Verlag Berlin Heidelberg New York in 1970.
Softcover reprint of the hardcover 1st edition 1970

Library of Congress Catalog Card Number 56-49162.

The use of general descriptive names, trade names, trade marks, etc. in this publication, even if the former are not especially identified, is not to be taken as a sign that such names, as understood by the Trade Marks and Merchandise Marks Act, may accordingly be used freely by anyone. Title No. 4755.

Contents

BÄSSLER, R.: The Morphology of Hormone Induced Structural Changes in the Female Breast. With 26 Figures 1

JELLINGER, K., SEITELBERGER, F.: Spongy Degeneration of the Central Nervous System in Infancy. With 15 Figures 90

HAMPERL, H.: The Myothelia (Myoepithelial Cells). Normal State; Regressive Changes; Hyperplasia; Tumors. With 29 Figures 161

Author Index 221

Subject Index 240

Institute of Pathological Anatomy, Johannes Gutenberg University, Mainz,
Direktor: Prof. Dr. H. BREDT

The Morphology of Hormone Induced Structural Changes in the Female Breast

ROLAND BÄSSLER

With 26 Figures

Table of Contents

I. Introduction	2
II. Development	3
1. Embryology of the Mammary Gland	3
2. Intrauterine Sexual Dimorphism	5
3. Development after Castration by X-Ray	5
4. Induction of Deformities by Hormones	5
5. Effect of Anti Androgens	6
III. Growth and Cytomorphology	7
1. Biometry of Normal Glandular Growth	7
2. Autoradiography and Biochemistry of the Mode of Proliferation of Epithelial Cells	8
3. Morphology of Proliferating Glandular Epithelium	11
IV. Effects on the Mammary Gland of Experimental Administration of Hormones	16
Ovarian Hormones	16
1. Oestrogen	16
2. Progesterone	23
3. Combined Action of Oestrogen and Progesterone	24
4. Histochemistry of the Connective Tissue During Hormone Action	27
5. Histochemical Enzyme Model	30
6. Electron-Microscopic Morphology of the Hormonally Stimulated Mammary Gland	32
Hormones of the Pituitary	38
1. Somatotropin (STH)	38
2. Adrenocorticotropin (ACTH)	39
3. Extract of the Anterior Lobe of the Pituitary	40
4. Transplants of the Anterior Lobe of the Pituitary	40
5. Mammogenic Effect of Transplanted Pituitary Tumours	41
6. Prolactin and the Morphology of the Pigeon Crop Test	41
7. Oxytocin	45
a) Galactokinetic Effect	45
b) Galactopoetic Effect	48
Hormones of the Adrenal Cortex	49
Testosterone	50
Thyroxin	52

Parathyroid Hormone and AT 10 54
Insulin 56
Relaxin 57
Summery 57
V. Pathology of Effects of Hormones on the Human Mammary Gland . . 57
  1. Pathomorphology of the Lobules of the Gland 58
  2. Morphology and Function of the Intralobular or Mantle- and Circumlobular or Supporting Connective Tissue 60
  3. Aetiology and Pathogenesis of Benign Dysplasias 63
  4. Galactorrhoea in the Human Mammary Gland 65
References 67

I. Introduction

Many morphological, physiological, and biochemical investigations have contributed to the classification of the endocrine regulatory mechanisms responsible for development and function of the mammary gland. These studies received their crucial impetus when the synthesis of the sex hormones had been achieved and from their experimental use. The history of the use of these drugs is thus also the history of the concept of control of the mammary gland by hormones. The individual factors and combinations of factors responsible for the normal growth of the glandular structure of the mammary gland, for its secretory function, and for its pathomorphology have been elucidated by systematic studies. The laws that have been discovered have led to a classification of reaction types and have made it possible for experimental observations to be compared with the responses of the human mammary gland. Current concepts of quantitative morphology and endocrinology have broadened our understanding of the mechanisms of the action of sex hormones on the mammary gland. Generally valid concepts of hormonal regulation of growth and metabolism have been derived from this.

The structural changes of the mammary gland, discovered in experimental work and reported initially in the gynaecological and anatomical literature, are now largely objects of research in the fields of endocrinology, galactology, and biochemistry. This explains why the literature on the subject is so dispersed. Recently, new aspects of fundamental research have arisen, chiefly concerning the sites of hormone action and intracellular enzyme induction by hormones.

It is my aim to present the essentials of the current views on changes of structure due to hormones, based on the reviews of the physiology by FOLLEY (1956), STEINBECK (1969), of the cytomorphology and anatomy by TURNER (1952), DABELOW (1957), MAYER and KLEIN (1961), the pathology of the breast by SCHULTZ (1933), GESCHICKTER (1948), HAAGENSEN (1956), GÖGL and LANG (1957), CUTLER (1961), and on the voluminous monograph by KON and COWIE (1961). Special consideration will be given to the results of electron-microscopic and histochemical investigations. The stress will be on results of experimental research, including some of the morphological aspects of dysplasia of the human mammary gland. Problems of experimental tumour pathology and of lactation will be covered only in so far as they are of importance for the explanation of the action of endocrines on the metabolism.

II. Development
1. Embryology of the Mammary Gland

The development of the mammary gland is essentially the same in monotremes, marsupials, and placentalia, independent of whether there are one or several pairs of glandular primordia. The embryology of the human mammary

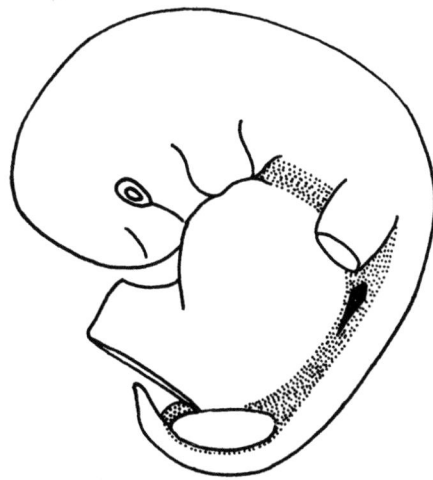

Fig. 1. Extent of galactic band (dotted) and milk-ridge (black line) in a human embryo, $11^1/_2$ mm long (32/33 days old). (After SCHMITT, 1898)

gland is similar to this phylogenesis, as the older descriptive morphological studies of KOELLIKER (1852), REIN (1882), BROUHA (1905), BERK (1913), LUSTIG (1915), and v. EGGELING (1927) have shown. Reconstructions by LUSTIG (1915), BROMAN (1927), and SPULER (1930), and histological studies by NEUMANN and OING (1929), THÖLEN (1949), and GRAUMANN (1950) have demonstrated that the glandular primordium differentiates continuously. This differentiation starts in human foetuses in the fifth week of germination with an epithelial thickening of the lateral wall of the trunk. It then passes into a phase of the development of individual primordia (Fig. 1). The following phases of development are distinguished:

1. *Milk-streak* (H. SCHMIDT, 1897; H. SCHMITT, 1898). A thickened band of epithelium, 2—4 layers high, develops at the lateral wall of the thorax and abdomen in human foetuses of 6—10 mm vertex-breach length (THÖLEN, 1949). This galactic band is the site of supernumerary primordia.

2. *Milk-line or Milk-ridge* (BROUHA, 1905; LUSTIG, 1915). The epithelium widens to 4—6 layers in the area of what later is to become the site of individual primordia, and the galactic band involutes, in foetuses measuring 9—15 mm (Fig. 1).

3. *Stages of hillock-, bud-shaped, or globular individual primordia.* The cell proliferations developing from the cranial part of the milk-ridge form small prominent hillocks, and then become depressed buds or globules in the mesenchyme. This happens during the 3rd and 4th months and is combined with an increase of local mesenchymal cells.

4. *A cone- or flask-shaped growth sector* with elongation of the epithelial primordium develops. Superficial desquamations of the epithelium cause the nipple groove to appear into which later the lactiferous tubules open.

5. The solid *epithelial proliferations* develop lumina in the 5th and 6th lunar months (THÖLEN, 1949). The primordium enlarges, and in foetuses of 15 cm length extends to the subcutis. At the end of pregnancy the peripheral ends of the proliferations enlarge and form terminal vesicles, usually filled with secretion (DABELOW, 1957).

This morphological analysis of the development of the mammary gland has been broadened by experimental work on embryos relating both to the initial phases of development (BALINSKY, 1950a, b; GRAUMANN, 1950; HARDY, 1950) and to the problems of sexual dimorphism and the induction of deformities by hormones (RAYNAUD, 1961).

The bud of the gland during the 3rd—5th foetal months consists of polygonal cells with chromatin-rich nuclei and is surrounded by a highly prismatic layer of cells (SPULER, 1930; HUGHES, 1950). — BALINSKY (1950) distinguished a phase of cell aggregation, a rest phase, and a phase of growth during proliferation. He made the notable observation that the mitosis index in the primordium was lower than in the surrounding epithelium. He concluded that the buds were formed by cell migration. The individual primordia, which are independent of each other, are formed by a mesenchymal inductor, the RNA-rich cells of which are supposed to be derived from Wolff's duct; they slowly lose their nucleic acid content. — GRAUMANN (1950) interpreted these interrelations to the surrounding mesenchyme during the budding stage as being due to a displacement of tissue fluid, because the epithelial cells of the budding stage are large and transparent and because the mesenchymal cells become denser.

2. Intrauterine Sexual Dimorphism

The question of the dependency of the embryonal development of the mammary gland on hormones has been investigated experimentally in explantates and histomorphologically:

According to BALINSKY (1950) skin explantates of ten days old mouse embryos had a globular stage of glandular development, which additions of hormone to the culture medium did not influence. — Similarly, HARDY (1950) had described developmental stages of the mammary gland in explantates of the chest wall of 10—13 days old mouse embryos that corresponded to the developmental stage of the 7th day. These observations indicate retardation, but neither inhibition nor stimulation.

The dimorphous histogenesis of the mammary gland appears in the mouse only after the 15th day of intrauterine development. The primordia in *female animals* are characterised by a narrower neck between bud and epidermis, with involution on the 16—17th day. This leads to the incorporation of the bud into the epidermis (RAYNAUD, 1961). The *male primordium*, on the other hand, shows a stronger circular mesenchymal reaction, which is of importance for further development and may be influenced by foetal testicular hormone (RAYNAUD, 1947; RAYNAUD, 1961) (Figs. 2a, b, c).

The results of these experimental studies indicate that the *early stages* (up to the 10—12th day) of the mammogenesis in the mouse are *independent of specific hormones*. The glandular development between the 12th and 14th day is in a highly *sensitive phase*, which has disappeared by the 15th day of development. The following observations provide evidence for this:

3. Development after Castration by X-Rays

When the gonads are treated with x-rays of 100,000—120,000 r on the 13th day, female foetuses show a degree of development of the primordium of the mammary gland that corresponds to that of the control animals. The glands of male foetuses behaved, on the other hand, like those of the female animals (RAYNAUD and FRILLEY, 1947, 1949; RAYNAUD, 1961). This means that the testes are responsible for the normal course of male development, i.e. separation of the epithelial buds from the epidermis and lack of an areola. — Gonadectomy in both sexes leads to female differentiation, indicating that this is a neutral, non-hormonal type (RAYNAUD, 1961).

4. Induction of Deformities by Hormones

Androgenic. When either pregnant mice or foetuses are injected with testosterone-propionate, the primordium of the mammary gland becomes masculinized (RAYNAUD, 1947a; RAYNAUD and RAYNAUD, 1954, 1961). It is concluded, that androgens normally prevent the development of nipples and extensive formation of mammary tissue in male fetuses (NEUMANN and ELGER, 1967). Sometimes it may cause athelia. Inhibition or lack of the endogenous androgens results in a female organogenesis of the mammary gland (ELGER and NEUMANN, 1966). The development of the gland of female animals is inhibited by androgens.

When *oestrogens* are injected into either mother animals or foetuses the development of both gland and nipple is stimulated. Arrest of mammogenesis in dose-dependency has also been observed, exhibiting as *amastia, micromastia* or *koilomastia* (pivot nipple) (RAYNAUD, 1947b, 1952). Also, secondary epithelial buds developed from primordia (Figs. 2D, E, F).

Injection of 40—150 mg oestradiol benzoate into the foetus produced 95% deformities, when the drug had been given on the 12—14th day. On the 15th day the deformity rate was a mere 5%. Injection into the mothers during the sensitive phase caused in dose-dependency derangements of the primordia:

50 mg oestrogen produced 5 % deformities of the mammary gland, 100—200 mg oestrogen 50%, and 500—1,000 mg oestrogen 90% (RAYNAUD and RAYNAUD, 1956).

Injection of *progesterone* (HOSHINO, 1966) in pregnant mice induce in female mice an inhibition in development of the duct system, but not athelia. The reaction in male mice is comparable with effects of anti-androgens. The mammary glands are developed like female mice.

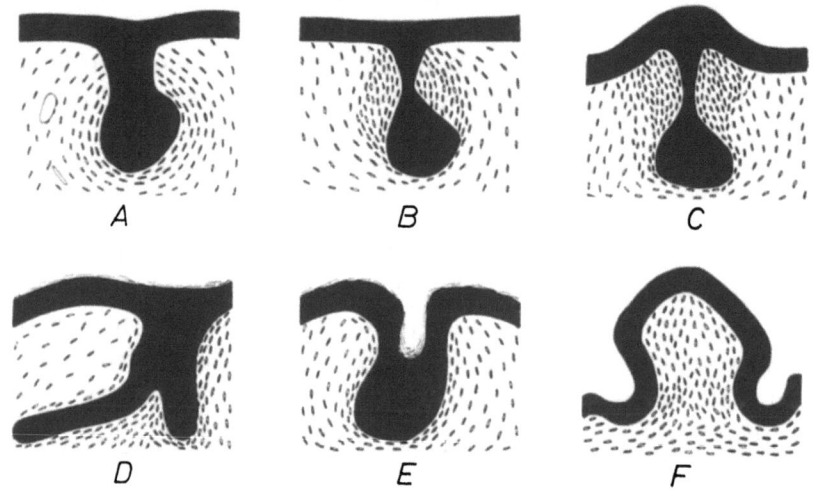

Fig. 2A—F. Schematic presentation of various types of development of the first inguinal glandular primordium of the mammary gland of the mouse (modified after RAYNAUD, 1947, 1961). A Female mouse, 15th day, 17 hours. B Male mouse, 15th day, 17 hours. C Female mouse, 15th day, 16 hours after treatment of the mother with testosterone. Development of narrow neck of the primordial gland and siting of mesenchymal reaction are very similar in B and C. D Female mouse, 18 days, thoracic bud with proliferation of two solid primordia of ducts after injection of oestradiol in foetuses on the 13th day. E Female mouse, 18 days, thoracic primordium after injection of oestradiol (75 mg) on the 13th day with production of an epithelial pocket with desquamated epithelium (coilomastia). F Female mouse, 18 days; suppression of development of mammary gland by injection of 94 mg oestradiol on the 13th day (amastia)

5. Effect of Anti-Androgens

When synthetic gestagenous steroids were studied, a substance with anti-androgenic action was isolated that was called cyproterone acetate (1, 2α-methylene-6-chloro-Δ4,6-pregnadiene-17α-ol-3,20-dion-17α-acetate). It became thus possible selectively to exclude testosterone in sex differentiation (HAMADA, NEUMANN, and JUNKMANN, 1963; JUNKMANN and NEUMANN, 1964; NEUMANN and ELGER, 1966; ELGER, V. BERSWORDT-WALLRABE, and NEUMANN, 1967). — Cyproterone acetate, when administered into the uterus, caused female differentiation of the mammary gland of male rat foetuses after the 13th day, with extensive epithelial proliferation and formation of an epithelial ridge corresponding to the nipple. This is evidence that *androgens of the foetal testis by themselves may inhibit the development of the mammary gland* (NEUMANN and ELGER, 1966). — Foetuses that were genetically male, and which had been feminized in utero by anti-androgens, behaved outside the uterus on combined hormone treatment like genetically female animals, began to lactate, and to form nipples (NEUMANN, ELGER and v. BERSWORDT-WALLRABE, 1966).

III. Growth and Cytomorphology
1. Biometry of Normal Glandular Growth

To the investigation of the tissue structure of the mammary gland has now been added the biometrical exploration of the structural changes that occur in the mammary gland under normal and abnormal conditions, resulting in further insights into morphogenesis and dynamics of function.

The earliest accounts of quantitative research are by GARDNER and STRONG (1935), VAN HEUVERSWYN, FOLLEY, and GARDNER (1939), FOLLEY, GUTKELCH and ZUCKERMAN (1939), and DUBOIS (1944), who had tried to study the growth of the mammary gland semi-quantitatively. RICHARDSON (1947, 1949, 1953, 1966, 1967) further developed these methods. Three quantitative aspects were presented: 1. The relationship between the growth of the mammary gland and the expansion of the body surface area. 2. The analysis of the extent of ramification of the lactiferous ducts, four steps of ramification and proliferation being stipulated (NANDI, 1958, 1959). 3. The determination of the total surface of the mammary gland. The relationship to the expansion of the body surface may be expressed by a formula. According to COWIE (1949), the mammary gland of the rat up to the 21st—23rd day develops isometrically compared with the body surface. Subsequently, growth becomes allometric under the influence of sex hormones and increases 3—5fold. This may be inhibited by ovarectomy. BENSON, COWIE, COX and GOLDZWEIG (1957) determined the volume of glandular tissue when they investigated the induced development of the mammary gland of the guinea pig. The assessment of the total surface of the secretory epithelium was based on a method developed by SHORT (1951) for the determination of the total surface of the pulmonary alveoli. This method has been used by RICHARDSON (1953) for the investigation of the mammary gland of the goat. CHALKLEY (1943) estimated the relative volumes of individual tissue components by relating, under the microscope, the areas of these components in histological sections to a system of specially arranged points. KIRKHAM and TURNER (1954) used biochemical methods for the quantitative assay of the glandular parenchyma. They assessed the increase or decrease of parenchyma by the increase or decrease of the numbers of cell nuclei, which, of course, are in proportion to desoxyribonucleic acid.

These quantitative methods had been used to assess the influence of hormones on the mammary gland and its morphological reactions. This was done by FOLLEY (1952, 1955), FLUX and MUNFORD (1957), BENSON, COWIE, COX and GOLDZWEIG (1957), and v. BERSWORDT-WALLRABE (1958a, b). The last author had studied in lactating mice, using volumetric, karyometric, and statistical methods, the involution of the gland under the influence of oestrogen.

Compared with the number of publications of quantitative studies about the effect of hormones, publications that describe quantitative studies of the structures of the mammary gland under physiological conditions, are sparse: SCHAIRER (1936) had differentiated the cell nuclei of the resting from those of the lactating cells by comparative measurements. WEBER, KITCHELL, and SAUTTER (1955) had determined the volume of the lobules in the mammary gland of the cow and had counted the alveoli of the individual lobules. — MOSIMANN (1957) measured the volume of cell nuclei in the epithelium of the mammary glands of goats and rats, in relationship to the state of function and after administration stilboestrol.

The writer and FLÖRCHINGER (1966a, b) had carried out systematic studies of the histometry of the mammary gland during normal functioning, during experimental galactostasis, and under the influence of an increased fluid supply, when Periston infusions had been given. By contrasting the findings in the periphery and the centre of the gland, of parenchyma and connective tissue, of height of epithelium and width of alveoli, certain correlative data about secretion, fluid transport, and absorption were obtained.

NICOLL's (1965) experiments have shown that mammary growth has no humoral autoregulation, so that there is no evidence for a feed-back mechanism by substances with mammotropic action. On the other hand, transplantations have indicated that there is a *regulating influence of local fat tissue* on glandular growth.

2. Autoradiographic and Biochemistry of the Mode of Proliferation of Epithelial Cells

Protein and nucleic acid synthesis in the mammary gland is subject to regulation by hormones; at the beginning of pregnancy these synthetic processes increase by several times their resting value. Post partum proliferation of the glandular epithelium is mainly due to prolactin, which regulates the production of cytoplasmatic proteins, DNA-synthesis, and cell proliferation (BALDWIN and MARTIN, 1968). Prolactin and cortisol are needed after hypophysectomy to stimulate RNA- and casein synthesis and the production of glucose-6-phosphate-dehydrogenase. This key enzyme increases 100fold 24 hours post partum; this indicates the shift of carbohydrate catabolism from the Emden-Meyerhof cycle to the oxidative pentose-phosphate cycle (GLOCK and MCLEAN, 1954; RAPOPORT, 1962). The intermediate metabolism is thus regulated to produce $NADPH_2$ for fatty acid synthesis to provide pentoses for nucleic acid requirements. Metabolic conditions for cell replenishment and cell differentiation are thus created by mammotropic substances.

The mammary gland is subject to hormonal stimulation, and during normal functioning belongs to the group of labile tissue elements, because desquamation in the lumina requires the perpetual replacement of cells. This replacement is done by the basal cells. Mitoses were observed only rarely, amitoses not at all (MAEDER, 1922; JEFFERS, 1935). The division into sequent phases of proliferation and differentiation (ALTMANN, 1966) suggests comparison with the endometrium. Proliferation and cellular differentiation of the epithelium are closely related in the mammary gland during pregnancy. Structural differences certainly narrow down as pregnancy goes on, compared with functioning, i.e. lactation, but they remain important, because the specific protein casein is synthesised in the post partum phase only.

According to *autoradiographic studies* the time needed for DNA-synthesis in the nuclei of epithelial cells of the resting mammary gland of C_3H/HeJ mice was 20.7 hours. When the mammary gland was stimulated for three days with oestradiol and progesterone, the S-phase lasted for 10.7 hours (BRESCIANI, 1964) only. After pretreatment for 2—3 weeks the time needed for synthesis was 8.8 hours (BRESCIANI, 1965). These observations demonstrate that ovarian hormones accelerate synthesis of DNA in the mammary gland. Both synthesis and synchronicity of chromosome duplication are affected by the hormones through co-factors. According to JERVELL, DINIZ, and MUELLER (1958) the rate of assimilation of C^{14}-O_2 into the nucleotides adenine, guanine, and uridine, is increased by oestrogen, before the amount of RNA increases. — From the point of view of cytomorphology this explains the increased chromatin content and the enlarged cell nuclei, which synthetize more protein and RNA, of hormone stimulated mammary glands. This has been demonstrated in model studies of functional nuclear swellings by STÖCKER (1962, 1964), SANDRITTER, FEDERLIN, and PFEIFER (1964). Comparative studies with double thymidine labelling by BANERJEE and WALKER (1967) gave the following results:

Table 1. *Time required for synthesis of DNA in the mammary gland*

Glandular cells of the lactiferous tubules	virgin C_3H-mice	20.7 hrs.[a]	S-phase
Pre-lactating breast	8th day of pregnancy	14.1 hrs.	S-phase
Pre-lactating breast	15th day of pregnancy	8.2 hrs.	S-phase
Pre-lactating breast	15th day of pregnancy	9.4 hrs.	S-phase
Lactating breast	2nd day	8.5 hrs.	S-phase
Transplant of pre-lactating breast (15th day)	in virgin mouse	21.5 hrs.	S-phase

[a] According to BRESCIANI (1964).

DNA-synthesis in the mammary gland increases 2—3fold during pregnancy and lactation. This is in conformity with the increase of cell reproduction and proliferation, compared with the resting gland. TRAURIG (1967a, b) has shown by autoradiographic studies that the distribution of epithelial proliferations in the mammary gland during pregnancy is bimodal. There is a maximum at the 4th day, at the time of implantation. A second peak on the 12th day coincides with the beginning of progesterone secretion of the placenta of the mouse.

During this phase of development the epithelium of the lactiferous tubules is identical with that of the epithelium of the lobules. During lactation the greatest number of labelled cells was found on the 2nd and 3rd day (TRAURIG, 1957b) (Fig. 3). During these days the secretory activity of the glandular epithelium also rises, and this is accompanied by enlargement of the terminal

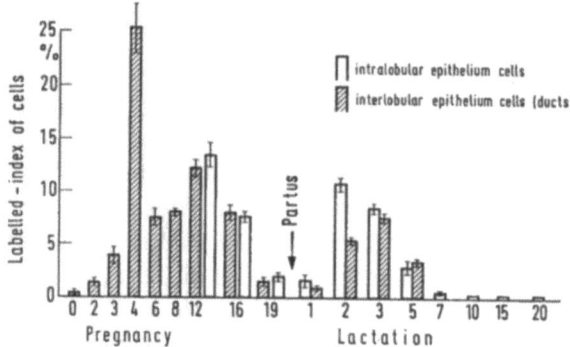

Fig. 3. Summary of autoradiographic examinations with H³-labelled thymidin of epithelial cells of the pregnant and lactating mammary gland of the mouse. (Modified after TRAURIG, 1967a, b)

buds of the lobules and formation of alveoli (BÄSSLER und FLÖRCHINGER, 1966a). The number of labelled myoepithelial cells is greatest too, on the 2nd, 3rd, and 5th day post partum, thus indicating their ability to proliferate. The fibroblasts of the intra- and interlobular stromas show the same behaviour.

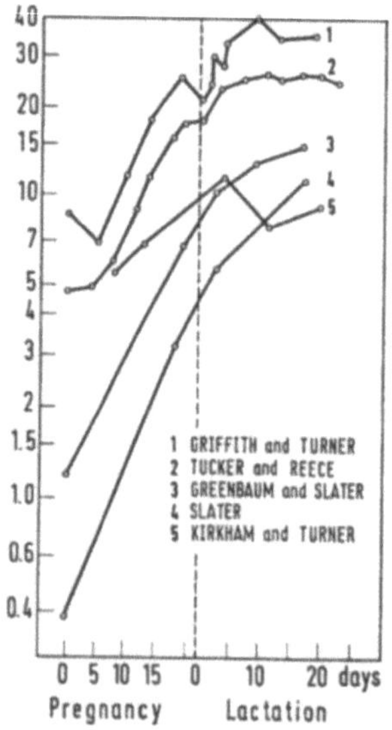

Biochemical studies of the DNA-content of the mammary gland during pregnancy and lactation have demonstrated that nucleic acids rise intensively and continuously, obtaining maximal values within the first 5—8 days of lactation (Fig. 4) (KIRKHAM and TURNER, 1953; GREENBAUM and SLATER, 1957; GRIFFITH and TURNER, 1957, 1961; MOON, 1962; NELSON, HEYTLER and CIACCO, 1962; TUCKER and REECE, 1963a, b, c; MUNFORD, 1964). When lactation lasts as long as 40—60 days, the DNA-content remains constant, whilst RNA decreases. The body weight of the young animal also diminishes (TUCKER and REECE, 1963b). During involution DNA and RNA greatly decrease within a few days. The effect of oestrogens, administered at this time, is accelerating, that of oestrogens together with progesterone inhibitory (TUCKER and REECE, 1963c; GRIFFITH and TURNER, 1961c). — Studies of experimentally induced growth (MOON, GRIFFITH, and TURNER, 1959; TUCKER and REECE, 1963d) underscore the significance both of the DNA-content as indicator of glandular growth and of the (simultaneous) increase of protein synthesis. —

Fig. 4. Summary of rise of DNA in the pregnant and lactating mammary gland according to different authors. (Modified after MUNFORD, 1964)

Discrepancies found in autoradiographic observations (TRAURIG, 1967) are due to the manner in which the glandular tissue has been prepared, because the admixture of connective tissue, fat, intramammary lymph nodes, and bloodvessels is usually not taken into account when the tissues are homogenised.

3. Morphology of Proliferating Glandular Epithelium

The epithelium of the lactiferous tubules and of lobules consists of a regular, palisade-type layer of cylindrical surface epithelia and of flat or cubical cells as basal layer (V. EGGELING, 1927; SCHULTZ, 1933; DABELOW, 1957).

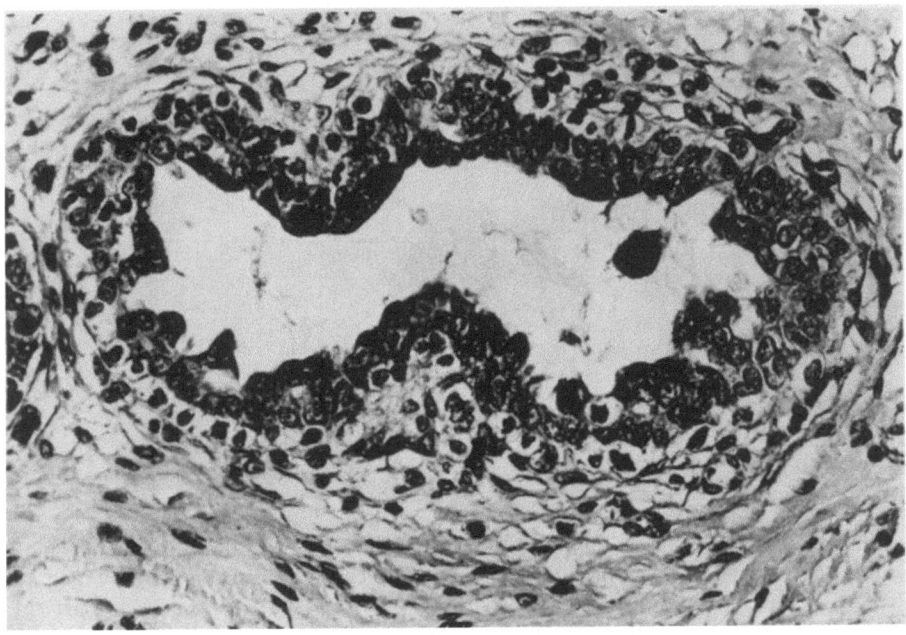

Fig. 5. Duct with considerable proliferation of epithelium and mitoses in gynaecomastia. Superficial cell layer dark, basal cell layer clear. Proliferation of histiocytes and fibroblasts in mantle tissue. Bouin, paraffin, enlargement 230 ×

The height of the epithelium is related to the width of the lactiferous tubules and lobules. Some of the basal cells contain myofilaments and constitute the system of myoepithelial cells. In the lumina of human and animal mammary glands droplets of a protein-containing secretion are often found, this being a product of apocrine secretory processes. The sex hormones, especially oestrogen, stimulate the glandular epithelium to proliferate. The epithelium becomes multilayered and forms buds and papillae, contingent upon the intensity of the hormonal stimulation. The epithelial cells differentiate more than normally into large clear cells and basophilic dark cells, the latter being situated superficially and surrounding the lumen (Fig. 5). The cells change further in that the nuclei enlarge, chromatin increases, and large nucleoli and mitoses emerge. The intracanalicular buds also consist of these cells. In the basal row of cells highly transparent cell plasma structures may be seen. GRAUMANN (1953) called these cells in the male mammary gland "clear epithelia", and VOGLER (1947) mentioned "clear cells" in Feyrter's sense.

When seen under the light microscope, epithelial proliferations are characterized by an irregular increase of cell layers, which may protrude into the lumen as individual cell buds or as groups of cells with small papillae. These proliferations reveal themselves, as in animal experiments, under the influence,

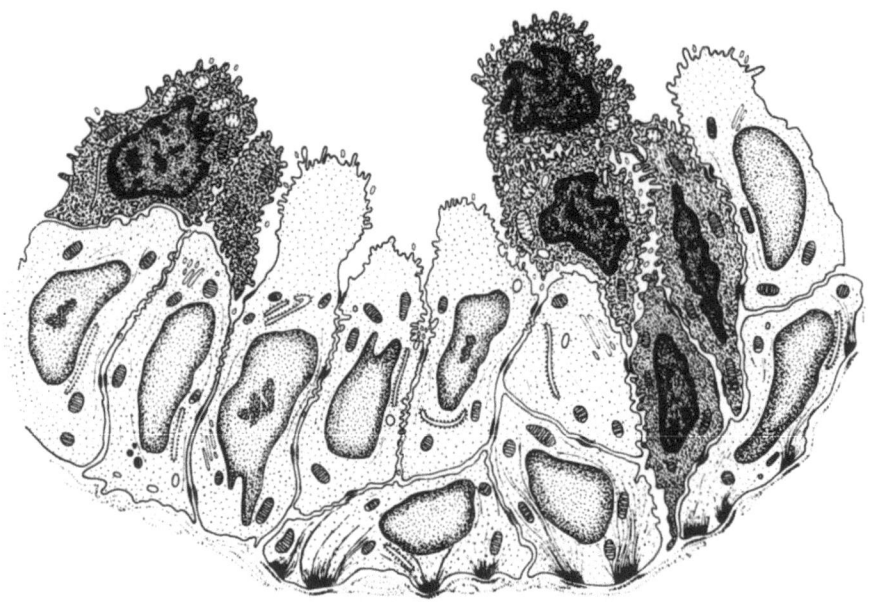

Fig. 6. Schematic representation of proliferation of cells in a duct in gynaecomastia, according to electron-microscopic findings. The clear cells contain filaments, which insert basally on hemidesmosomes. Superficially they form budshaped processes of the cytoplasm. — Dark cells and cells with intercellular dehiscences and regressive changes are also present (superficial cells)

of exogenous or endogenous oestrogen, as evidenced by the occurrence of gynaecomastia after application of oestrogen (Fig. 5): the proliferating epithelium consists of a basal layer of transparent cells with mitoses, which are covered by several layers of basophilic epithelia, and which protrude as pseudopapillary cell groups into the lumen. Individual cells desquamate, and there is a little secretion. In the stroma loosening and cellulation are seen. — According to CASPERSSON (1950) the basophilia of the cytoplasm of the dark superficial cells indicates a large amount of RNA and of ergastoplasm as morphological expression of intensive protein synthesis. —

This microscopical picture may be contrasted with a schematic representation of electron-microscopic findings in gynaecomastia. BÄSSLER and SCHÄFER (1968, 1969a) claim that the shape and structure of clear basal cells and basophilic superficial cells become evident when hormone induced proliferation (Fig. 6) occurs.

Electron-microscopic examination of the mammary gland and of carcinomas of the mammary gland (HAGUENAU, 1959; HAGUENAU and ARNOULT, 1959) have revealed cell forms that have been divided into A and B types. WAUGH and VAN HOEVEN (1962) have questioned this categorization and have thought the A cells to be artefacts. BUSCH and MERKER (1968) have claimed that the dark (A) cells in carcinomas are the outcome of supravital reactions to the fixing compound. BERGER (1964), on the other hand, still believes in the A-B grouping in fibrocystic mastopathy and in carcinomas. — My own investigations of the cytomorphology of the female and male mammary gland, of gynaecomastia, and of highly differentiated and anaplastic carcinomas have led me to classify the epithelial cells as follows:

1. The *A-cell* is a cell that is rich in ribosomes and therefore appears dark in the electron-microscope (Fig. 7). The nucleus is rich in chromatin and partly lobulated. There is very little ergastoplasm. This type corresponds to the basophilic form in the light microscope. — The isomorphism of this type, the lack of regressive changes, and the siting in groups indicate that these cells are part of the epithelium and occur chiefly under the influence of proliferation. The action of oestrogen on the mammary gland (BÄSSLER and FORSSMANN, 1964) and on the uterus (ROSS and KLEBANOFF, 1967) in experiments seems to show that the high ribosome content of these cells is the response of protein synthesis to stimulation by hormones.

2. The *B-cell* or *Chief cell*, which numerically preponderates, has a clear, transparent cytoplasm, a round or oval nucleus, and smooth cell membranes. These cells are held together in groups by desmosomes, and microvilli occur as differentiation products of the surface of the lumen. They contain fewer ribosomes than A-cells. The chief cells of the normal female and male mammary glands have no or sparse fibrillar cytoplasmatic structures, although proliferating cells and tumours often contain filaments of 50—80 Å diameter (Fig. 7).

My own observations have demonstrated that the chief cell is the essential structural element in the acini of female and male mammary gland (BÄSSLER and SCHÄFER, 1969b). Its content of ribosomes and filaments varies greatly, so that this cannot be used as such for the classification of these cells. I believe that the occurrence of filaments and of a dense felt of fibres in the cell plasma is an indication of a differentiation process. The ability of these cells to produce fibres is ubiquitous and is used when the cells proliferate. These cytoplasmatic filaments morphologically and dimensionally correspond to those of myoepithelial cells. The fibres in the myoepithelium are denser and contractile. In the chief cells the cytoplasmatic fibrils present structures that correspond to tonofilaments as stabilizing structures, as found in other epithelial cells also in the endothelium of lymph and blood capillaries (SCHIPP, 1968). The occurrence of filaments in the cytoplasm does *not justify the designation of all cells that contain fibrils as myoepithelial cells*, because this term includes the ability to contract and a special localization.

Large clear cells that have the morphological properties of chief cells also predominate in the lactiferous tubules and acini of the mammary glands of rats. In experimental work when sex hormones are given cell forms develop with a variety of para- and metaplasmatic inclusions (compare p. 35).

3. *The myoepithelial cells*, which rest upon the basal membrane as elongated cell bodies (Fig. 8), are regular elements of the excretory ducts, of acini, and of alveoli. The cell nucleus usually protrudes within the cell groups and rests

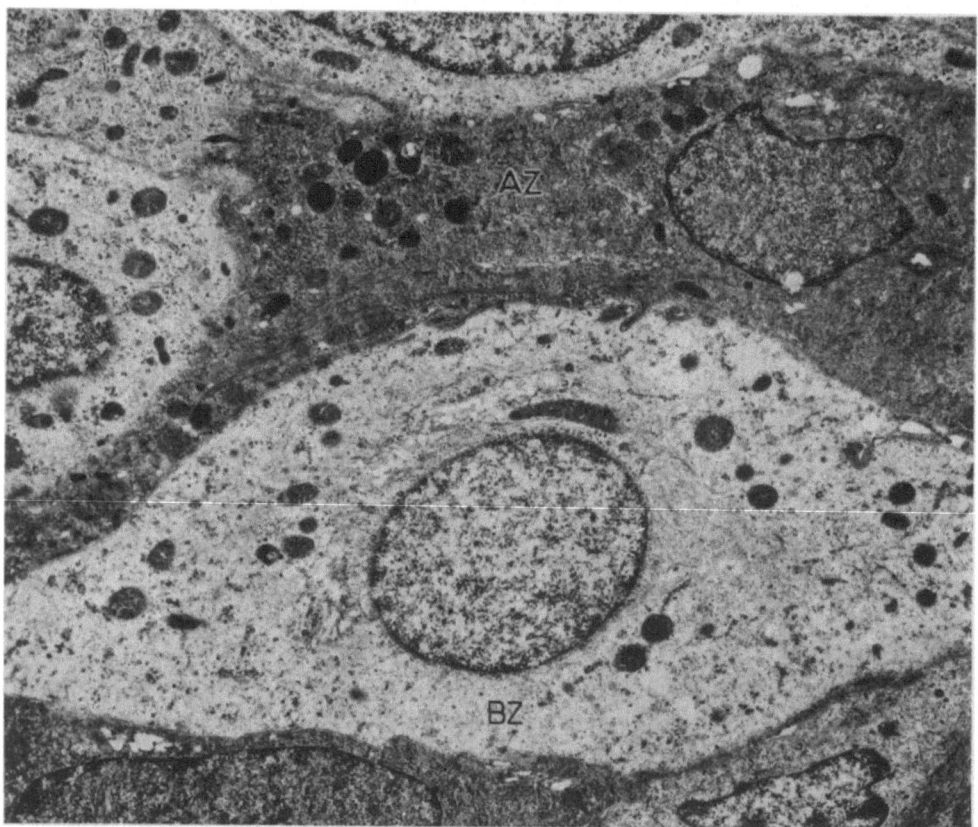

Fig. 7. Group of cells with dark A-cell (*AZ*): cytoplasm is rich in ribosomes and has bordering filaments. There are also clear B-cells (*BZ*): transparent cytoplasm, circumnuclear filaments, serrations with neighbouring cells. From a lobular carcinoma of a female. Record no. 1829/67: em. magnification 3,000; in the figure 9,600 ×

upon them like a shell upon the snail. When enlarged (lactation, congestion of secretion) the cell is flattened to a ribbon and is only recognizable by its parallel bundles of filaments. The first description of their electron microscopic structure in the female mammary gland was given by LANGER and HUHN (1958); this was followed by the papers by TAKAHASHI (1958) and HAGUENAU (1959). It was possible to present the functional phases of myoepithelial cells by selective representation by impregnation with silver (HAMPERL, 1940; KUZMA, 1943; RICHARDSON, 1949/50; and LINZELL, 1952, 1955) and by determination of alkaline phosphatase with the azo-dyestuff method (BÄSSLER, SCHÄFER, and PAEK, 1967; BÄSSLER and BRETHFELD, 1968).

4. These cell types seen at the luminal surface of the cell groups are called *superficial cells*. They possess wide intercellular spaces, indicating a loosening of the cellular structure. They possess, moreover, an optically dark cytoplasm, rich in ribosomes, with wide fissures of the ergastoplasm. The mitochondria are usually swollen. The cytoplasmatic changes are evidence of regressive alterations. These, together with their localization and the formation of inter-

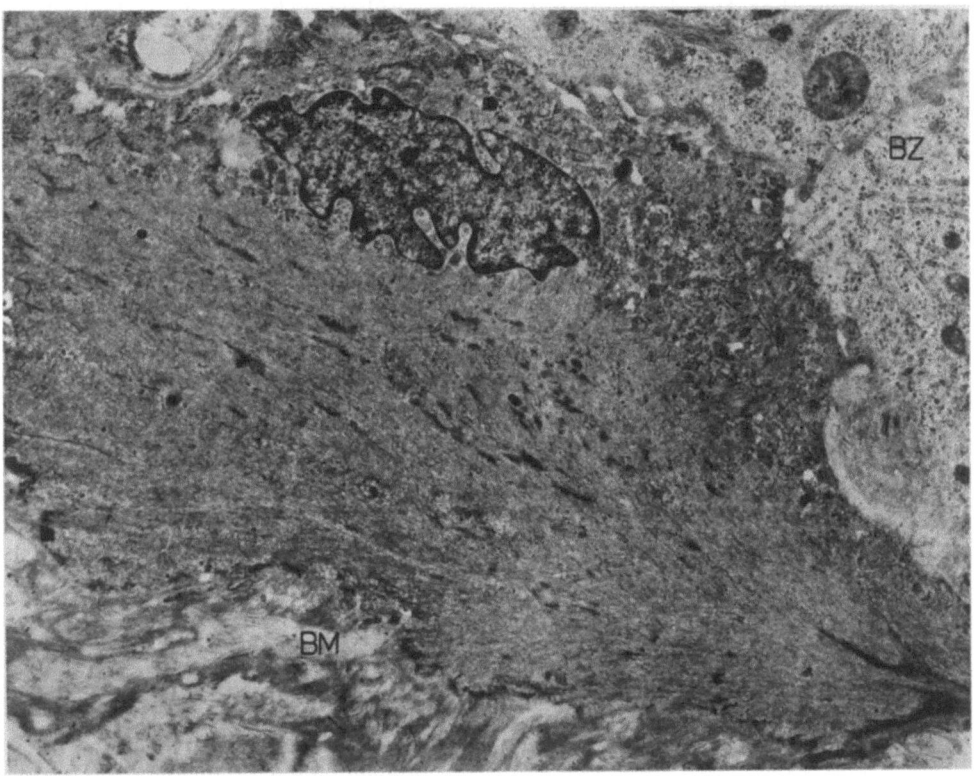

Fig. 8. Myoepithelial cell of the female mammary gland with dense fibrils, spotted densities, and hemidesmosomes. The nucleus is lobular, turned towards the epithelial cells and surrounded by organelles. Basal membrane structures (*BM*). At the margin a B-cell (*BZ*). Record no. 1832/67; em. magnification 3,000; in the figure 9,600 ×

cellular dehiscences, indicate a detachment from the cell group. Some groups of cells may remain in contact with the epithelial surface and may form epithelial buds or bridges, which protrude into the lumen. They are characteristic for gynaecomastia and are the typical outcome of experimental administration of oestrogen (Fig. 6). These superficial cells are therefore thought to be an indication of increased proliferation of the epithelium under the influence of hormones. The intensity of cell replacement is correlated with the degree of regressive changes in the cytoplasm of these cells.

Electron-microscopic findings of the human mammary gland may be compared from a cytomorphological point of view with the proliferations induced by hormones in animals. The mammary gland of the virgin rat contains clear cells, rich in ribosomes, too. But after three days of treatment with oestrogen (5γ/d) cells of differing basophilia appear in the loosened epithelium with intercellular gaps, which probably belong to one of the above categories. The cell types are not found in regular layers. The clear chief cells and the dark A-cells are found in equal numbers both in the base of the acinus and in the intermediary zone.

I believe that the development of these polymorphous cells, which differ in their ribosome content, is due to proliferation of the glandular epithelium, caused by hormones, especially by oestrogen.

IV. Effects on the Mammary Gland of Experimental Administration of Hormones
Ovarian Hormones
1. Oestrogen

Earlier investigations have shown that the mammary glands of different species react differently to oestrogen, when the hormone is administered in physiological doses. They may react either with proliferation of lactiferous tubules or with growth of tubules and simultaneous development of alveoli. FOLLEY in a comparative study (1956) demonstrated similar morphogenetic effects on certain species, when oestrogen was administered continuously (Table 2). Tissue response changes, however, when large doses are given continuously.

Table 2. *Effect of oestrogen on the mammary glands of different species*

1. Type: rat, mouse, rabbit, cat	→ growth of tubules, low-grade development of alveoli
2. Type: guinea pig, monkey, goat, cow	→ growth of tubules, intensive lobulo-alveolar development
3. Type: dog, ferret	→ low-grade growth of tubules

At first, differing statements about the hormone induced development of the mammary gland were made (LAQUEUR and DE JONGH, 1928; WEICHERT, BOYD, and COHEN, 1934). Out of this developed with increasing experimental experience a unitary concept of the mechanism of action. The essential parameters for the assessment of hormonal stimulation are the ages and weights of the animals, time of application, previous castration, hypophysectomy, and adrenalectomy (triple operation), single injections or depot effect, and duration of hormone supply.

In *newborn rats* oestrogen causes no glandular growth in the first and second weeks post partum, even when large doses ($100\ \gamma$/day) are given. In the third week, however, the lactiferous tubules dilate and form buds, when doses as small as $\frac{1}{10}\gamma/d$ are given (ASTWOOD, GESCHICKTER, and RAUSCH, 1937). — LEWIS and TURNER (1941) and AHRÉN (1959) discovered a morphological test for the minimum dose of oestrogen that would produce proliferation of the lactiferous tubules in castrated adult rats. The first named authors gave 0.25 γ—1 γ/d stilboestrol, the second named 1 γ/d as minimum dose. But even 10 γ/d induced limited growth of alveoli. TRENTIN and TURNER (1947) and CURTISS (1949) had obtained similar results when administering oestradiol propionate. REECE and LEATHEM (1945) had no success with the same drug.

The mammary glands of non-castrated rats grew intensively when oestradiol propionate was applied topically (LEONHARD and REECE, 1942). This was ineffectual if preceded by hypophysectomy (LEONHARD and REECE, 1942). — In rabbits and men unilateral topical inunction of follicular hormone (1,000 IU for 14—22 days) caused hyperplasia of the mammary gland with enlargement of the areola, and in men gynaecomastia (KUNERT, 1951).

Injections and implantations. The majority of experiments that had been carried out on castrated rats (WERNER, 1938; FAUVET, 1940; LEWIS and TURNER, 1941; WATTENWYL, 1949; TRENTIN and TURNER, 1947; CURTISS, 1949; LYONS, 1951; SMITH, 1955; AHRÉN, 1959; MOON and TURNER, 1960; McDONALD and REECE, 1962; reviews by MEITES, 1959a, and JACOBSOHN, 1961) showed that oestradiol dipropionate, oestradiol benzoate, and stilboestrol, in varying dosages and given by injection for up to 30 days, caused development of lactiferous tubules with formation of buds and development of alveoli of different widths. — Together with LIESER (1954) I demonstrated that the proliferation of the glandular system depended upon dose and duration of action: administration of 5 γ/d of oestradiol propionate (Progynon oleosum, Schering) resulted on the 20th and 50th day in increasing development of lactiferous ducts with dilatation, overgrowth of epithelium in the form of small papillomas, and lateral outgrowths. Large doses (50 γ/day) produced after 20 days multiple cysts, which enclosed a secretion containing both protein and fat. This oestrogenic effect was weak in non-castrated animals (HEROLD and EFFKEMANN, 1936), which instead showed proliferation and lobuloalveolar overgrowth, followed by an increase of circumcanalicular and intralobular connective tissue.

Even larger doses of oestrogen (30—200 γ/d) and the longer lasting treatment (20 to more than 300 days) caused the glandular tissue to react with proliferation and dilatation of the tubules, with formation of cysts and overgrowth of epithelium. The results of my own investigations are shown in Fig. 9. They demonstrate the regularity with which these effects occurred in castrated and non-castrated female rats. The studies of McEUEN, SELYE and COLLIP (1936), ASTWOOD, GESCHICKTER and RAUSCH (1937), HEROLD and EFFKEMANN (1937), ASTWOOD and GESCHICKTER (1938), BIEDERMANN (1938), EMGE (1938), and GRUMBRECHT (1940) report the same results. — The relationships in time between the effect of oestrogen and morphogenesis were given

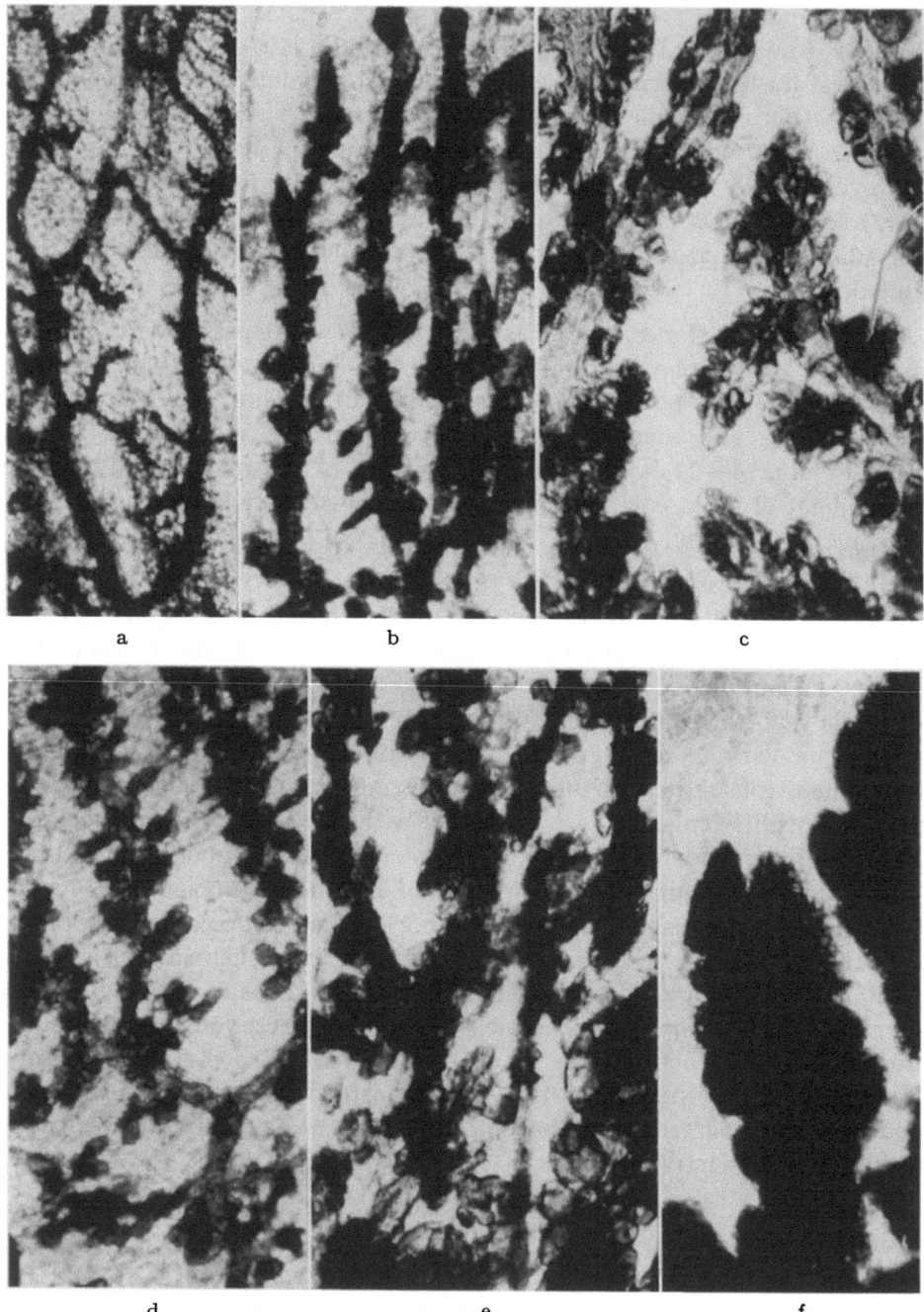

Fig. 9a—f. Morphology of the female mammary gland (rat) after treatment with hormones. a Castrated control animal. b Castrated, 5 γ/20 d Progynon: little dilatation of ducts, development of lateral arborization. c Castrated, 5 γ/50 d Progynon: considerable dilatation of ducts with increasedly developing lateral arborization. d Normal animal, 50 γ/20 d Progynon: regular branching of ducts and intensive arborization. A tendency to formation of lobuli. e Normal animal, 50 γ/50 d Progynon: general dilatation of ducts with dilated adventitious branchings. f Castrated, 10 mg/17 d Proluton: intensive and regular formation of lobuli. Formalin, alumcarmine, magnification 10 ×

by EISEN (1942) (implantation of oestradiol propionate, 1—20 mg for up to 27 months): the sequence was:

Proliferation of the tubular system	26th day
Secretion	40— 60th day
Dilatation of ducts	60— 90th day
Formation of cysts of up to 1 cm diameter	90—150th day
Fibrosing	150—180th day

The changes that occurred afterwards seemed to be comparable from a pathogenetic point of view with *fibro-cystic mastopathy*, by concensus of all authors, when treatment had been continued for a long time.

Influence on the oestrogenic activity by other drugs. Castration and adrenalectomy diminished the oestrogenic effect (TRENTIN and TURNER, 1947). After thyroidectomy the tubules developed energetically. When thyroxin and oestrogen were given after castration and thyroidectomy, the tubules grew and showed proliferation at the ends and sides (LEONARD and REECE, 1941). Combinations of the drugs and protamine-zinc-insulin (AHRÉN, 1959) given to castrated, hypophysectomized rats resulted in little proliferation only. — Oestrogen (0.1 mg) together with desoxycorticosterone acetate (5 mg/10 d) caused lobular development in castrated rats. Doubling of the dose was ineffective (SMITH and BRAVERMANN, 1953).

The same hormones are ineffective after hypophysectomy [LEONARD and REECE (1941)]. — LYONS, JOHNSON, COLE and LI (1955), LYONS LI and JOHNSON (1957), and LYONS, LI and JOHNSON (1958) carried out systematic studies to show that STH when given together with oestrogen had a definite proliferating effect on the lactiferous tubules after castration and hypophysectomy. When adrenalectomy was performed at the same time, oestrogen, STH, and desoxycorticosterone acetate caused proliferation of the lactiferous tubules, equal to that of normal 30—40 days old rats. After triple operation oestrogen, desoxycorticosterone acetate, STH, progesterone, prolactin, and prednisolone, all administered at the same time, caused uniform lobuloalveolar differentiation of the gland. — Oestradiol in conjunction with either acetylcholine or epinephrine equally produced a lobular and alveolar glandular structure with secretion (MEITES, 1959).

The *mouse* reacts to oestrogen with growth of the lactiferous tubules, proliferation, and formation of alveoli. — In non-castrated animals dose-dependent proliferations are produced with alveolar differentiation that often is quite considerable (GARDNER, SMITH, and STRONG, 1935). Smaller doses of oestrogen (up to 10 mg/week) produce better development than large quantities (50 mg/week), which produce tumours after 220 days (GARDNER, 1941). TRENTIN and TURNER (1948) gave oestradiol benzoate for three days. This caused production of buds, but to only a sixth of the extent of that produced by the injection treatment, taking the development of the tubules as control standard. Growth of ducts, budding with secretion, and development of alveoli were evoked after castration (DAANE and LYONS, 1954). Castration and hypophysectomy prevented development (GARDNER, 1940; TRENTIN and

TURNER, 1948; FERGUSON and VISSCHER, 1953; FERGUSON, 1956). — Oestrogen and extract of the anterior lobe of the pituitary (in mouse units with mammogenic action) gave different, though positive reactions in different strains of mice (MIXNER and TURNER, 1957), which indicated different sensitivities for oestrogen (MÜHLBROCK, 1948). Thyroxin given together with oestrogen and progesterone greatly increased the development of the mammary gland (MIXNER and TURNER, 1942c). According to MIXNER and TURNER (1942b) the effect of desoxycorticosterone acetate and oestrogen was about a third of that of progesterone. This combination when given to male hypophysectomized mice caused intensive proliferation (GARDNER, 1940), as did the combination of oestradiol propionate and purified prolactin (GARDNER and WHITE, 1941). — FERGUSON (1956) calculated that the rate of growth was normal with oestrogen, progesterone, prolactin, and STH, and that this was not increased by addition of ACTH and thyroxin.

FRAZIER and MU (1935) and LEWIS and TURNER (1941) had found in rabbits that oestrogen caused development of ducts with lobulation. According to SCHARF and LYONS (1941) five weekly injections of oestrogen (30—960 IU) caused gradual formation of ducts, of lobuli with secretion, and of cysts. LEWIS and TURNER (1942b) published their comparative investigations of the effect of percutaneous oestrogen on growth. According to JACOBSOHN (1954) the anterior lobe of the pituitary is prerequisite for the effect of ovarian hormones on the mammary gland. — According to recent observations by NORGREN (1966) the optimal dose lies between 2.5—5 mg/d when administered for 28—45 days. Larger quantities of oestrogen cause disorders of growth and of differentiation.

Second group: Guinea pigs, monkeys, cows, goats.

The reaction to oestrogen of the mammary tissues of these species is characterized by growth of the lactiferous tubules and lobulo-alveolar proliferation of the parenchyma.

This had been thought to be due solely to the effect of oestrogen (TURNER and GOMEZ, 1934; NELSON, 1937). LEWIS and TURNER (1942a) remarked on the dose dependency of lobulation; COWIE (1951) and SMITH and RICHTERICH (1958) pointed to the long duration of the experiments, which caused extensive formation of alveoli.

Local application had similar results (NELSON, 1941). HÖHN (1957) had shown recently that a progesterone that originates in the adrenal cortex was likely to be of importance for the lobular and alveolar development of the mammary glands of these species, because in castrated and adrenalectomized animals treatment with oestrogen caused proliferation of the tubuli only. BENSON, COWIE, COX and GOLDZWEIG (1957), too, had to use a combination of oestrogen and progesterone to obtain optimal development. — GARRETT and TALMAGE (1952) have reported on potentiation by relaxin.

Experimental studies of the mammary glands of *monkeys* by FOLLEY, GUTKELCH, and ZUCKERMAN (1939), GARDNER (1941), CHAMBERLAIN, GARDNER and ALLEN (1941; local application), GESCHICKTER and SPEERT (1941), and

SPEERT (1948) have provided evidence that oestrogens may produce a mammary structure that is completely ductular and lobuloalveolar. It is tempting to ascribe to this process in primates a special *significance for the pathology of the human mammary gland*. In long-term experiments, lasting seven years and seven months, with non-castrated and castrated rhesus monkeys (GESCHICKTER and HARTMAN, 1959) the lobular structure remained intact. Islets of pale epithelium, ectasias of the lobules, secretion, and fibroses, as regressive changes, began to appear. Although stimulation with oestrogens continued for years, no carcinomas were observed.

In ruminants the effect of oestrogen has been examined chiefly on the udder of *goats*.

MIXNER and TURNER (1943) had found that stilboestrol disturbed the development of the mammary gland, producing cysts and papillary proliferations of the epithelium. This became less obtrusive when progesterone was administered at the same time. COWIE, FOLLEY, MALPRESS, and RICHARDSEN (1952), BENSON, COWIE, COX, FLUX and FOLLEY, (1955) in comparative studies of the influence of both hormones in varying dosages have demonstrated abnormal folds and papillae of the alveolar epithelium when large doses of oestrogen were given, even when given together with progesterone. When smaller doses of oestrogen and progesterone were given the reactions became milder, so that the substance was considered essential for the development of the udder (BENSON, COWIE, FOLLEY and TINDAL, 1959).

The *udder of the cow* behaves similarly and for physiological development requires both oestrogens and progesterone (SYKES and WRENN, 1950, 1951; REINEKE, MEITES, CAIRY, and HUFFMAN, 1952; MEITES, 1960; FOLLEY, 1956). When oestrogen alone was given to cows, irregular structures of the alveoli were produced, which were characterized by small compressed and by ectatic-cystic areas.

The last group of species is distinguished by the fact that oestrogens have no or hardly any effect on the development of the mammary gland. *Ferrets and bitches* belong to this group. GARDNER (1941) had found in experiments with oestradiol benzoate that the lactiferous tubules of bitches grew only slightly or not at all even though the drug had been applied for up to 109 weeks.

The effect of *oestrogens* on the *mammary gland of male rats* was studied, so that the structural changes of gynaecomastia might be imitated. In my own experiments (BÄSSLER and SCHÄFER, 1968) the mammary glands of young male rats responded to Progynon ($10\,\gamma/d$) after five and 10 days with growth of tubules and proliferation of the adventive-buds (Fig. 11). The same treatment applied to castrated animals resulted in intensive proliferation with production of small alveoli, a picture that simulated that of the female hormone-stimulated breast (Fig. 9). This development of the mammary gland is essentially determined by the antagonistic effect of testosterone. This statement may be used to clarify the pathogenesis of hormonally stimulated arborization in gynaecomastia, a process based on relative or absolute preponderance of oestrogens or of compounds with oestrogenic effect.

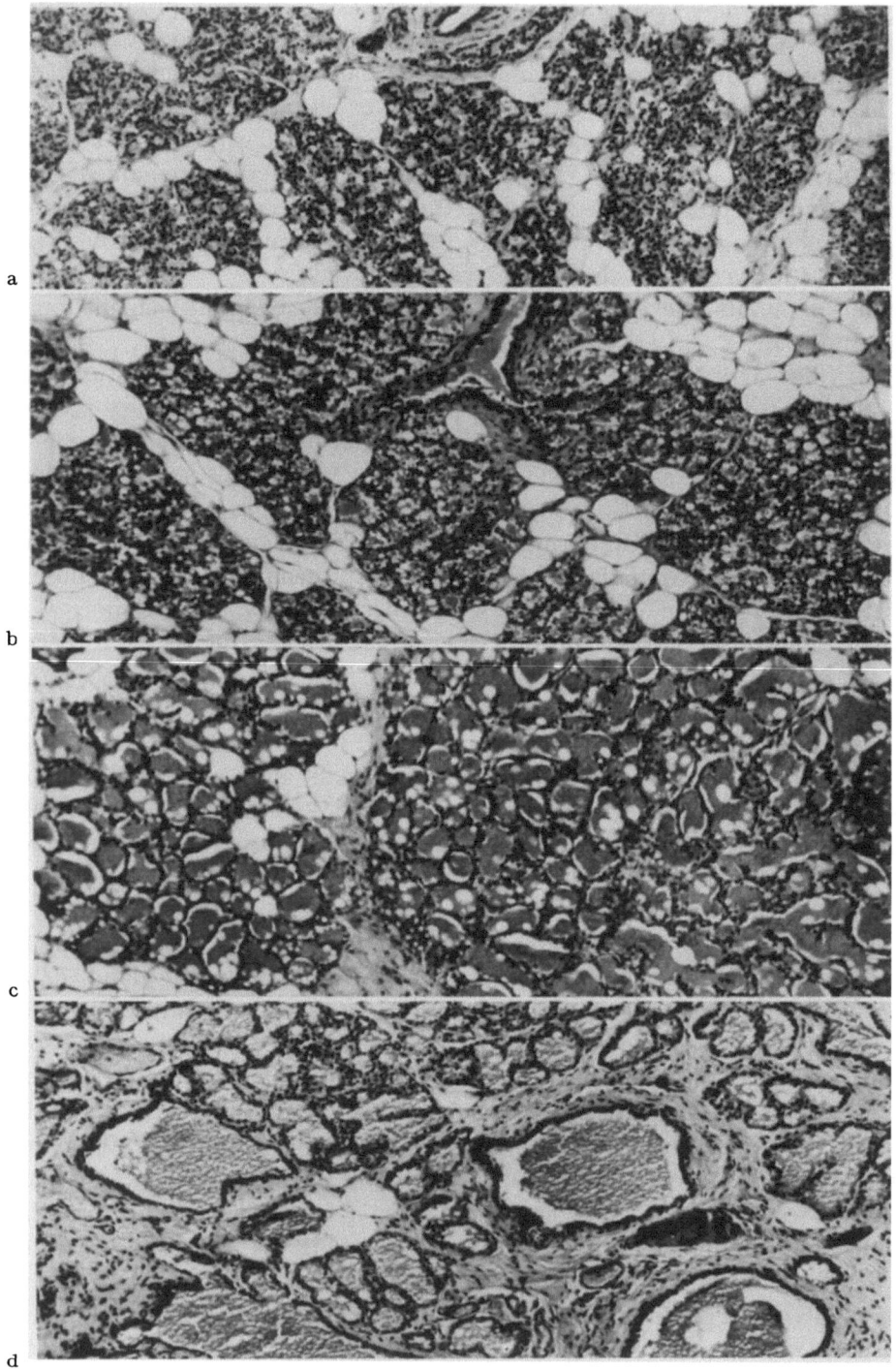

Fig. 10a—d. Effect of oestrogen, progesterone and prolactin on the mammary glands of castrated rats. a Lobular proliferation of the mammary gland with little secretion and formation of fat in the glandular epithelium after treatment with 5 γ Progynon and 5 mg Proluton for 15 days. b Greater lobular proliferation and secretion after 15 days

2. Progesterone

There is no doubt about the importance of corpus luteum hormone and follicular hormone for the normal development of the breast. There are, however, differences of opinion about the effects of progesterone. Dosage is the best criterion of morphogenetic action on the parenchyma of the mammary gland. The lower limits of effective dosage are 5 mg/d (10 days) for rats according to SELYE (1940a, b) and 2.4 mg/d (68 days) for guinea pigs by BENSON, COWIE, COX and GOLDZWEIG (1957). No doubt, these doses are far greater than the normal amounts which are used in combination with oestrogens, so as to obtain a steady lobulo-alveolar differentiation.

GARDNER (1940) gave to hypophysectomised *mice* 0.125—0.25 mg of corpus luteum hormone, but only weak growth of tubules resulted. TRENTIN and TURNER (1948) mentioned slight terminal budding and dilatation of tubules. Experiments by DAANE and LYONS (1954) were unsuccessful. MIXNER and TURNER (1942a), however, observed a lobulo-alveolar development after a dose of 6 mg in 57.7 % of experimental animals. The same authors (1941a) obtained similar dose-dependent results with the orally active drug pregneninolone.

CORNER (1930), NELSON (1936), and SELYE, BROWNE and COLLIP (1936) denied that 4 mg/d of progesterone had any effect on the mammary gland of the *rat*. ASTWOOD, GESCHICKTER, and RAUSCH (1937), ASTWOOD and GESCHICKTER (1938), LYONS (1951), and SMITH (1955) on the basis of their experimental results also doubted that progesterone had an isolated effect. SELYE (1940a, b), GESCHICKTER and BYRNES (1942), CHAMORRO (1944), and AHRÉN (1959a) by greatly increasing the usual dose were able to induce a development of the mammary gland with lobulation, that simulated the picture of late pregnancy. SELYE (1940) underscored the compact structure of the lobuli and went so far as to call progesterone *the* steroid hormone with the best production of acini. CURTISS (1949) alone was unable to confirm SELYE's finding in a similar experimental arrangement and pointed out the differences between isolated animals and those kept in groups. SMITHCORS and LEONARD (1943) obtained growth impulses of the mammary glands in castrated and hypophysectomized rats with 10—30 mg/d, given for 10 days, provided the hormone injections were given immediately after operation (LEONARD, 1943).

Together with LIESER (1964) I had found in juvenile castrated female rats that the tubular structure of the breast had remained unchanged after 20 days of treatment with 1 mg/d progesterone. Only the circumtubular connective tissue had increased. Large doses (10 mg/d) produced lobuli in dense stratification, which simulated the picture of late pregnancy (Fig. 9f).

---

of treatment with 5 γ Progynon, 5 mg Proluton, and finally treatment with prolactin 2 mg/d for three days. c Considerable secretion with development of dilated alveoli. Same pretreatment, followed by six days of 2 mg/d prolactin. d Lobules with diminished secretion and retention, cysts and dilated excretory ducts with circumcanalicular fibrosis. Same pretreatment, followed by 12 days of 2 mg/d prolactin

In *rabbits* (NORGREN, 1966) and *guinea pigs* small doses of progesterone were also ineffective (SMITH and RICHTERICH, 1958). COWIE (1951) compared the dose and proliferation effects and, like BENSON, COWIE, COX, and GOLDZWEIG (1957), obtained an effect on the growth of the tubular system only with 2.4 mg/d, given for 68 days.

3. Combined Action of Oestrogen and Progesterone

The results of these investigations indicate that neither oestrogen nor progesterone alone will produce a condition of uniform development and secretion of the mammary gland. Obviously, suitable combinations of the drugs might be tested to ascertain the optimal quantities of each hormone that would be appropriate normally for each animal species (Figs. 9, 10, 12a, b).

MIXNER and TURNER (1941a, 1942a, b) reported the quantitative relationships for the optimal development of the mammary gland of the *mouse* as being 1 mg progesterone and 40—1,200 IU oestrogen. High environmental temperatures (35°C) and thyroidectomy reduced the activities of the drugs. Experiments on non-castrated animals (TRENTIN and TURNER, 1948) and castrated mice (MIXNER and TURNER, 1957) also indicated species-dependent reactions. The findings of DAANE and LYONS (1954) and ANDERSON, BROOKRESON, and TURNER (1961) underscore the syntropic lobulo-alveolar reaction, which was also observed in hypophysectomized male animals (GARDNER, 1940). MIXNER and TURNER (1943) gave a ratio of 1:75—250 oestrogen to progesterone as lobuloalveolar growth factor (see Table 3).

The mammary gland of the *rat* behaves similarly (NELSON, 1936; ASTWOOD and GESCHICKTER, 1938; MIXNER and TURNER, 1941b). FAUVET (1940) in view of WERNER's (1940) work took the view that it was possible to produce a functioning mammary gland with oestrogen alone, but that this development took too stormy a course in experimental work. Only synchronous protrated influence made organic development possible. Subsequent studies by CURTISS (1949), LYONS (1951) and by FOLLEY (1940, 1947, 1952, 1956) confirmed that in rats the complete and proper development of the mammary gland was possible only by combined treatment. SMITH (1955), BENSON, COWIE, FOLLEY, and TINDAL (1959), — who pointed to the uniformity of growth — AHRÉN (1959a), LINZELL (1959) and MEITES (1959a) confirmed these findings. MOON, GRIFFITH and TURNER (1959) pointed to age, interval between injections, and duration as special factors in the assessment of these experiments. MCDONALD and REECE (1962), AHRÉN and JACOBSOHN (1956), and AHRÉN and ETIENNE (1958) discussed questions of dosage. — KIRKHAM and TURNER (1954), SMITH and RICHTERICH (1959) used the ratio of 3—5 mg progesterone to 1.0 mg oestradiol benzoate and observed at optimal differentiation that enzyme and DNA-values rose only little even when administration of the hormones was continued. In the state of maximal differentiation there is thus a rest phase of proliferation.

Morphology of Hormone Induced Structural Changes in the Female Breast 25

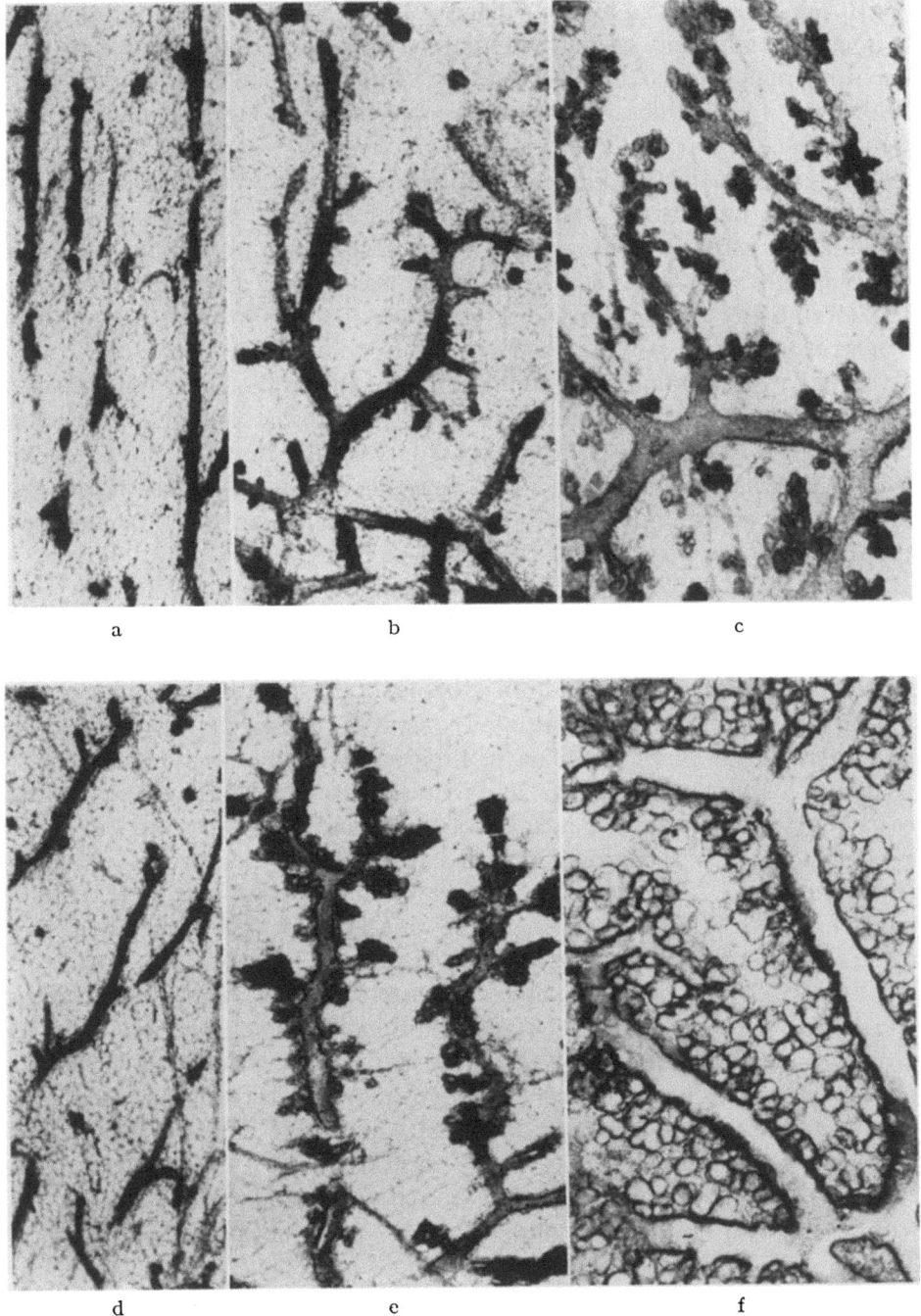

Fig. 11 a—f. Morphology of the male mammary gland (rat) after treatment with hormones. a Control animal, castrated. b 10 γ/5 d Progynon: dilatation of duct system and formation of broad lateral branches, small lobules. c 10 γ/10 d Progynon: strong lobular development with dilated alveoli, milk ducts, and secretion. d Control animal, not castrated. e 10 γ/5 d Progynon: proliferation of the tubular system and development of small lateral branches. f 10 γ/10 d Progynon: lobular and tubular development of glands with dilatation of lactiferous ducts. — Formalin, alumcarmine, magnification 10 ×

Hypophysectomized animals reacted to the combination of hormones only if injection treatment began immediately after operation. Additional desoxycorticosterone had no noticeable effect (SMITHCORS and LEONARD, 1943). — LYONS (1951, 1953) observed after hypophysectomy only insignificant formation of buds.

All dosage ratios are ineffective in castrated and hypophysectomized rats (AHRÉN and JACOBSOHN, 1956; AHRÉN and ETIENNE, 1958; AHRÉN, 1959). — When 2 mg oestradiol benzoate and 6 mg progesterone were given to castrated, thyroidectomized, and parathyroidectomized rats, the mammary gland proliferated and DNA increased after 19 days (v. BERSWORDT-WALLRABE and TURNER, 1960).

COWIE (1951) found in systematic studies that the ratio for *guinea pigs* was 50—100 mg oestrogen and 600—2,400 mg progesterone. BENSON, COWIE, COX and GOLDZWEIG (1957) a few years later found that the gland developed maximally when a ratio of 1:20—100 was given. They noted that the quantities of the drugs as well as the ratio were of importance, in that amounts of less than 0.1 mg oestrogen caused formation of cysts.

SCHARF and LYONS (1941), LYONS and McGINTY (1941), and YAMAMOTO and TURNER (1956) found similar results in *rabbits*. The proliferated glandular fields could only be distinguished from those during pregnancy by incomplete lobuli in the periphery. NORGREN (1966) obtained optimal lobular differentiation by administering graduated doses of oestrogen (5—20 mg/d) and progesterone (1—5 mg) for 28 days. Progesterone alone was ineffective.

COWIE, FOLLEY, MALPRESS and RICHARDSON (1952) found in castrated *goats* that combinations of hexoestrol and progesterone resulted in uniform development and secretion, provided the dose of oestrogen (0.25 mg/d) remained small. An increase to 1 mg/d produced cysts and epithelial proliferation. BENSON, COWIE, COX, FLUX and FOLLEY (1965) obtained similar results in castrated virgin goats, and BENSON, COWIE, COX, FOLLEY, and HOSKING (1965) obtained similar results after daily injections of oily solutions and of depot preparations. The oily solutions that were administered daily proved more effective than crystalline depot suspensions. After complete hypophysectomy the drugs were ineffective. After castration and hypophysectomy hexoestrol, progesterone, prolactin, and STH induced lobulo-alveolar development (COWIE, TINDAL, and YOKOYAMA, 1966). SYKES and WRENN (1951), HANCOCK, BRUMBY, and TURNER (1954), and TURNER, YAMAMOTO, and RUPPERT (1956) studied the udders of *cows* and showed the importance of progesterone for the uniform development of a proficient udder.

The empirically obtained *optimal ratios for the lobulo-alveolar development of the mammary gland* are presented in Table 3.

Comparative studies by SOEMARWOTO and BERN (1958) of the *vascularization of the mammary gland under the influence of sex hormones* in C_3H/He Crgl mice have shown impressive differences. Vascularization during the genital cycle did not change as shown by injections of Indian ink and by making thick sections translucent. It increased during pregnancy and lactation, however,

Table 3

Species	Ratio of oestrogen: progesterone	Authors
Rat	1:1,000—5,000	KIRKHAM and TURNER (1954)
	1:3,000—5,000	SMITH (1955)
	1:4,000—5,000	MCDONALD and REECE (1962)
Mouse	1:75—250	MIXNER and TURNER (1943)
Rabbit	1:10—40	LYONS and MCGINTY (1941), SCHARF and LYONS (1941)
	1:67	YAMAMOTO and TURNER (1956)
Guinea Pig	1:20—100	BENSON, COWIE, COX, GOLDZWEIG (1957)
Goat	1:140	BENSON, COWIE, COX, FLUX and FOLLEY (1955)

and under the influence of oestrogen and progesterone capillary plexus formed around tubules and adventitious buds. This indicates that there is a correlation between hormonal action, vascularization, and development of the gland, and that this correlation may be cancelled by hypophysectomy and ovarectomy.

4. Histochemistry of Connective Tissue During Hormone Action

After puberty in man the mesenchymal portions of the mammary gland differentiate into loose intralobular connective tissue, called "mantle tissue" by BERKA (1911). This is particularly concerned with the hormonally induced changes of the glandular apparatus. The coarsely fibred, collagenous connective tissue surrounds tubules and lobules and acts as supportive tissue in anchoring the body of the gland in the Fascia pectoralis and in the corium (GRUBER, 1921; DIECKMANN, 1925; SCHULTZ, 1933; DABELOW, 1957). In disorders of the mammary gland multiple histopathological changes of structure occur in connective tissue, which exhibit as secretion of fluid, oedematous-mucoid swellings of this stroma, and hyalinisation. The depositions of fluid observed in fibrocystic mastopathy and carcinoma were called "oedema lakes" by RATZENHOFER (1951), RATZENHOFER and SCHAUENSTEIN (1952a, b). They contain 1—6 g-% protein, mainly albumin, thought to derive from permeable blood-vessels and presenting precursors of the fibrillar and hyaline collagen. This permanent invasion of fluid with abnormal proteins is of great importance in mastopathy (RATZENHOFER, 1951).

Histochemical studies have been restricted to the recognition of mucopolysaccharides: according to KURU (1909) and SYLVEN (1938) the stroma is not metachromatic. In contrast, investigations by CONSOLANDI (1947), OLIVI and BARBIERI (1952), IHNEN and PEREZ-TAMAYO (1953) have shown low-grade positive reactions. VERONESI and CANDIANI (1955) have described PAS-positive deposits in the lactiferous ducts, metachromatic material and mucicarmine staining components. DEMPSEY, BUNTING and WISLOCKI (1947) and BUNTING (1950) had found metachromasia in mantle tissue that was at

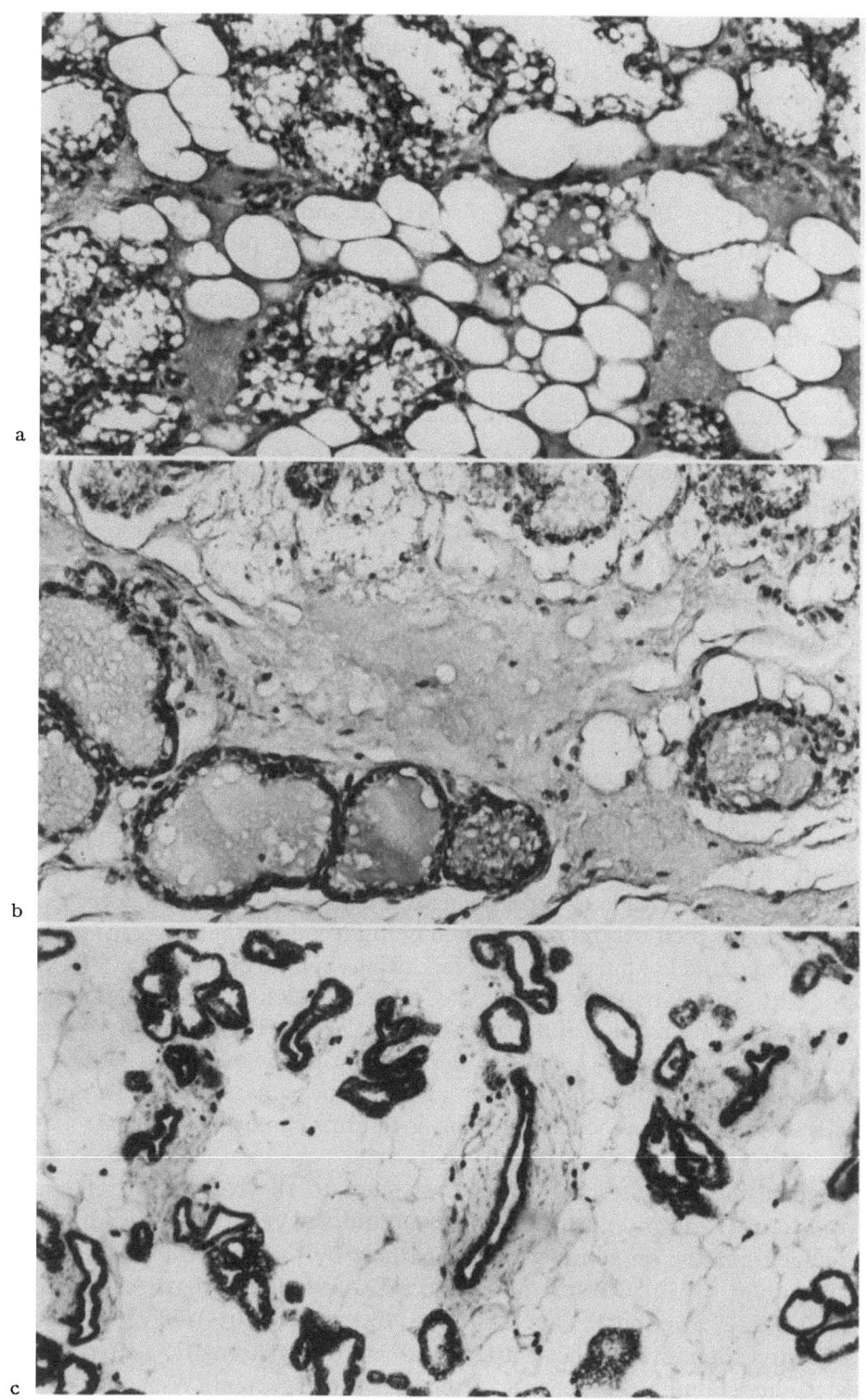

Fig. 12a—c

least partially stable for testicular hyaluronidase. Systematic studies by OZZELLO and SPEER (1958) showed positive PAS- und Hale-reactions with metachromasia to toluidine blue in the intralobular and circumductal connective tissue. The intensity of the reactions depended upon the menstrual cycle in so far as the time of strong oestrogen activity was related to a rise of acid mucopolysaccharides. Correspondingly, this effect was reduced in the menopause.

New histochemical investigations by LEUSCHNER (1969) demonstrates deposits of metachromatic and periodine reactive substances in solid-scirrhous carcinoma of the mammary gland indicating growth activity.

SCHULZE (1968) had tested histochemically the relationships between mucopolysaccharide content and sex hormone. She had found that castrated rats showed a rise of acid muco-polysaccharides after treatment with oestrogen. CHAIN and DUTHIE (1940), DURAN-REYNALS, BUNTING, and VAN WAGENEN (1950), VITRY (1953), OZELLO and SPEERT (1958) reported similar observations. Progesterone, on the other hand, inhibited the mesenchymal action of oestrogen (ASBOE-HANSEN, 1958, 1959). I was able to confirm this in the animals that had not been castrated and had not received additional progesterone. Animals that had been pretreated for 10—20 days with hormones started to secrete profusely, and developed distension of the glandular alveoli, cysts, and congestion of the secretion. As treatment proceded, homogenous and finely granulated deposits occurred in the intra- and interlobular connective tissue, which after acetylation and saponification reacted positively, but to varying degrees, to PAS and Hale (Fig. 12a, b). In view of the pathology of the human mammary gland in hormonally induced dysplasias and in involution after lactation it may thus be assumed that these deposits are present in the preformed mesenchyma and, like vascular albumins (RATZENHOFER and SCHAUENSTEIN, 1952), are of importance for the fibrosing of glands (BÄSSLER, SCHULZE and SCHRIEVER, 1970).

The increase of *mast cells*, which settle in the circumductular and lobular mesenchyma when the connective tissue develops further on stimulation by hormones is thus explicable (Fig. 12c). The mast cells, first demonstrated and counted in the mammary gland of man and in dysplasias by HIGUCHI, (1930) are formed in the "mantle tissue", i.e. the cytogenous stroma, and are supposed to increase in the transitional area between carcinomatous and healthy tissue, and in lactation and mastopathy. They are said to be scarce

Fig. 12a—c. Mucopolysaccharide and mast cell presentation in the stroma of mammary gland after hormonal stimulation. a Castrated rat after treatment with Progynon (5 γ) and Proluton (1 mg) for 10 days. Lobular proliferation of gland and intensive secretion. Homogenous dense deposits in the circumlobular connective and fat tissue. Saponification and PAS, magnification 70×. b Normal animal after the same treatment. The terminal sectors of the gland are filled with secretion, in the connective and fat tissue homogenous, cloudy deposits are seen. Acetylation and PAS, magnification 230×. c Castrated rat after treatment with 5 γ/50 d oestrogen. Tubular proliferation and dilated ducts. Staining with toluidine-blue, mast cells represented in peritubular stroma (black dots). — Magnification 90×

in fibroadenoma and fibrosis and are unsystematically arranged in carcinoma (LEUSCHNER, 1969).

5. Histochemical Enzyme Model

Enzymes have been demonstrated so far mainly in tissue homogenates. The assay has been related to problems of the synthetic activity of the mammary gland during pregnancy, lactation, and involution (HANSEN and CARLSON, 1961; MUNFORD, 1964). Histotopochemical studies have been comparatively neglected and have been limited to demonstrations of alkaline phosphatase activity (DEMPSEY, BUNTING and WISLOCKI, 1947; VERNE, 1951; PERRINI, 1952; SILVER, 1954; HOLMES, 1956).

In recent histochemical enzymatic studies of the infantile, juvenile, and proliferating mammary glands under the influence of sex hormones topical enzyme models have been demonstrated, which depend upon the duration of action (PAEK, 1967; LANI, 1967; BÄSSLER and PAEK, 1968): *alkaline* and *acid phosphatase* and also *glucose-6-phosphatase* are localized in the base of the epithelial cells, especially of the myoepithelium, and form ribbon-shapped reaction products in infantile and juvenile animals and after hormone stimulation (Figs. 13a, b). It is possible by means of azodye selectively to stain the myoepithelial cells. The behaviour of this cell system may thus be studied in the growing gland and during phases of physiological functioning (Fig. 13b) (BÄSSLER and BRETHFELD, 1968). Irrespective of the galactokinetic importance of the basket cells the localization of the phosphatases in the basal boundary zone towards the vascular mesenchyme points to their importance for the uptake of substances from the blood stream. Electronmicroscopic histotopochemical findings have shown selective visualisation in the cell membranes (Fig. 15a), with basal folds also showing strong positive reactions (Fig. 15b). GIRARDIE and WOLF (1967) had thought that this localization indicated active transport of fluid by pinocytosis. — *Glucose-6-phosphatase* biochemically liberates glucose in the cell and is the primary source of fatty acid synthesis in nonruminants (FOLLEY and MCNAUGHT, 1961). The localization shown in Fig. 13a thus marks the site where phosphate groups are split off and where glucose enters the base of the epithelial cells.

An increase of acid hydrolytic enzyme activity, specially *acid phosphatase*, during the period of involution is revealed by electron microscopy, histo- and biochemically (HELMINEN, ERICSSON and ORRENIUS, 1968; BRANDES, ANTON and BARNARD, 1969; ZARZYCKI, PERYT, KLUBINSKA, HJAC and ZAK, 1969). The results indicate the activity of lysosomes in areas of focal cytoplasmic degradation in the glandular and macrophage-like cells.

Adenosine triphosphatase is localized exclusively in the mesenchymal parts of the mammary gland, especially in blood-vessels, nerves, and lymph nodes. It shows differences of reactions only when there is congestion of milk with increased fluid outflow. MEIER-RUGE (1966) and HOLZNER and KAUFMANN (1965) have described in carcinoma of the breast rises of intensity of ATP-ase, whereby a kind of negative picture of the tumour tissue is created.

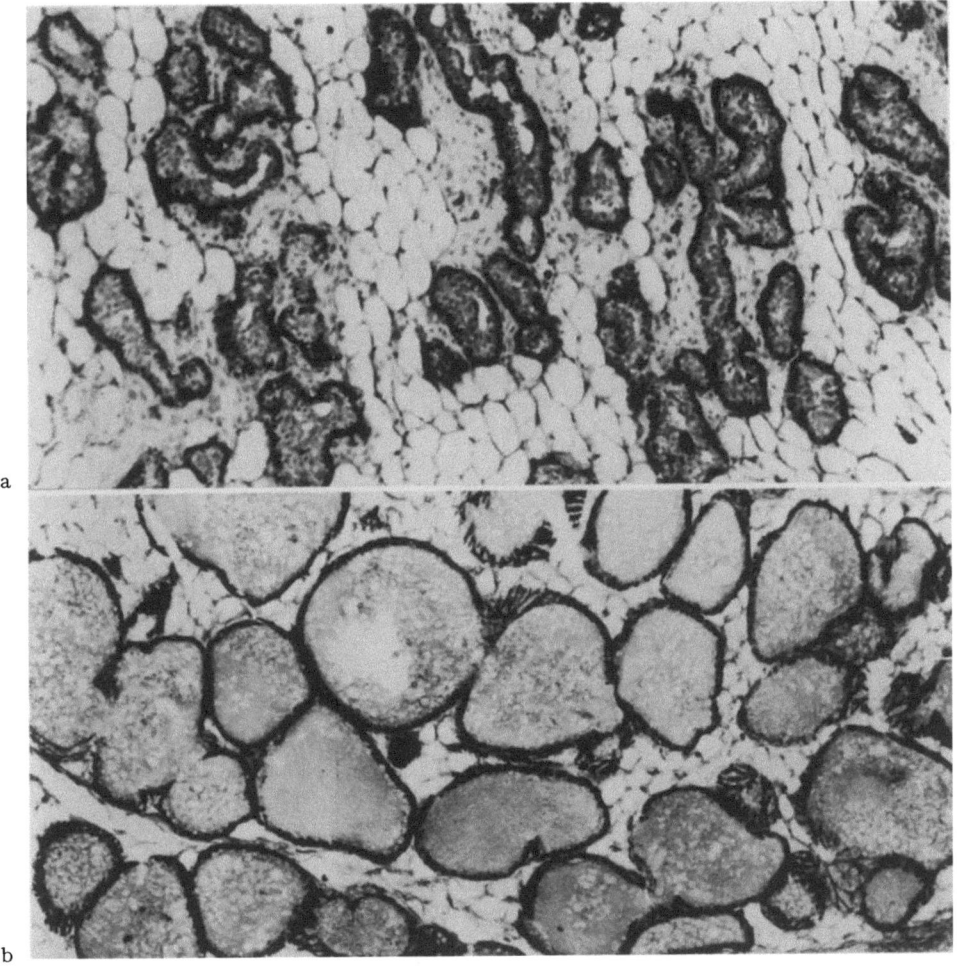

Fig. 13. a Demonstration of glucose-6-phosphatase in the base of proliferating tubules after treatment of a castrated rat with oestrogen for five days (magnification 90 ×). b Alkaline phosphatase (azodye method) in the base, especially in the myoepithelium of dilated and secreting alveoli. Treatment of a castrated rat with oestrogen and progesterone (1 : 1,000) for 10 days. Magnification 90 ×

5-nucleotidase possesses only insignificant activity in the epithelial cells and rises only little under the influence of hormones. The same applies to *succinodehydrogenase* and *glucose-6-phosphate-dehydrogenase*, the key enzyme for the pentose-phosphate cycle (GLOCK and MCLEAN, 1954).

When the mammary glands of castrated animals were stimulated with oestrogen and progesterone the intensity of the enzymatic reaction products rose, remained high up to the fifth day, and then levelled out. Continued administration of hormone caused no further change. In other words, on the fifth day the hormonally induced cell metabolism had reached a constant level (Fig. 14a, b). *The effects of oestrogen dominated*, and were not greatly increased by progesterone and prolactin. — When the mammary gland had been pretreated and had proliferated, and prolactin was injected for several days, retention of secretion in the alveoli and epithelial caused a reduction of enzyme activity.

The development of the mammary gland during pregnancy and lactation is related to a general increase of enzyme activity. Involution is related to a reduction of activity, as is to be expected. The metabolic and catabolic pro-

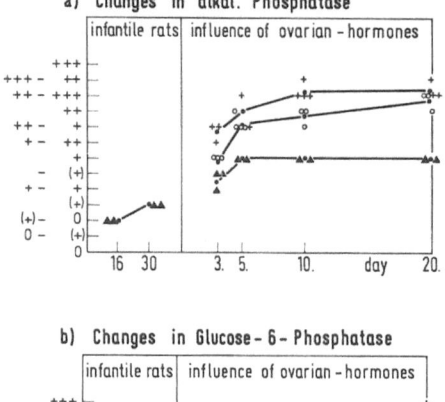

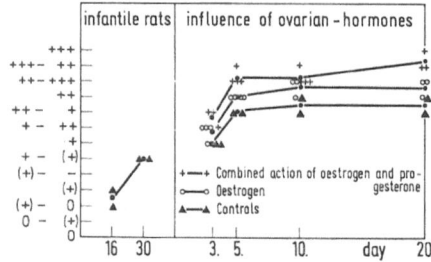

Fig. 14. The histochemical changes of enzyme activity under the influence of oestrogen and progesterone (PAEK, 1967)

cesses in glandular and fat tissue are marked by great activity of non-specific esterases (BÄSSLER and BRETHFELD, 1968).

FISCHER and SCHAEFER (1967) and SCHAEFER and FISCHER (1968) observed oestrogen-dependent activity of alkaline phosphatase in subcutaneous fibroblasts. They had also found that phosphatase activity was influenced by sex, castration, time and dosage of hormone treatment. These observations seem to point to neosynthesis of this enzyme, which is stimulated by oestrogen and directed by messenger RNA.

6. Electron-Microscopic Morphology of the Hormonally Stimulated Mammary Gland

Under *normal conditions* the glandular cells of young animals are characterized by their cubic shape, which becomes prismatic when they are in superficial position. The cytoplasm is relatively poor in differentiation products and surrounds an ordinary oval nucleus. The epithelial surface may protrude hemispherically or sometimes tongueshaped, into the lumen. It possesses

Morphology of Hormone Induced Structural Changes in the Female Breast 33

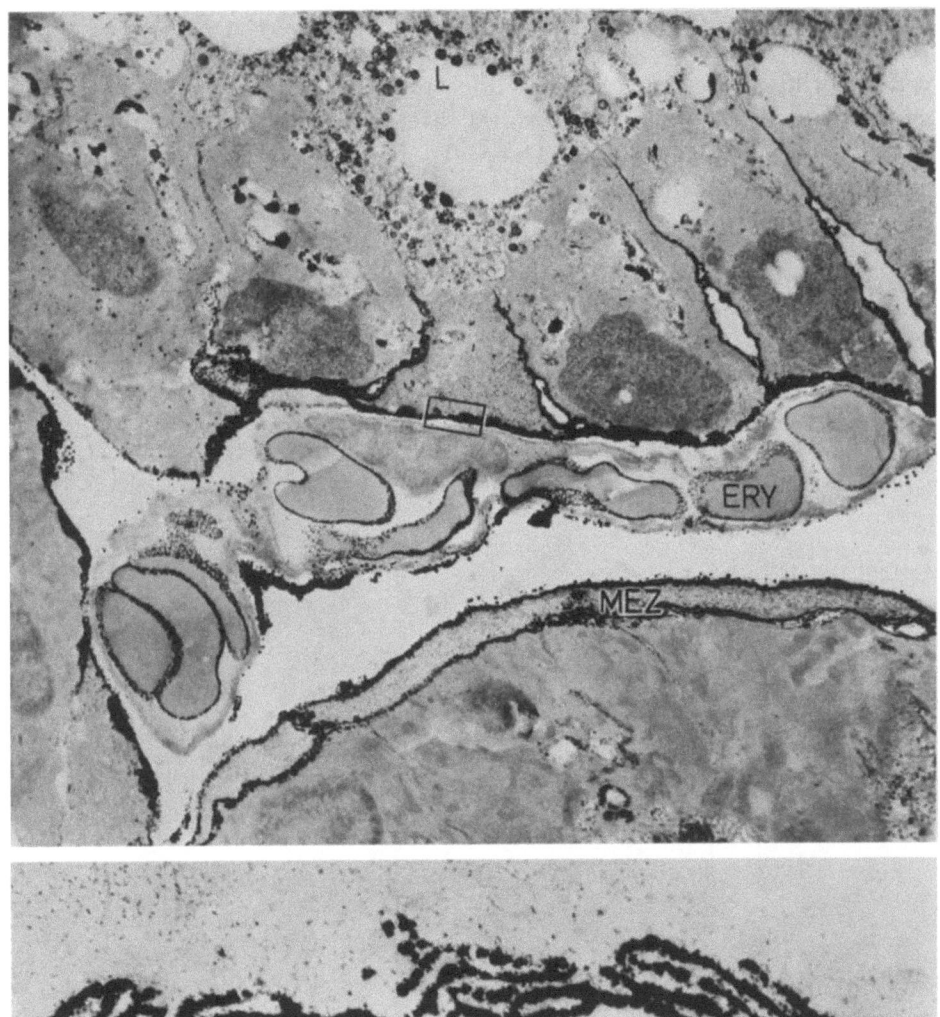

Fig. 15. a Electronmicroscopic representation of the siting of alkaline phosphatase (azo-method) in the lactating mammary gland. The reaction products are shown as black deposits in the cell membranes, myoepithelium (*MEZ*), partly in the lumen of the gland (*L*) and in the membrane of erythrocytes (*ERY*). Record no. 1299/68; em. magnification 2,400; in the fig. 5,525 ×. b Enlargement of sector of the basal membrane of a glandular cell with basal folds, which are characterized by reaction products of the azodye method. Record no. 1292/68; em. magnification 13,500; in the figure 31,050 ×

microvilli of various sizes. The large microvilli frequently become detached and together with parts of detached cells form a detritus that partially fills the small lumina (Fig. 16). At the apical end of these gaps are found basal folds, indentations, desmosomes of the cell membranes, and also thickened ridges, which serve to hold the cells together against pressure or tension forces, arising from secretion or retention, which may deform the groups of cells. During the resting state of the epithelial cells the energy carriers for synthetic activity, the mitochondria, are small and sparsely distributed in the ribosome-rich cytoplasm. The Golgi field, which consists of small gaps and small vesicles and is optically empty, lies beside the nucleus. Near the

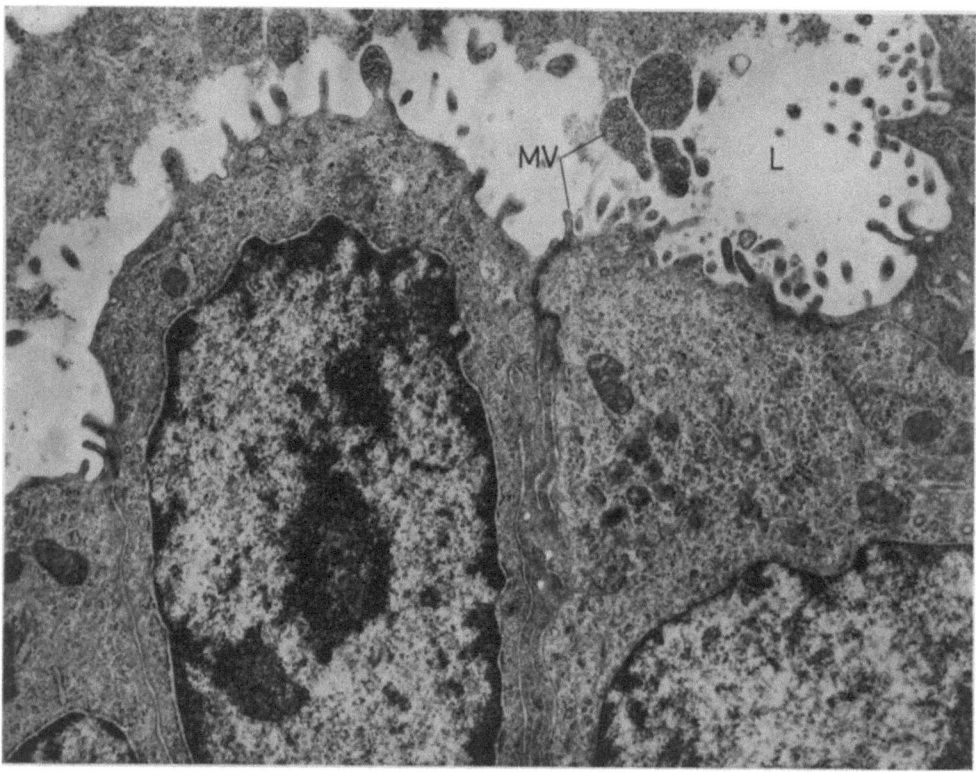

Fig. 16. Glandular epithelium of the mammary gland of a juvenile rat with regular cytoplasmatic structure. On the surface microvilli (*MV*) of varying size, some in the stage of constriction. In the lumen (*L*) detritus and remnants of secretion. In the cell plasma ribosomes and a few mitochondria. Record no. 1384/68; em. magnification 7,500; in the figure 18,000

epithelial base small fat vacuoles, occasionally also short pairs of lamellae of the endoplasmatic reticulum may occur.

The action of *oestrogen* may be recognized morphologically after two days by proliferation of the epithelium with intercellular gaps, and by desquamation of superficial cells. The content of ribosomes in the cytoplasm increases; an ergastoplasm develops with lamella that are widely set apart; the nuclei are dark and have a large nucleolus. — After treatment with oestrogen for several days epithelial proliferations goes together with increasing differentiation of the cytoplasm, which shows large swollen mitochondria of the matrix and crista type (THOENES, 1964). The cytoplasm becomes more transparent and contains numerous fat vacuoles, which are surrounded by mitochondria or by ergastoplasmatic lamellae (Fig. 17). Fat synthesis is at first localized in the base of the cell. This is also the site of lysosomes, phagolysosomes, siderosomes, and vesicular bodies, which appear as results of hormonal action. After treatment

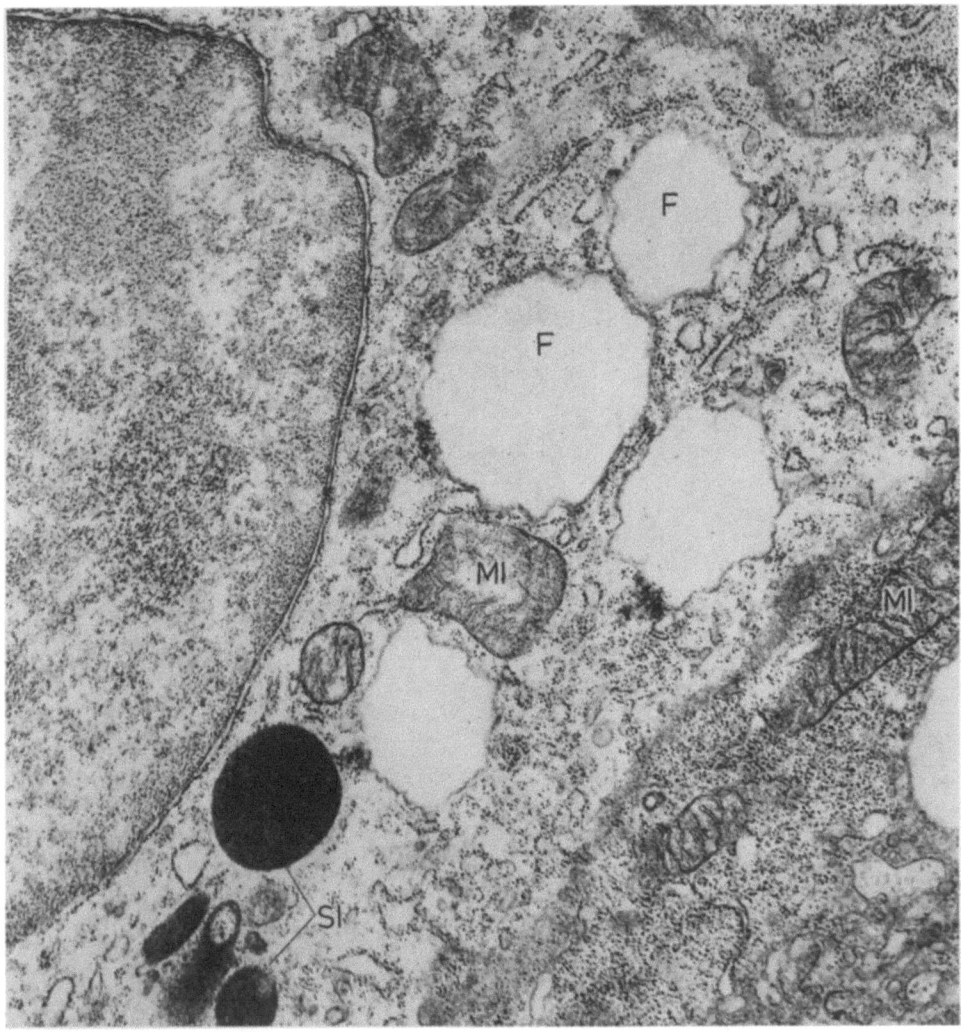

Fig. 17. Sector of cytoplasma and nucleus of a glandular epithelial cell of the mammary gland after castration and treatment with oestrogen for 10 days. In the perikaryon several fat droplets (*F*), large mitochondria (*MI*) and siderosomes (*SI*). Record no. 892/66, em. magnification 8,000; in the figure 26,400

for 20 days fat synthesis is nearly ubiquitous. Fat issues in the form of small droplets into the enlarging lumen of the gland. These droplets consist of small round fat particles and larger confluent particles (Fig. 18). The Golgi field also increases in size, but always remains free from secretion products. The casein synthesis characteristic for lactogenesis does not occur after experimental treatment with oestrogen and progesterone.

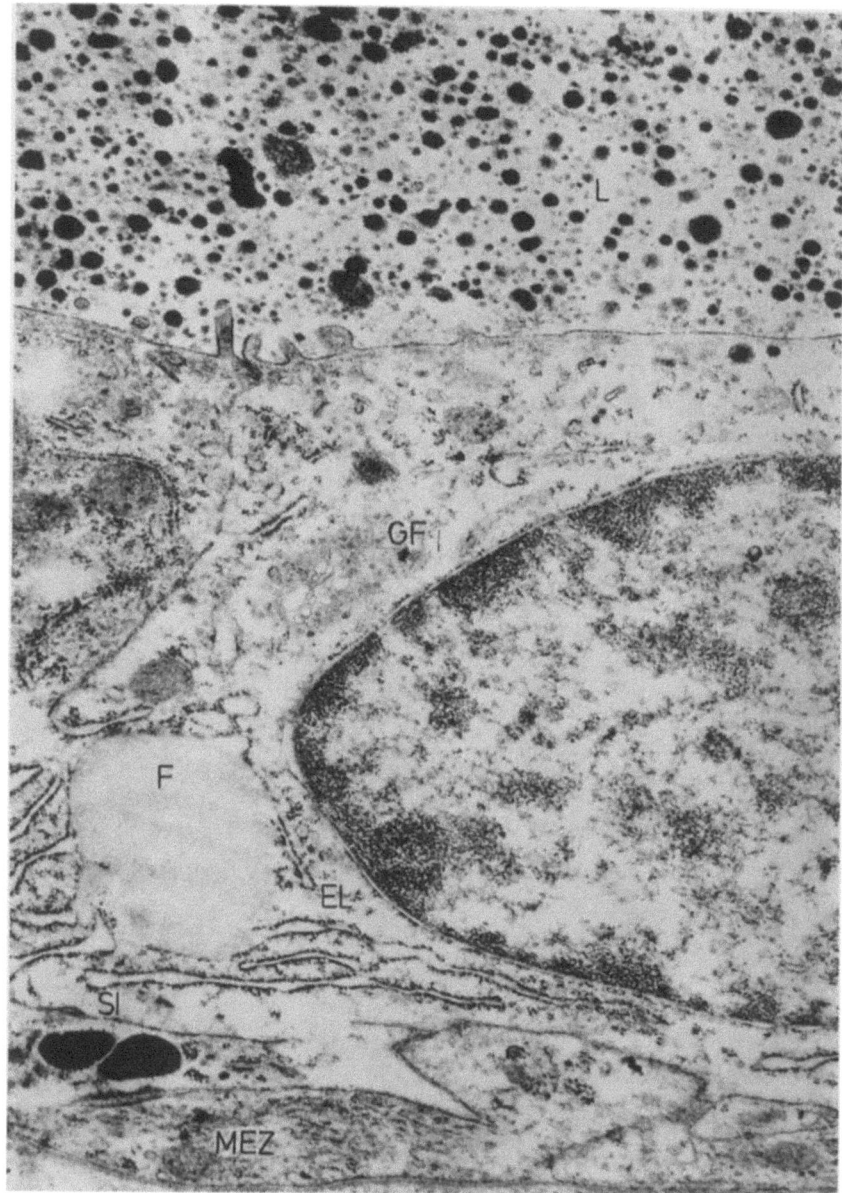

Fig. 18. Partial reproduction of the wall of a glandular alveolus after treatment of a castrated rat with oestrogen for 20 days. In the lumen (L) massive small fat droplets; the cytoplasm is transparent. Small Golgi field (GF); basally a few ergastoplasmatic lamellae (EL) and fat droplets (F), siderosomes (SI) and myoepithelial cells (MEZ). Record no. 971/66; em. magnification 7,000; in the figure 19,600

Combinations of oestrogen and progesterone differ cytomorphologically in that they produce much more fat. This starts during the first days after injection. After 10 days small droplets will fill the whole cell plasma. The nuclei become deformed and the lumina of the acini become narrower, so that eventually a pregnancy-like state will result (CHENTSOV, 1964; BÄSSLER and FORSSMANN, 1964; SUETINA, CHENTSOV, SMIRNOVA, and SAMOILOV, 1966). — WELLINGS, and NANDI (1968) succeeded in producing a cell picture in mice that corresponded to normal lactogenesis with synthesis of milk proteins, after triple operation and treatment with oestrogen, progesterone, cortisone, STH, and prolactin.

Unusual lamellated lipoid-rich deposits in droplet form with multitudinous transformations to fat droplets were observed after combined oestrogen-progesterone treatment, when corpus luteum hormone preponderated.

From a cytomorphological point of view the structural changes in the glandular epithelium of the mammary gland caused by ovarian hormones are characterized during the first days of administration mainly by an increase of ribosomes, mitochondria, and greater denseness of ribonucleoproteins. An endoplasmatic reticulum then forms, and fat synthesis starts, at first in the base of the cell and then involving the whole of the cytoplasm. Secretion of fat as droplets and retention of secretion may follow on continued stimulation. Recent studies by O. STEIN and Y. STEIN (1966) have supplied information about the high velocity of turnover of triglycerides in the mammary gland. The authors have proved by electron-microscopic autoradiography, that the inclusion of esterified substances into fat globuli takes place 1—3 minutes after injection of labelled fatty acids. The site of reaction is the endoplasmatic reticulum, with mitochondria assisting. Protein synthesis that was assessed in lactating mammary glands by the same method with tritium-labelled leucine took 30 minutes from injection until labelled protoproteins accurred in the Golgi field (WELLINGS and PHILP, 1964; VERLEY and HOLLMANN, 1964; FISKE, COURTECUISSE and HAGUENAU, 1967).

The *biochemical mechanisms* of action of the oestrogens are known in some of their essential aspects. The receptor organs used were uterus, vagina, and the anterior lobe of the pituitary, in which oestrogens form a receptor-hormone-protein complex, which triggers off further metabolic reactions. Activation of RNA in the target organ is in the fore. A specific m-RNA is formed, and its information is transferable. The m-RNA is the matrix for the synthesis of specific proteins, which as enzymes direct the cellular metabolism so that energy may be obtained and building elements be synthetized (LAURITZEN, 1965; DELLWEG, 1967). KARLSON (1961, 1962, 1963) had demonstrated the relationship between hormones and gene-conditioned metabolic processes on the model of the hormone ecdyson, which causes insects to cast off their skin. These relationships have also been used to explain other interactions.

JENSON and JACOBSON (1962), KING, GORDON, and INMAN (1965), KING, GORDON, COWAN, and INMAN (1966) have demonstrated by means of labelled steroids the passage of oestrogens through the cytoplasm into the nucleus in the uterus, pituitary, and in a carcinoma of the mammary gland. They have stressed that there is a direct reaction to DNA-synthesis. According to observations by BEATO and DIENSTBACH (1968) the duration of DNA-synthesis remained constant, independent of whether oestrogen or progesterone had been administered previously. EISENFELD and AXELROD (1965) and GORSKI, NOTEBOOM, and NICOLETTE (1965) described an increase of RNA- and protein syntheses and mechanisms of attachment in the target organs. Androgens, too, caused an increase of RNA (KOCHAKIAN, 1964; WILLIAMS-ASHMAN, 1965).

SEGAL and SCHER (1967) reviewed comprehensively the partial processes of the action of oestrogen on the uterus. These are already known from the biochemical and morphological points of view and may be used as explications of the structural changes in the epithelial cells of the mammary gland induced by hormones.

Hormones of the Pituitary

1. Somatotropin (STH)

Formerly the question whether the site of mammogenic action of STH was at the glandular parenchyma had remained unanswered. LYONS, LI, and JOHNSON (1957) had observed lobulo-alveolar differentiation of the mammary gland of castrated and hypophysectomized rats, when ovarian hormones, prolactin, and STH simultaneously acted upon the gland. Later investigations of the same authors (1958) showed that the mammary gland developed gradually, depending upon mutually complementary combinations of hormones:

Table 4

a) Hypophysectomized		→ delicate system of ducts, no buds
b) Hypophysectomized + ovarectomized	+STH	→ Proliferation of terminal buds and ducts
c) Hypophysectomized + ovarectomized adrenalectomized	+STH +oestrone	→ Strong terminal buds -proliferation, ectasia of ducts
d) Hypophysectomized + ovarectomized + adrenalectomized	+STH +oestrone +DOCA	Proliferation of ducts, formation of terminal buds
e) Hypophysectomized + ovarectomized + adrenalectomized	+STH +oestrone +DOCA +progesterone +prednisolone + prolactin	→ Lobulo-alveolar growth
f) Hypophysectomized + ovarectomized + adrenalectomized	+STH +oestrone +DOCA +progesterone +prednisolone +prolactin (i. m. and locally)	→ Lobulo-alveolar differentiation and secretion

STH thus directly stimulates the duct system and the terminal buds, a stimulus that is supported by oestrogen even after adrenalectomy. After triple operation the glandular tubules develop fully when desoxycorticosterone acetate is given. When the six hormones are administered a status praelactans is produced, during which prolactin gives the impulse towards secretion (LYONS, LI, JOHNSON, 1958). COWIE and LYONS (1959) obtained the same results.

TALWALKER and MEITES (1961) treated virgin rats, 3—4 months old, with cattle STH and cattle prolactin. Some of the animals were castrated and adrenalectomized and received hormone three times daily for 10 days: after administration of 2 mg STH there was considerable growth of tubules with arborization of the glands and formation of buds. After 30 IU prolactin the tubules also grew. Combined administration (1.33 mg STH and 20 IU prolactin) resulted in proliferation of lactiferous tubules and dense lobulo-alveolar development, corresponding to that of pregnancy. The results of triple operation and the combined administration were extensive growth of ducts and lobulo-alveolar development of the mammary gland. MEITES (1965) had similar results and found in castrated and adrenalectomized rats that STH was of importance mainly for the upkeep of growth of ducts. Together with prolactin it promoted the formation of lobuli.

Investigations of the mammogenesis of hypophysectomized *mice* as compared with that of rats showed considerable differences of reactions of the mammary tissues in several strains of mice. HADFIELD (1957), and HADFIELD and YOUNG (1958) had not observed after hypophysectomy proliferation in response to ovarian hormones alone when they had used strain 2AG. Prolactin or STH alone had also not resulted in proliferation by the combination had. — FLUX (1958) had described intensive growth of ducts in CHI mice on administration of STH with oestrogen and progesterone and lobulo-alveolar growth with prolactin. NANDI (1958a, b) reported after triple operation on C_3H/He Crgl mice that normal growth of ducts occurred only when ovarian hormones, STH, and corticoids were given. When additional progesterone and prolactin acted together with the other hormones alveoli were produced, but secretion was only demonstrated when the ovarian steroids were no longer given. NANDI had also found that in this strain STH replaced prolactin in all phases of mammary development and secretion. The author concluded that progesterone was of greater importance for the development of lactiferous tubules in mice than in rats.

2. Adrenocorticotropin (ACTH)

There are varying assessments of the influence of ACTH on the growth of the glandular structure of the mammary gland: NELSON (1941b) had observed increased growth of the mammary gland in rats after treatment with ACTH; after adrenalectomy administration of ACTH had been unsuccessful. FLUX (1954b) had doubts about these findings. He thought that the crude extracts containing ACTH had been impure, as there had been no changes in castrated mice treated with 0.5—2.0 IU ACTH. The growth of animals that had been pretreated with oestrone, and who had developed lateral outgrowths of the lactiferous ducts, was inhibited by accessory injections of

ACTH. — No changes were found in castrated mice after treatment with ACTH for 21 days (FLUX and MUNFORD, 1957). SELYE (1954a), on the other hand, observed intensive development of the mammary gland and secretion in castrated rats, who had been pretreated with oestradiol, following administration of large doses of ACTH (25 JU twice daily for eight days). Continuing these studies JOHNSON and MEITES (1955) had found after treatment of castrated rats with ACTH for 10 days that the lactiferous ducts had proliferated, and that limited lobulo-alveolar differentiation and secretion had occurred.

3. Extract of the Anterior Lobe of the Pituitary

STRICKER and GRUETER (1928) were the first to study the lactogenic action of extracts of the adenohypophysis. The possible induction of glandular proliferation by administration of extracts of the anterior lobe had been investigated in later studies. According to MIXNER and TURNER (1942a) these extracts are able to increase the action of oestrone in castrated mice and to produce lobulo-alveolar growth. The same authors (1941b) also reported the synchronous influence of raised environmental temperatures (35°C), which decreased the effect of oestrone and progesterone. Extracts of the anterior lobe prevented this decrease. — Investigations by LEWIS, GOMEZ, and TURNER (1942) had shown that it took 16—30 days of treatment to stimulate the growth of ducts in castrated rats, various extracts from pregnant and non-pregnant cattle being used. GOMEZ and TURNER (1937) had obtained the same results. — SYKES and WRENN (1950) had experimented on cows with extract of anterior lobe, which was administered together with diethylstilboestrol and progesterone, and which produced normally shaped lobuli and numerous alveoli at the end of five months. DAMM and TURNER (1961) had found that administration of extract of the anterior lobe and oestradiol benzoate had caused considerable growth of ducts and lobuli in castrated mice. This did not, however, reach the extent seen in the mammary gland during pregnancy. Experiments with the initial residue of the anterior lobe extracts (after removal of tropic hormone) resulted in an increase of DNA in the mammary gland. Extracts from the initial residue, denoted "mammogen C", also triggered off an increase of DNA.

4. Transplants of the Anterior Lobe of the Pituitary

When homologous transplants of the pituitary of 60-day-old female mice were implanted into the inguinal region of mice of similar age, some of whom had been castrated, the non-ovarectomized animals showed lobulo-alveolar growth 120 days later around the transplant. BARDIN, LIEBELT, and LIEBELT (1962) had found some formation of buds in castrated mice. This is a direct mammogenic impulse towards local growth. When transplantation into the anterior chamber of the eye was carried out (BARDIN and LIEBELT, 1964), the mammary glands reacted with lobulo-alveolar proliferation. In hypophysectomized mice with transplants only ducts, but not lobuli, developed further. — Simultaneous intramammary transplants of the pituitary and intraocular transplants of the ovary in mice showed after five months the following picture: ovarian transplants had the same effect as stimulation with oestrogen. Transplants of the anterior lobe of the pituitary produced structures that corresponded to combined oestrogen-progesterone treatment. Both transplants together produced lobulo-alveolar proliferation with little secretion (BROWNING, WHITE and GIBBS, 1964). Further studies of this group of research workers (1965) with the same experimental methods showed that hyperplastic nodules were more common after transplantations than in animals with replanted ovaries or ovaries in situ. — BROWNING and WHITE (1965) reported the local stimulating influence of transplants of the pituitary and of the ovaries on proliferation and secretion of the mammary gland.

5. Mammogenic Effect of Transplanted Pituitary Tumours

CLIFTON and FURTH (1960) and TALWALKER and MEITES (1961, 1964) had postulated that tumours of the anterior lobe of the pituitary contained more STH, ACTH, and prolactin and were able to produce full lobulo-alveolar growth of the lactiferous ducts. These studies confirmed the predictions after 40 days or eight weeks.

6. Prolactin (Mammotropin, Luteotropin, Lactation Hormone, Galactin) and the Morphology of the Pigeon Crop Test

STRICKER and GRUETER'S (1928, 1929) discovery considerably advanced knowledge of the physiology of milk secretion as lactationlike secretion was started in castrated, pseudopregnant rabbits, in bitches, sows, and cows by administration of total extracts of the adenohypophysis. RIDDLE and BRAUCHER (1931) identified and isolated this lactogenic protein and called it "prolactin". The authors demonstrated a substance in the adenohypophysis of pigeons, which regulates the proliferative and secretory activity of the crop epithelium. RIDDLE, BATES, and DYKSHORN (1932, 1933) worked out experimentally the basis of the action of prolactin on the pigeon crop as test object. The crop proliferation test in young pigeons is still the best method for the assay of units of prolactin (JUNKMANN, 1957). The structural changes of the crop epithelium are a simple model of morphogenetic hormone action, which may be used to conceptualize similar mechanisms of action in the mammary gland and which is characterized by proliferation and secretion.

Morphology of prolactin action in the pigeon crop proliferation test. The crop of columbides — compared with other bird species — has changed its function, in so far as it serves not only for storage and predigestion of food, but in and during breeding it supplies a milky secretion, rich in fat, for the nourishment of the young. The term "crop milk", which is still used today, was coined by HUNTER (1786), who was the first to investigate these secretory processes. LITWER (1926) proved the holocrine mode of secretion, and lately

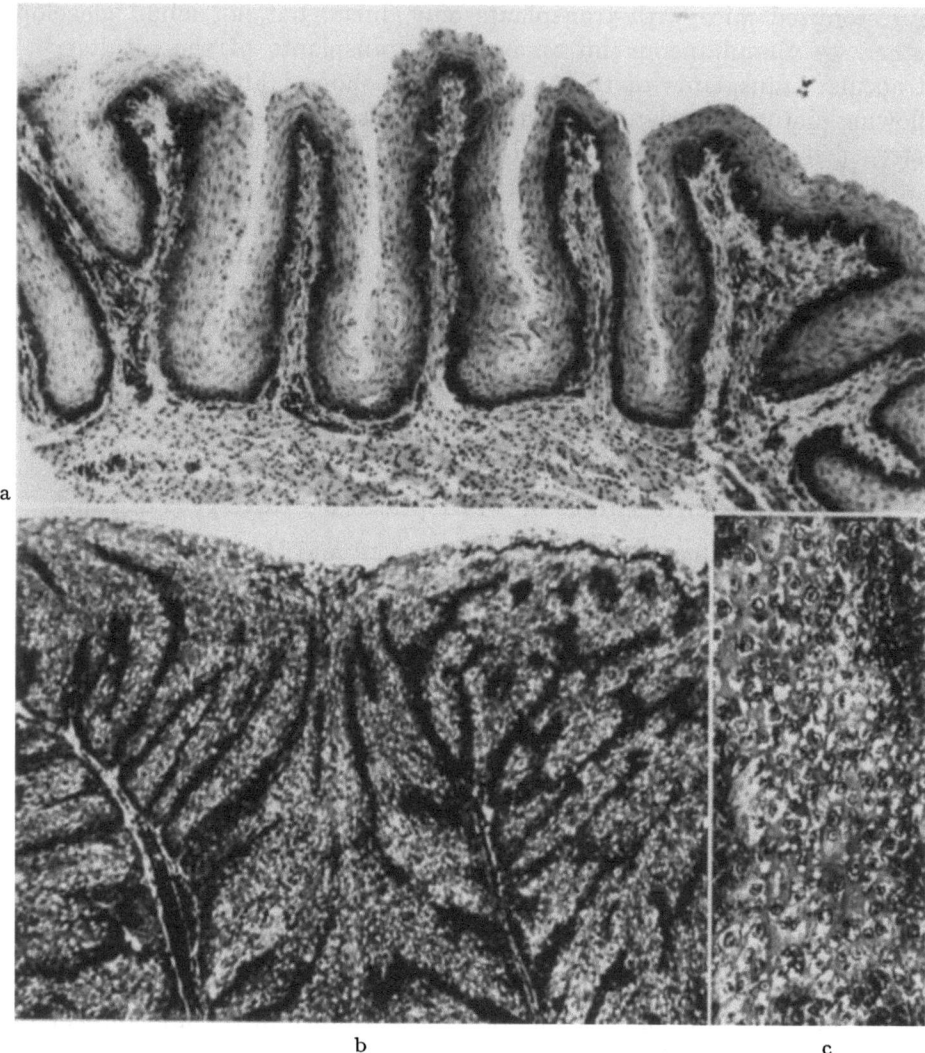

Fig. 19a—c. The effect of prolactin on the pigeon crop. a Resting crop epithelium with formation of folds in the lateral areas of the crop. Formalin, paraffin, HE, magnification 90×. b Hyperplasia of crop epithelium with formation of papillary structures and desquamation of superficial cell structures, 90 hours after administration of prolactin (25 IU), subcutaneously in the region of the crop. In the stroma dilated capillaries. Formalin, paraffin, HE, magnification 90×. c Enlargement of sector shows transparent gaps in the cytoplasm of the epithelium due to formation of fat droplets. Formalin, paraffin, HE, magnification 230×

WEBER (1962) has analysed morphologically the various functional phases of the crop epithelium and has found that there are no morphological differences between normal secretion during care of the young and experimental induced secretion of crop milk. Under the influence of prolactin the epithelium of the lateral areas of the crop proliferates, producing a wide epithelial band that is penetrated by septa, which carry blood-vessels. In the individual cells of this band there are mitoses, changed shapes of nuclei and nucleoli, extrusion of nucleoli, and formation of fat droplets. The essential characteristics of hormonal action are proliferation, synthesis of fat, and desquamation (holocrine secretion), as shown in Fig. 19.

Electron-microscopic investigations by BÄSSLER and FORSSMANN (1964), FORSSMANN (1965) and by DUMONT (1965) have demonstrated that the cells of the resting crop epithelium have the cytological properties of a syncytium with basal, spinous, and disjoint strata. Under the influence of prolactin the ribosomes in the cytoplasm of the epithelial cells of the basal and spinous strata increase greatly. DUMONT (1965) had also observed polysomes. The increasing basophilia of the cell plasm is concurrent with this early reaction. The basophilia may be observed in the microscope. It goes together with the synthesis of neutral, unsaturated triglycerides in droplet form. After 20 hours the mitochondria increase in size and lose their matrix contrast (FORSSMANN, 1965). The intensive micropinocytosis of the cell membranes and of the capillary endothelium and the increased vascularization of the stroma of the proliferating epithelium clearly seen under the microscope, indicate an intake of precursors of fat synthesis. The epithelial cells, held in place by numerous desmosomes, loosen their connections as stimulation with prolactin continues. The intercellular gaps increase, so that space for intercellular transport of substances is created. When the cells, loaded with fat droplets, part from their neighbours and perish, the gaps near the surface are filled with fragmented microvilli and cell detritus. The detachment of the epithelium at its natural boundaries and the subsequent cytolysis are the criteria of holocrine secretion (BARGMANN, FLEISCHHAUER, KNOOP, 1961), the product of which is the white crop milk indicating the action of prolactin.

LYONS and CATCHPOLE (1933a, b), CATCHPOLE and LYONS (1933), CATCHPOLE, LYONS, and REGAN (1933) were the first to report the promotion of lactation by prolactin in mammals (guinea pigs, rabbits, heifers). They called the purified substance "lactation hormone" or "mammotropin". In further studies of the lactogenic effect by GARDNER and TURNER (1933) the terms "galactin" and later "lactogen" were used. — LYONS (1942) and later MEITES and TURNER (1947) and BRADLEY and CLARK (1956) convincingly demonstrated a direct influence on the glandular parenchyma in pseudo-pregnant rabbits by intracanalicular instillation of prolactin in different doses: those sectors of the gland treated with prolactin reacted with considerable secretion and enlargement of the alveoli, whilst the other sectors showed no reaction. It was impossible to decide with certainty whether endogenous hormones of the anterior pituitary were of importance for lactogenesis. The question therefore arose whether prolactin was *the* lactogenic hormone or merely part of a lactogenic hormonal complex. This concept that had been conjectured by FOLLEY and YOUNG (1941) and underscored by FOLLEY (1956) had been supported by experiments of NANDI (1958a, b) because milk secretion in mice was triggered off by STH and cortisol after triple operations. FOLLEY (1956) and COWIE and FOLLEY (1961) therefore believed that secretion of milk was due to a pituitary lactogenic hormone complex, the essential and limiting component of which was prolactin.

MEITES and SGOURIS (1952, 1954) had shown in castrated rabbits and LANI (1968) in rats that oestrogen, progesterone, and prolactin had a mutually stimulating and inhibiting action at different quantitative ratios. The antagonism was relative, in other words, dependent upon the individual components. The same goes for lactation, which is inhibited when the activators for mammogenesis, i.e. oestrogen and progesterone, are more powerful than the stimulus for secretion, i.e. prolactin, and vice versa (VOSS, 1958).

Comparative histological and histochemical studies of this problem by LANI and BÄSSLER (1967) and LANI (1968) have demonstrated that castrated rats, when pretreated with ovarian hormones and then received simultaneously oestrogen, progesterone, and prolactin, had smaller alveoli and produced less secretion than control groups, to whom prolactin alone had been given after pretreatment lasting for 15 days. The variations in amounts of secretion are depicted in Fig. 10. Fig. 10d clearly shows that the amount of secretion has caused formation of cysts and fibrosing of the intralobular stroma. These are consequences of congestion of secretion. — Simultaneous histochemical investigations of phosphatases and dehydrogenases have shown no differences of reaction between animals that had received either ovarian hormones only or these and prolactin together. At the end of hormone treatment enzyme activity usually decreased, because increasing congestion of secretion had caused cell compression and cytolysis.

Secretion (*galacto-* or *lactopoesis*) may be maintained only if pituitary function remains undisturbed. Hypophysectomy stops secretion within 24 hours. Even after 4—8 hours alterations of metabolism may be observed in vitro. These changes may be detected biochemically. They correspond to the involutional phase of the mammary gland (BRADLEY and COWIE, 1956). The amounts produced in experimental galactopoesis obtained with combinations of hormones reached only 30% of those of normal lactation (BENSON, COWIE, FOLLEY and TINDAL, 1959).

Recent studies of active placental compounds are of importance for mammo- and lactogenesis, because substances with qualities similar to prolactin and STH may be obtained (AVERILL, RAY and LYONS, 1950; CANIVENC and MAYER, 1953; RAY, AVERILL, LYONS, and JOHNSON, 1955). — HIGASHI (1962) had described two active glycoproteins of the placenta with a molecular weight of 80,000 and 45,000 and with prolactin-like effects on pigeon crops. JOSIMOVICH and MCLAREN (1962) had described similar effects of serum and placenta proteins. These stimulated the crop epithelium and milk secretion and were immunologically related to STH. — RIDDLE (1963), in a review of prolactin, pointed to the growth and weight-promoting effects of prolactin, which related to accessory sex glands and which sensitized the prostate and the seminal glands to androgen (PRICE and WILLIAMS-ASHMAN, 1961). COLE and HOPKINS (1962) in comparative enzymatic studies on mammary tissue after prolactin action for 14 days reported significant rises of activity of succino-dehydrogenase, alkaline phosphatase, β-glucuronidase, DNA, and nitrogen. —

In view of the numerous observations of the biological activity of prolactin, the question of its biochemical entity and specificity of action has been raised recently. In immunological studies by HAYASHIDA (1962), using the agar diffusion technique of OUCHTERLONY, human prolactin reacted very similarly to STH.

Anti-STH serum contains antibodies both against STH and prolactin. It may be assumed that both compounds consist of one molecule only. The observation that prolactin may promote growth and that STH may be lactogenetic (RIDDLE, 1963) is supported by experimental studies by FORSYTH, FOLLEY and CHADWICK (1965): it was shown by means of the intraductal rabbit test and the pigeon crop test that human STH was strongly lactogenetic. The crop epithelium reacted to a lesser degree than the mammary gland of the rabbit. On the basis of these results it is at present under discussion whether the growth hormone is the solely hypophyseal lactogen.

Questions of the hypothalamic inhibition of synthesis and incretion of prolactin cannot be dealt with here.

7. Oxytocin

Experimental experience indicates that this hormone of the posterior lobe of the pituitary is of no importance for mammogenesis. The stimulating influence of oxytocin on the system of myoepithelial cells and on the discharge of prolactin of the adenohypophysis is considerable according to recent observations, so that two effects and sites of action ought to be distinguished.

a) Galactokinetic Effect

The path of secretion from the site of production of the glandular alveolus up to the mamilla is several centimetres long both in man and animals. Negative sucking pressure is too small to overcome this distance. In the human infant it is 4—14 cm initially. During continuous stimulation by sucking it may rise to 140 cm water (VOLKMANN, 1951), so that sucking can move milk from the lactiferous ducts and sinuses only. A vis a tergo is needed for the outflow of greater quantities of secretion from the periphery of the gland. This is supplied by the functioning of the myoepithelium of the alveoli and the small lactiferous tubuli. This cell system, which has arisen out of the glandular epithelium has special functions (WATZKA, 1955). It is the receptor and transformer of the oxytocin effect on the glandular alveolus. For the *mechanism of milk outflow* the term "milk let down" (for the oxytocin effect "milk let down factor") has been used, which according to FOLLEY (1947, 1956) and COWIE, FOLLEY, CROSS, HARRIS, JACOBSOHN, and RICHARDSON (1951), should be replaced, however, by the term *"milk ejection reflex"*, as it is preceded by active cell work.

The structural formula of oxytocin, an octopeptide, was discovered in 1953, and the compound was synthetized in the same year by DU VIGNEAUD *et al.*

(1953a, b). It is produced in the paraventricular nucleus. The hormone reaches the posterior lobe of the pituitary as neurosecretion (BERDE, 1959). The short duration of action, with a half-life time of approx. three minutes (SAAMELI, 1961), 9.7 minutes after blocks of the kidneys (CHAUDHURY and WALKER, 1957), is due to an inactivating enzyme, oxytocinase. The oxytocinolytic property of an aminopeptidase of the plasma during pregnancy increases up to delivery and then immediately decreases to its initial value (BERDE, 1959). BERDE and CERLETTI (1960) obtained two reaction types in the lactating mammary gland by pharmacological doses: intravenous individual injection caused a short rise of mammary internal pressure; long-term infusion after a latency period of about one minute caused a tonic reaction with persistent rise of pressure or rhythmic variations of pressure. The effect may be temporarily interrupted by adrenaline.

The secretion and the activity of oxytocin are maintained by a neurohumoral reflex arc, which is triggered off by tactile stimuli of the suckling young animal at the mamilla and which enters the hypothalamus as an afferent nerve arc. Oxytocin is liberated there via the neurohypophysis. It acts by humoral pathways on the myoepithelia, these were called the motor apparatus of the mammary gland by ZAKS (1962). This explains the synergic action. — Two further reflex arcs were proposed by ZAKS (1962): a segmental, short arc for the varying dilatation and contraction of the lactiferous ducts during milk transport and a cortical arc to explain psychic influences on secretion. —

Description of *the morphology of the oxytocin action* is subject to knowledge of the myoepithelial cells and their normal behaviour. Their structure was elucidated microscopically by selective staining methods or in-vivo observations (LINZELL, 1955). HAMPERL (1940) and KUZMA (1943) had used silver impregnation to discover abnormality of these cells. It became possible then to assess the myoepithelia directly by silvering of their basal membrane. By means of direct silvering they were shown by RICHARDSON (1949) in the udder of the goat, and by LINZELL (1952, 1955) in the alveolar wall. DEMPSEY, BUNTING, and WISLOCKI (1947), SILVER (1954), LEESON (1960), BÄSSLER, SCHÄFER and PAEK (1967), and BÄSSLER and BRETHFELD (1968) have obtained similar results by the essay of alkaline phosphatase, using the azodye method (GÖSSNER, 1959) and taking into account the varying functional stages of the alveoli (Fig. 20). The changes of structure of the myoepithelial cells during pregnancy were shown to have a uniform pattern, in that delicate cell processes increased in size during lactation, but became denser during involution. The increase of size in congestion of milk may lead to rupture of the cell processes, which then surround sectors of the alveolar surface only. In experimental work under the influence of sex hormones myoepithelial cells developed with the same enzyme-histochemical and morphological properties as during normal functioning.

The area occupied by myoepithelial cells increases concurrently with the enlargement of the alveoli during pregnancy, lactation, and acute galactostasis. During involution this is reversed. Under the influence of oxytocin the alveoli

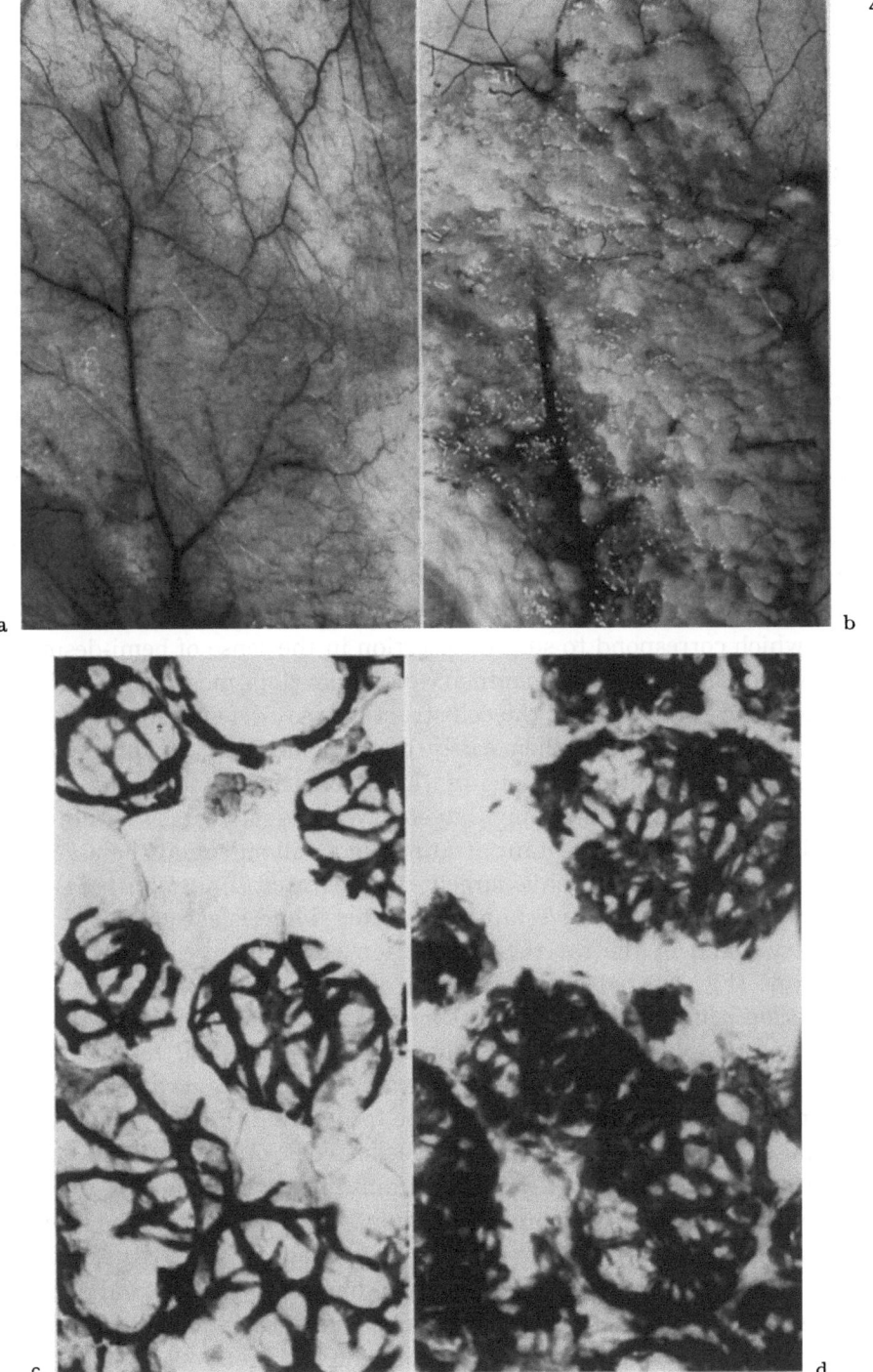

Fig. 20. a Lactating abdominal mammary gland of the rat with considerable vascularization. b Condition after syntocinon injection, two minutes after beginning of injection. Contraction of circumscribed areas of the gland and dilatation and filling with secretion of the prominent glandular fields. Representation of myoepithelial cells by determination of alkaline phosphatase (azodye method). c Lactation with dilated alveoli. d Contracted state of the myoepithelium after injection of syntocinon. Broad irregular cell structures and diminished alveoli. Magnification 245 ×

diminish in size, whilst the myoepithelium increases in area to one-third more than during lactation.

Electron-microscopic investigations of the myoepithelium of the mammary gland by TAKAHASHI (1958), LANGER and HUHN (1958), HAGUENAU (1959), and MURAD A. v. HAAM (1968) were restricted to morphological analysis of these cell types, which resemble those of the salivary glands (TAKAHASHI, 1958; MYLIUS, 1960; TANDLER, 1965; TAMARIN, 1966), of the eccrine sweat glands (HIBBS, 1958; MUNGER, 1961; TERZAKIS, 1964; ELLIS, 1965), of the apocrine sweat glands (TAKAHASHI, 1957; MUNGER, 1964, 1965), of HARDER's gland (CHIQUOINE, 1958), and of the extraorbital lacrimal gland (LEESON, 1960a, b).

The fine structure of the narrow cords of cells, which surround the alveoli, is characterized by its myofilaments, which enclose the nuclei. The mean diameter of the filaments is 50—90 Å. It is of similar dimensions both in the mammary gland and in the salivary gland (TAMARIN, 1966) and of the same dimensions as in actin fibres, as determined by NEEDHAM and SHOENBERG (1964). Contrast-rich cords, which recall the Z-membranes of the skeletal musculature, are interlaced with the filaments. Dense bundles are seen along the cell membranes which correspond to sites of insertion in the sense of hemi-desmosomes. The motor cell system of the mammary gland develops most abundantly during lactation, and differences in the cell structure that depend upon the degree of filling of the alveoli may then easily be recognized. Even during transient conditions of stasis cross-sections of the myoepithelia may hang saddlewise between extended and "drooping" alveoli. When galactostasis is more permanent, these cells form a resistant stratum that still surround the alveoli, even though the glandular cells have largely disintegrated (BÄSSLER, 1961).

In experiments when oxytocin is administered and is acting on the lactating mammary gland of the rat the contraction effect manifests itself under the microscope (Fig. 20a, b) by a retraction of circumscribed glandular areas and by secretion being packed in the lactiferous ducts, which may show variciform distension. Histologically and histochemically alveoli and lobuli shrink and interstitial oedema may develop (Fig. 20c, d). Irregularities of alveolar contours prove electron-optically to be prolapse of the cytoplasm, which protrudes between contracted myoepithelial cells. As there is no proper coordination between contraction and simultaneous secretion in experiments these phenomena appear more conspicuous than normally. The contraction stimulus, when observed in the electron microscope, manifests itself by denseness of the intracellular myofilaments, leading to retraction and serration of the sites of insertion at the cell membrane. The cords of cells surrounding the alveoli shorten, and the diameter of the alveoli is therefore lessened. Emptying of the alveoli is followed by fresh synthesis of milk products and secretion into the alveolar lumen.

b) Galactopoetic Effect

SELYE (1934), BENSON and FOLLEY (1956, 1957a, b) and DESCLIN (1956a, b) found that oxytocin may inhibit the involution of the mammary gland.

Experience indicates that it is unlikely for oxytocin to act directly on the mammary glandular cells. It may thus be assumed that prolactin stimulates by indirect action, because under identical condition this hormone in particular produces the same results (BENSON, COWIE, FOLLEY and TINDAL, 1959). This is supported by the fact that the effect is not observed in hypophysectomized animals (BENSON and FOLLEY, 1956b, 1957).

The angioarchitectonic relationships between the hypothalamus, the stalk of the pituitary, and the adeno- and neurohypophysis suggest the regional "portal" circulation as an explanation for the direct influence of neurohypophyseal substances on the adenohypophysis (GREEN and HARRIS, 1946/1948). GROSVENOR and TURNER (1957a, b) were opposed to these assumption, because of the fall of the level of prolactin when excretion of milk ceases, i.e. when involution begins.

Hormones of the Adrenal Cortex

HÖHN's (1957) experiments have provided evidence for the importance of the steroids of the adrenal cortex for growth and differentiation of the mammary gland: guinea pigs react to administration of oestrogen by formation of lobuli; after adrenalectomy, however, only by proliferation of ducts. Numerous investigations have shown the variations of responses of the mammary gland to hormones of the adrenals, supposed to depend, according to AHRÉN and JACOBSOHN (1957), upon the initial hormonal condition of the species and also upon the chemical structure of the hormones.

SELYE (1954a) was the first to demonstrate the synergic reaction to cortisol (500 mg/d) and oestradiol (5 mg/d) in ovarectomized rats. There was maximal development of gland, maximal secretion, and maximal dilatation of the alveoli, corresponding to the lactation phase. Administration of hydrocortisol acetate (0.5 mg/d) alone to noncastrated rats produced proliferation of ducts after gonadectomy and adrenalectomy there was only slight growth of the mamillae. When oestradiol was administered simultaneously, the gland was developing markedly (SELYE, 1954b). — FLUX (1954) had observed both antagonistic and synergistic reactions of the hormones of the adrenal cortex: cortisone inhibited the growth of castrated mice when they had been pretreated with oestrone. After administration of desoxycorticosterone acetate (DOCA) the growth stimulus, initiated by oestrogen, became more intense. — MUNFORD (1957) reported dose-dependent reactions, in that combinations of oestrone and small quantities of cortisol caused greater glandular growth than cortisol.

According to JOHNSON and MEITES (1955) non-castrated rats react to cortisol or cortisone with proliferation of ducts and lobuli. Both formation and excretion of secretion were more intense when cortisone had been given. The findings of JOHNSON and MEITES (1956) seem to support the assumption that cortisone will promote lactation and that hydrocortisone acetate will cause a proliferating mammary gland of pregnancy to secrete on the 16th—19th day

(TALWALKER, NICOLL and MEITES, 1961). Cortisone may inhibit involution after weaning in lactating rats (JOHNSON and MEITES, 1957).

Other points of view have been presented by AHRÉN and JACOBSOHN (1957) in extensive studies. They had shown that cortisone stimulated increase in size and increased proliferation of duct epithelium in hypophysectomized animals, although differentiation was not normal, even when ovarian hormones were given in addition. — Nonhypophysectomized rats merely secreted without there being growth; this occurred only when ovarian hormones were administered in addition. These observations indicate that cortisone chiefly promotes the growth of alveoli and secretion, although the intensity of the metabolic action of cortisone limits any inhibitory effect or deformity of the gland (COWIE and FOLLEY, 1961). — Hydrocortisone acetate in late pregnant rats induce an increase of RNA but not of DNA (FERRERI and GRIFFITH, 1969).

SMITH and BRAVERMAN (1953) have described experiments carried out on immature rats after castration. They found dosedependent reactions on combined treatment. Earlier investigations on mice gave similar results (GARDNER, 1940; LEONARD and REECE, 1942; SMITHCORS and LEONARD, 1943). — The results of these investigations show that steroids also have a direct mammotrophic effect. Experiments on the synergic action of various combinations of hormones have shown that the development of the mammary gland is encouraged by simultaneous application of adrenal cortical hormones.

Testosterone

LAQUER (1943) was the first to demonstrate the effect of male sex hormones on the mammary gland of *non-castrated female rats*. He brought together experimental animals (2.5 mg testosterone propionate every other day; a total of 25 mg in 20 days) and young animals, aged 6—10 days. Four of the six experimental animals were able to breastfeed their adoptees on the second and third day after the start of the injections. The author by comparative histological investigation pointed to the similarity of the mammary structure in pregnancy, lactation, and on stimulation by testosterone, when a status praelactans was obtained. After administration of 40 mg testosterone and suckling of the young animals for 10 days the mammary glands could not be distinguished from normally developed lactating glands. — With increasing dosage and duration of administration the production of both acini and secretion increased. At the same time progressive atrophy of the corpora lutea was observed, which counteracted secretion. — LAQUEUR and FLUHMANN (1942) further investigated the action of testosterone on the genital cycle, when proliferation of ducts and acini was observed during oestrus. — According to FORBES (1942) the testosterone effect is not noticeable in prepubertal animals.

Numerous studies of castrated rats are in existence, based on work by MCEUEN, SELYE and COLLIP (1936), who compared mammary development in male animals. On the 48th day of life non-castrated controls showed regular development of small buds, alveoli, and secretion. This has been confirmed by

Astwood, Geschickter and Rausch (1937). The castrated animals had small glandular tubuli without the characteristics of secretion and proliferation.

Further experimental studies of similar arrangements have produced similar results (Table 5). The drugs were administered by the intramuscular or circumalveolar (local) routes.

Table 5

Single dose	Duration of administration	Alveoli	Cysts	Authors
0.05 mg	21 days	(+)	—	Ahrén and Etienne (1959)
0.15 mg	21—23 days	+—	—	Ahrén and Hamberger (1962)
0.2 mg	23 days	+		Selye, McEuen and Collip (1936)
	15 days	++		Reece and Mixner (1939)
0.3 mg	21—23 days	++		Ahrén and Hamberger (1962)
0.4 mg	18 days	++		McEuen, Selye and Collip (1936)
0.5 mg	8—30 days	++	(+)	Ahrén and Etienne (1959)
	60 days	+++	(+)	Astwood, Geschickter and Rausch (1937)
0.75 mg	21—23 days	+++		Ahrén and Hamberger (1962)
1.00 mg	25 days	+++		Nelson and Merckel (1937)
1.50 mg	21—23 days	+++		Ahrén and Hamberger (1962)
2.50 mg	30 days	+++	+	Ahrén and Etienne (1959)
2.50 mg	10 days	+++	++	Meyer (1967)
5.0 mg	5 day	++	+++	Meyer (1967)

Increasing individual doses given to female and male castrated rats, the duration of the experiment being alike, caused increasing lobulo-alveolar development of the mammary gland, secretion, and — with larger doses — formation of cysts. — Meyer (1967) and I were able to achieve this after five days, having injected large doses. We believe this to be due to the secretory impulse that starts immediately (Fig. 21a). Female animals reacted with simultaneous dosedependent production of udders.

Studies by Hamberger and Ahrén (1964) have shown that the stimulation of the glandular parenchyma by testosterone depends on intact function of the adrenal cortex: after adrenalectomy male sex hormone was effected only when cortisone was administered as well. Oestrogen as a substitute failed. Adrenalectomized and hypophysectomized animals did, however, react to combinations of STH and testosterone. — Similar investigations by Jacobsohn and Norgren (1965) in adrenalectomized and gonadectomized rats resulted in lobulo-alveolar growth only provided oestrogen (0.05 mg) and cortisone acetate (0.125 mg) were added to testosterone (0.1—0.2 mg).

There seems to be general agreement that the mammary gland of hypophysectomized rats is not stimulated although large doses may have immediately been given (McEuen, Selye and Collip, 1937; Leonard and Reece, 1942; Leonard, 1943). The last author merely mentioned hyperplasia of ducts and swelling of nuclei.

This was quite different after castration and hypophysectomy and treatment with testosterone: REECE and LEONARD (1942) and AHRÉN (1959a, b) mentioned hyperplastic ducts and epithelia, and DONOVAN and JACOBSOHN (1960) described also a coloured secretion. This is in conformity with observations of my own (Fig. 21 b). — A large number of further combinations of the compounds did not induce lobulo-alveolar differentiation of the mammary

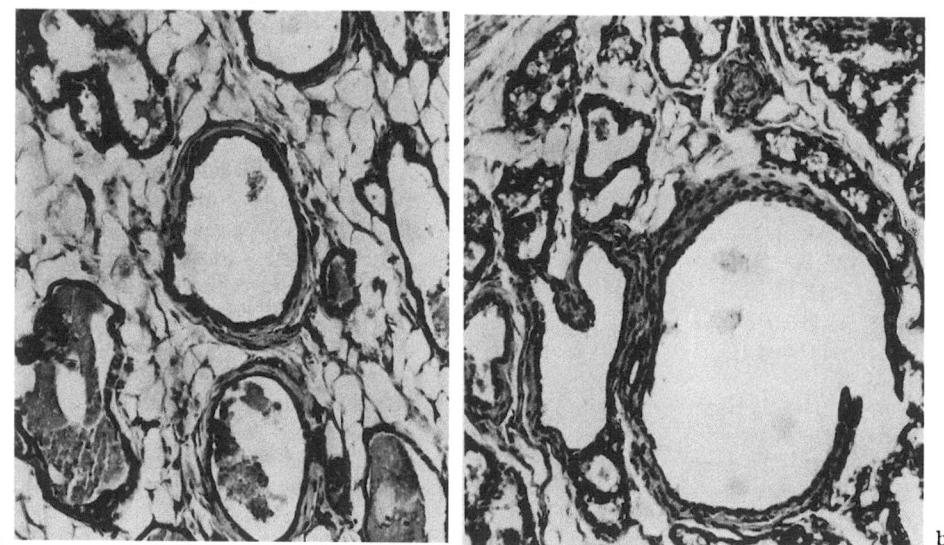

Fig. 21 a and b. Action of testosterone on the mammary gland of castrated female rats. a Strong lobular hyperplasia with formation of cysts and secretion after 2.5 mg/5 d. b Dilatation of duct, formation of alveoli and lobuli with secretion and castrated, hypophysectomized animal after treatment with testosterone (0.5 mg/10 d). Formalin, paraffin, HE, magnification 230 ×

gland after the preliminary operations, except when testosterone was administered together with STH (REECE and LEONARD, 1942; AHRÉN, 1959a, b). The following combinations produced hyperplasia of lactiferous ducts and of epithelial cells with variable amounts of secretion:

Table 6

Combinations of hormones	Alveoli	Hyperplasia of ducts	Secretion	Authors
Testosterone + Insulin	−	+	−	AHRÉN and ETIENNE (1959)
Testosterone + Insulin + Cortisone	−	+	+	DONOVAN and JACOBSOHN (1960)
Testosterone + Insulin + Cortisone + Thyroxin	−	+	(+)	DONOVAN and JACOBSOHN (1960)
Testosterone + Insulin + Cortisone + Oestrone	−	+	+	JACOBSOHN (1962)
Testosterone + Prolactin	−	+	++	AHRÉN (1959b)

BENGTSON and NORGREN (1961) studied the effect on *rabbits*. The authors had combined testosterone and oestrogen at different dosages and a time of observation of up to 56 days, and described differences in arborization and secretion of the glands.

HEUVERSWYN, FOLLEY and GARDNER (1939) and FLUX (1954) described in *mice* proliferations of the tubular system with buds in castrated and non-castrated animals. Alveoli were not observed. Testosterone had no stimulating effect in mice after castration and hypophysectomy (FERGUSON and VISSCHER, 1953; DORFMAN and SHIPLEY, 1956). Androgen together with extracts of the pituitary or STH promoted the growth of the mammary gland. Experiments by ARHELGER and HUSELY (1951) demonstrated the antagonism between androgen and oestrogens by implanting vaginal tissue into male animals, castrating some and treating them for four weeks with oestrogens (0.5 g/d). Proliferation of the mammary gland was found only in castrated animals, in whom the action of oestrogen had not been abolished by endogenous androgen. The implanted vaginal skin reacted with keratinisation and formation of mucous membrane, as was to be expected.

BOTTOMLEY and FOLLEY (1939) studied mammary glands and udders of immature castrated and non-castrated guinea-pigs. They pointed to the proliferation of ducts and production of alveoli and also to the fact that the position of the hydroxyl groups on C_3 or C_{17} and the double bonds in the androgen molecule were of importance for the development of the udders.

FOLLEY, GUTKELCH and ZUCKERMAN (1939) found production of alveoli only when rhesus monkeys received large doses (1.69 g for 151 days). VAN WAGENEN and FOLLEY (1939) had the same results with castrated female rhesus monkeys.

Thyroxin

The hormone of the thyroid gland belongs to a group of active compounds that influence the general metabolism and thus by indirect action proliferation of the mammary gland or that by stimulation of other hormones promote the secretion of the mammary gland. According to LEONARD and REECE (1941) and MEITES (1959a) the development of the mammary gland, ectasia of the ducts, and formation of buds may be increased in rats by thyroidectomy, whilst in mice hypothyroidism appears to inhibit the development of the gland (FOLLEY, 1952, 1956). On the other hand, CHEN, JOHNSON, LYONS, LI and COLE (1955) and LYONS, LI and JOHNSON (1958) pointed out that rats showed no signs of thyroxin deficiency after hypophysectomy, adrenalectomy, thyroidectomy, and administration of oestrone, progesterone, STH, prolactin, and STH. The action on the gland is thus indirect, not direct. — Measurements of DNA (MOON and TURNER, 1960) in castrated rats with mild hyperthyroidism gave higher values in mammary glands that had been stimulated by ovarian hormones than in controls with undisturbed thyroid function. GRIFFITH and TURNER (1961b) reported that thyroxin produced similar growth-promoting stimuli, which produced a development of the mammary gland in pregnant animals that was 22% greater than in rats that had not been pretreated with thyroxin. — Jacobsohn (1959, 1960) had described in castrated and hypophysectomized rats increased development of ducts under the influence of thyroxin after administration of oestrone and progesterone. The importance of hormonal synergism for glandular growth was the object of further studies by Donovan and Jacobsohn (1960a, b). According to Gomez and Turner (1937) small doses of thyroxin are ineffective in hypophysectomized animals. — Mixner and Turner (1942c) had found that glandular differentiation was 25% greater in mice who had been given optimal doses of thyroxin than in euthyroid controls. — Moon (1962) had treated castrated and thyroidectomized rats with ovarian hormones following equal pretreatment. He obtained a significant rise of DNA values of the proliferated mammary gland and a change of morphological structure by progressive treatment with thyroxin. Oestrone, progesterone, and thyroxin started secretion in the lobuli and thus produced a picture of early lactation. The synchronous rise of the LTH level when thyroxin was administered justified the assumption that thyroxin promoted both the production and the secretion of lactogen and somatotropin. — This was supported by in-vitro studies by Nicoll and Meites (1963). The authors were able to increase prolactin secretion of explantate cells of the adenohypophysis by thyroxin, but not by insulin. Recent observations of the pathogenetic relationship between disorders of the mammary gland and the thyroid gland have shown a positive syntropism between proliferating mastopathy and disorders of the thyroid gland, together with an increase of the survival rate of carcinoma of the mammary gland (Humphrey and Swedlow, 1964). — According to epidemiological studies the number of carcinomas of the mammary gland will increase under conditions of iodine deficiency and hypothyroidism (Eskin, Bartuska, Dunn, Jacob and Dratman, 1967). These authors found in experiments that iodine deficiency potentiated the simultaneous effect of oestrogen on the mammary gland of rats, whilst testosterone triggered off an increase in cellular and cystic hyperplasia. The typical morphological findings, characterized by cysts, epithelial proliferation, and secretion, were further intensified by iodine deficiency and propylthiouracil. When the mammary gland was stimulated by hormones in the same manner, different functional states of the thyroid gland caused different glandular structures in cystic hyperplasia. The authors were able to prove statistically that carcinoma of the mammary gland increased when endemic goitre with hypothyroidism increased. Vice versa, the number of carcinomas of the mammary gland in conjunction with thyrotoxicosis was smaller than when in conjunction with euthyroidism or myxoedema.

Parathyroid Hormone and AT 10

The high mineral content of milk, especially the content of calcium, the level of which is 10 times higher than in the blood, makes it appear likely that the epithelial bodies have an influence on lactation. Cowie and Folley

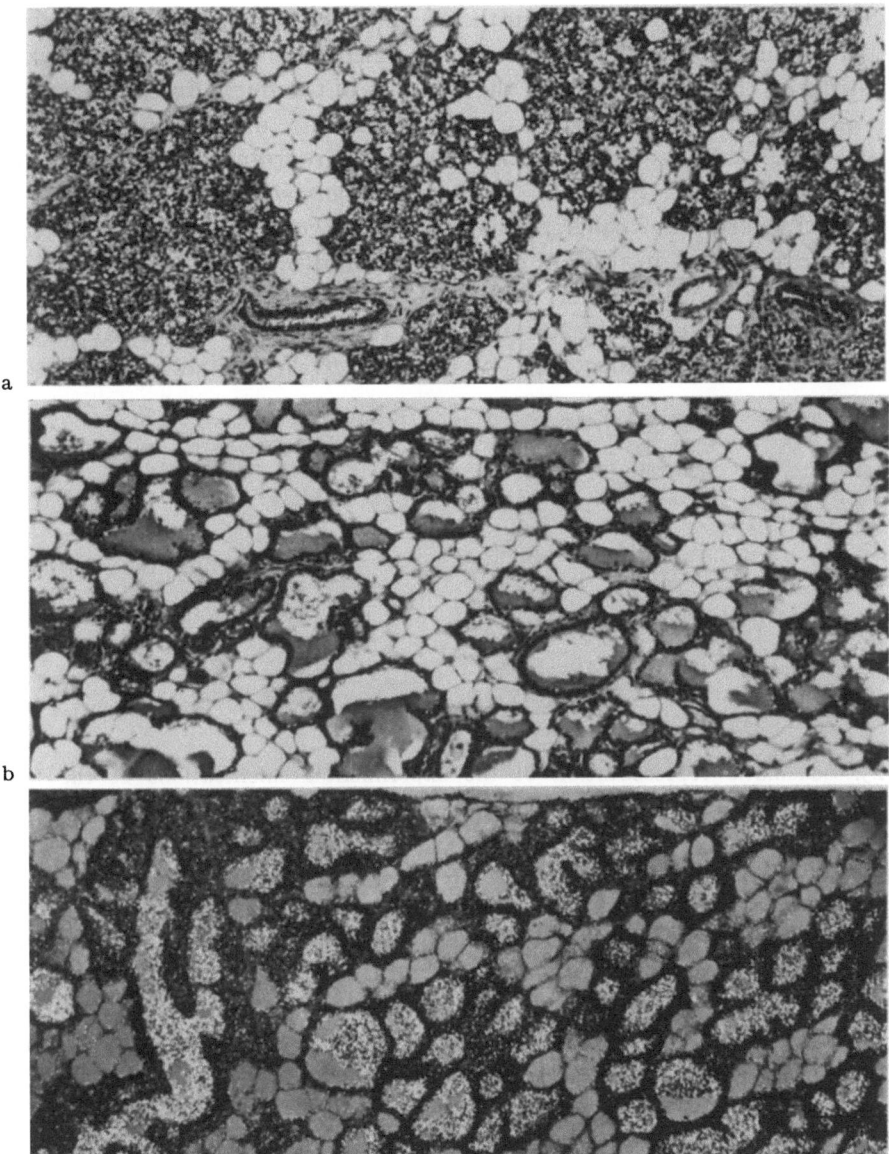

Fig. 22a—c. Effect of AT 10 on the mammary gland after stimulation with hormones. a Castrated female rat. Lobular proliferation with synthesis of fat and little secretion after treatment with 5 γ Progynon and 50 mg Proluton for 10 days. Formalin, paraffin, HE, magnification 90×. b Castrated female rat. Lobular proliferation and intense secretion with formation of alveoli filled with secretion after treatment with 5 γ Progynon and 50 mg Proluton and AT 10 for 10 days. Formalin, paraffin, magnification 90×. c Sector with representation of calcium enrichment in the secretion after Voigt in semi-polarized light. Alcohol, paraffin, Voigt's staining, magnification 90×

(1945) had found that secretion after parathyroidectomy alone decreased nearly as much as when the thyroid gland had been removed simultaneously. MUNSON (1955) observed 24 hours after parathyroidectomy a rise of calcium in milk with decrease of calcium in the serum. MOSIMANN (1955) had described increased calcium contents of milk after lactation had been started artificially by oestrogen. The enlargement of the volumes of the nuclei in the parathyroid gland indicates increased activity under the influence of hormones. — According to DJOJOSOEBAGIO and TURNER (1964a), dihydrotachysterol is a substitution of parathyroid function. Comparisons between parathyroid extracts, dihydrotachysterol, and calciferol have shown a general increase of lactation due to increased mobilization of serum calcium and increased intake of feeds (DJOJOSOEBAGIO and TURNER, 1964b). Combinations of dihydrotachysterol (AT 10), oestrogen, and progesterone, given to rats after ovarectomy, thyroidectomy, and parathyroidectomy (v. BERSWORDT-WALLRABE and TURNER,

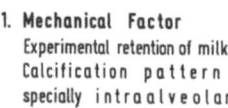
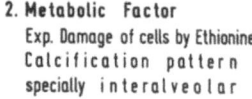
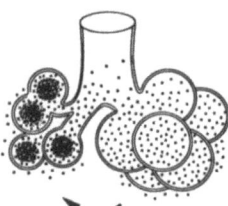
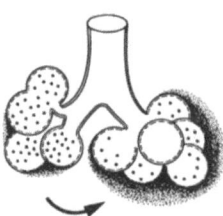

Fig. 23. Schematic representation of the experimental calcifications of the female mammary gland

1960a, b) and parathyroid extracts (DJOJOSOEBAGIO and TURNER, 1964c), raised the DNA content of the mammary glands. BRANDT and BÄSSLER (1968, 1969) had found in the mammary gland of the rat that had been stimulated by oestrogen and progesterone an increase of secretion by AT 10 on the 10th day of injection to the extent that alveoli developed, which were full of secretion (Fig. 22). The calcium content of the secretion was strongly positive, as shown histochemically (Fig. 22c). These studies demonstrate the stimulating action of AT 10 on secretion in the lobuli. This relates both to lobular distension and to the changed qualitative composition of the secretion. The importance of AT 10 for calciphylactic reactions of the mammary gland in experiments and for calcifications in the human mammary gland has been the object of recent studies by BRANDT (1968). According to the author two types of calcification may be distinguished: *intra-alveolar calcification* after *congestion of secretion* and *interstitial calcification* after experimental metabolic *cell damage*. I was able to produce the last in experiments by means of ethionin (Fig. 23).

Insulin

Insulin belongs to the group of hormones that are not directly mammogenic. It promotes proliferation and differentiation of the mammary gland when combined with other hormones. Experimental studies have shown that oestrogen, progesterone, prolactin, STH, and further hormones are necessary to trigger off complete development of the gland (BENSON, COWIE, FOLLEY and TINDAL, 1959). On the basis of observations by SALTER and BEST (1953) regarding a possible mammogenic effect of insulin in hypophysectomized rats AHRÉN and JACOBSOHN (1956, 1957), AHRÉN and ETIENNE (1958), and AHRÉN (1959a) have shown that insulin, when administered for a long time, is able together with ovarian hormones to stimulate growth of the tubules. It may be assumed that insulin enters beneficially into the general metabolism and that it increases the reactivity of mammary tissue towards oestrone and progesterone. Cortisone diminishes this effect, thyroxin increases it (AHRÉN and JACOBSOHN, 1956; JACOBSOHN, 1959, 1961).

Relaxin

Relaxin, most of which is produced in the ovary and which becomes active during pregnancy, is supposed to influence the development of the mammary gland (SMITH, 1954). Little is known about its effect on secretion. According to COWIE (1961) relaxin diminishes the milk yield of goats after castration and pretreatment with oestrone and progesterone. It is also assumed that this hormone is of importance for the contraction of the myoepithelium in sheep, but not in cows and rats.

Summary

Present opinion is that the morphogenesis of the female breast is regulated by a complex of hormones, the direct and indirect action of the various substances being complementary. The essential hormones are those of the ovary, *estrogen* and *progesterone*, and the *pituitary secretions*, *prolactin*, *STH* and *ACTH*. An indirect mammotrophic effect is exerted by thyroxine, insulin and the glucocorticoids by stimulating the metabolism in general. The full development of the mammary gland is achieved by the synchronous operation of this hormonal complex, not by any single hormone.

The *proliferation of the duct system* is triggered by estrogen, STH and the adrenocortical steroids.

Lobular-alveolar development is due to the synergic action of the ovarian hormones, STH, steroids and prolactin. Secretion of prolactin is stimulated by estrogens, thyroxine and steroids (STEINBECK, 1969).

V. Pathology of Effects of Hormones on the Human Mammary Gland

It is reasonable to expect that the results of the many experimental investigations of hormonal mechanisms of regulation of the mammary gland would explain disorders of the human mammary gland. This has formerly been taken into account to a small extent only, because the study of the actions of hormones on lactation and their therapeutic control was the primary concern.

Obviously, the physiology and the biochemistry of the various phases of nutritive function of the mammary gland have developed to a greater extent than those of disorders of the mammary gland. In comparison, endocrinological premises, by which the pathological developments of the human mammary gland may be interpreted, are still unsatisfactory. Difficulties of morphological interpretation arise from the great variability of the various reaction types of the lobuli and also because there is a lack of attempts at matching in individual cases hormonal status and structural changes. For this reason pathogenetic interpretations depend largely on analogies from animal experiments and on laws obtained by comparison of similar events by generalizing induction (M. HARTMANN, 1956). Morphogenetic patterns have been constructed from investigations of different species, which have then been transferred to human pathology. These patterns are co-ordinated with disorders of the human mammary gland, which are due to endocrine dysregulations. Pathomorphogenetic analysis of dysplastic mammary disorders must take into account the structural and functional individuality of this organ, the pathoclisis of which coincides with the phases of hormonal stimulation, and the possibilities of dysregulations during sexual maturation and involution. An essential precondition for pathohistological assessment would be a type classification of glandular structure, related to age and statistically verifiable, mainly of microscopic units which would serve as measure. The lack of this is at present balanced by general morphological findings, and the "harmonious" regular structure of the epithelium and the stroma of the lobuli is used as criterion. LETTERER (1948) has coined the terms "concordance" for the normal and "discordance" for the disordered structure of the gland, in adaptation from the terms used for changes of the endometrium. The disorders may concern the whole organ or parts only. The local dysregulations pertain to individual gland structures that have their own terminal flow path and are interpreted as localized misguidance of hormonal impulses. It remains open whether the terminal flow path or the whole of the angioarchitecture of the mammary gland are responsible for local dysplasias. The frequency of the localization of disorders of the mammary gland in the upper outer quadrant has not been explained and may well be a consequence of the particular type of vascularization of this region of the gland.

It is important, too, for morphological assessment to determine whether the mammary gland is stimulated by accessory endocrine in the state of tubular or lobular differentiation. The strength and quality of the hormones is, of course, also of importance. Metaplasia of the gland from a tubular to a lobular structural pattern or from a functionless phase to a state of secretory activity, when retention of secretion will cause dilatation and cysts, is the rule. The reverse changes are also observed.

1. Pathomorphology of the Lobules of the Gland

The changes of lobular structure, which frequently occur in benign dysplasias of the mammary gland and are essentially due to endocrine dysregulation, are shown schematically in Fig. 24. Classification depends upon the mode of metaplasia of the lobuli.

1. *Regressive changes.* These are characterized by diminution of the size of the lobuli, associated with intralobular fibrosis of the mantle tissue and with broadening of the basal membrane. The epithelial parts up to the peripheral sectors of the lactiferous ducts atrophy. The terminal buds may be taken into

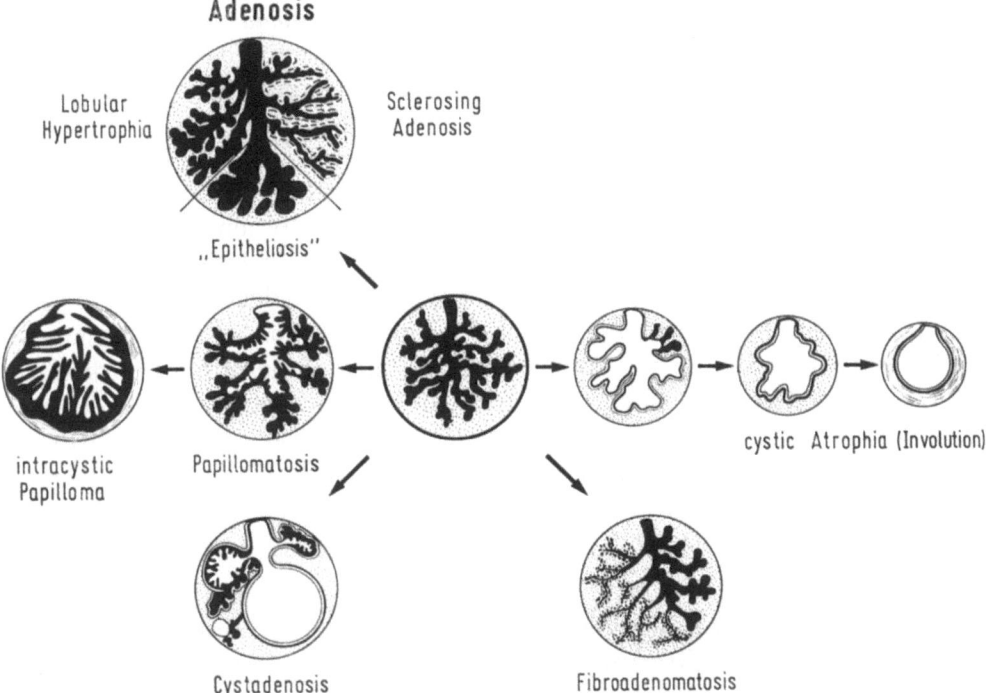

Fig. 24. Schematic representation of progressive and regressive changes in the glandular lobules of the mammary gland

the wall by increasing dilatation of the duct, and thus may then be transformed into a smooth-walled cyst. (Regarding delineation between dilatation and cyst, see BÖHMIG, 1952, 1964.) Type: senile atrophy, fibro-cystic mastopathy.

2. *Progressive changes.* This group is characterized by hyperplasia of the lobules with maintenance of their fundamental structure. The increase of epithelial components justifies the concept of adenosis, although differences in shape and order of magnitude should be allowed for.

a) *Lobular adenomatous hyperplasia* due to increase of regular or dilated adventitious proliferations. This is normal during pregnancy.

b) *Sclerosing adenosis* due to enlargement and confluence of lobules. Proliferation of myoepithelial cells and of the intralobular stroma whilst the glandular epithelium is maintained or atrophies (epimyothelial proliferation). (HAMPERL, 1940; FOOTE and STEWART, 1945; URBAN and ADAIR, 1949.)

c) *Epitheliotic or adenomatous intralobular proliferation of epithelium* with isomorphic solid, cribriform or papillomatous structures. Dilatation of terminal tubules and sectors of lobules, enlargement of lobular volume (BÖHMIG, 1964). DAWSON (1933) called this "epitheliosis" as against adenosis. Type: Schimmelbusch's adenosis; fibro-cystic mastopathy. Intermediate type between benignancy and malignancy. Delimitation towards lobular carcinoma (FOOTE and STEWART, 1941; NEWMAN, 1963, 1966; BÖHMIG, 1964; BÄSSLER, 1968).

3. Papillary adenosis of the lobules and of the tubular system. Commonly found in abnormal lobules. — Papillomas of the lactiferous ducts are found usually as circumscribed tumours in the large ducts near the mamilla (JONES, 1955).

Papillomatosis of the whole of the tubular system is unusual. Proliferation of the epithelium is then preceded by enlargement of large and small lactiferous ducts and is frequently accompanied by apocrine secretion. The ducts, which extend funnel-like, dissemble the lobular structure by inclusion of the terminal buds. Type: fibro-cystic mastopathy, papillary cystadenomas, macromastia.

4. Combined metamorphosis of lobules with formation of cysts. Commonly, proliferative and regressive changes coexist: metaplasia of lobules, dilatation of ducts and formation of cysts with apocrine secretion, also oedematous swelling of the mantle tissue. Type: mastodynia, fibro-cystic mastopathy.

5. Proliferation of mantle tissue with maintenance of the lobular structure or metaplasia (atrophy, proliferation), indicating hormonal stimulation. Type: fibroadenoma, angiomesenchymal macromastia types. Gynaecomastia.

2. Morphology and Function of the Intralobular or Mantle- and Circumlobular or Supporting Connective Tissue

Local proliferation of mesenchymal cells of the subepithelial connective tissue in the stage of budding between the 3rd—4th embryonal months is the first inductive reaction of the stroma to the proliferating epithelium. With increasing development of the gland the circumductular mesenchyma loosens, becomes transparent, rich in cells, and in the mammary gland of the newborn presents the essential portion of the stroma, surrounded by small terminal vesicles of collagenous fibres which lie only behind the fatty tissue and in the intermediary zone. When "witch's milk" is secreted, this portion of the mesenchyma is nearly completely replaced by the proliferating and extending glands, as happens later during pregnancy and lactation. When secretion of "witch's milk" ceases and the glands involute, the loose connective tissue is replaced by collagenous connective tissue, which in both sexes becomes that element of the gland that determines its shape (BÄSSLER, 1958a). At the beginning of sexual maturity the ducts and later the lobules are surrounded by a type of mesenchyma that is very similar to that present at the time of birth. BERKA (1911) distinguished this intralobular surrounding tissue from the rest of the interlobular supporting tissue of the mammary gland, which serves to shape and fix the body of the gland. The qualitative and quantitative changes of the structure of the mammary gland under normal conditions are shown in the schematic illustration (Fig. 25).

Mantle tissue is a special and reactive type of mammary glandular mesenchyme, the development and regression of which mirrors the phases of hormonal activity. Its extensive vascularity and ability to produce cells are of importance for normal and abnormal interactions. Its multifarious pathogenetic properties may be summarized as follows:

1. Mantle tissue differentiates under the influence of mammotropic hormones, especially of oestrogens and, as Fig. 25 shows, is biomorphic. It is the

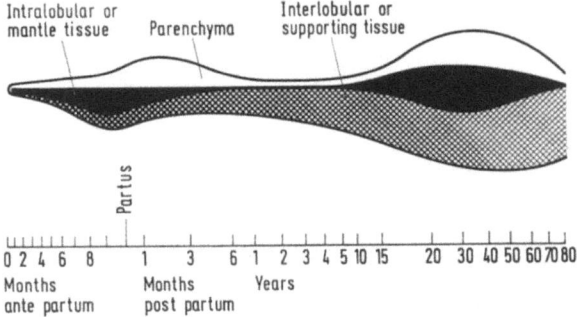

Fig. 25. Schematic representation of the quantitative and qualitative changes of the structure of the mammary gland under normal conditions

site of reaction for reversible oedematous swellings during the *menstrual cycle* (ROSENBURG, 1922; DIECKMANN, 1925; LITTEN, 1926; LUCHSINGER and CENTANO, 1927; KUECKENS, 1929; TAYLOR, 1936; MASSHOFF, 1955) and a *zone of growth* (guide path according to DABELOW, 1933, 1934, 1941) for the proliferating epithelium.

On pathological stimulation mantle tissue appears characteristically as a circumtubular or lobular mesenchymal envelope in gynaecomastia, macromastia of puberty (virginal hypertrophy), mastodynia, fibro-cystic mastopathy, and in several types of macromastia (Fig. 26).

2. Mantle tissue is able to *produce blood cells* during the whole of life (cytogenic stroma of the mammary gland). In the newborn transient, but regular *foci of haemopoiesis* may be observed (GRUBER, 1921), and in erythroblastosis intensive and persistent haemeopoiesis may be present (BÄSSLER, 1958b). — In *haemoblastosis* haematopoiesis may arise anew at any age and cause extensive infiltrates (SEIFERT, 1952).

3. Mantle tissue as the site of *inflammatory* reactions develops cellular infiltrates in *circumductal* (periductal) *mastitis*, plasma and giant cells in *plasma cell mastitis* (ADAIR, 1933; CUTLER, 1933) and specific granulomas in miliary tuberculosis, for example.

4. Mantle tissue is the site of the development of *fibroadenomas*. These tumours are therefore thought to be hyperplasms of the mantle tissue and glandular structures. This is supported by the facts that they occur in the fertile phase of women and that they have a tendency to sclerosing during age.

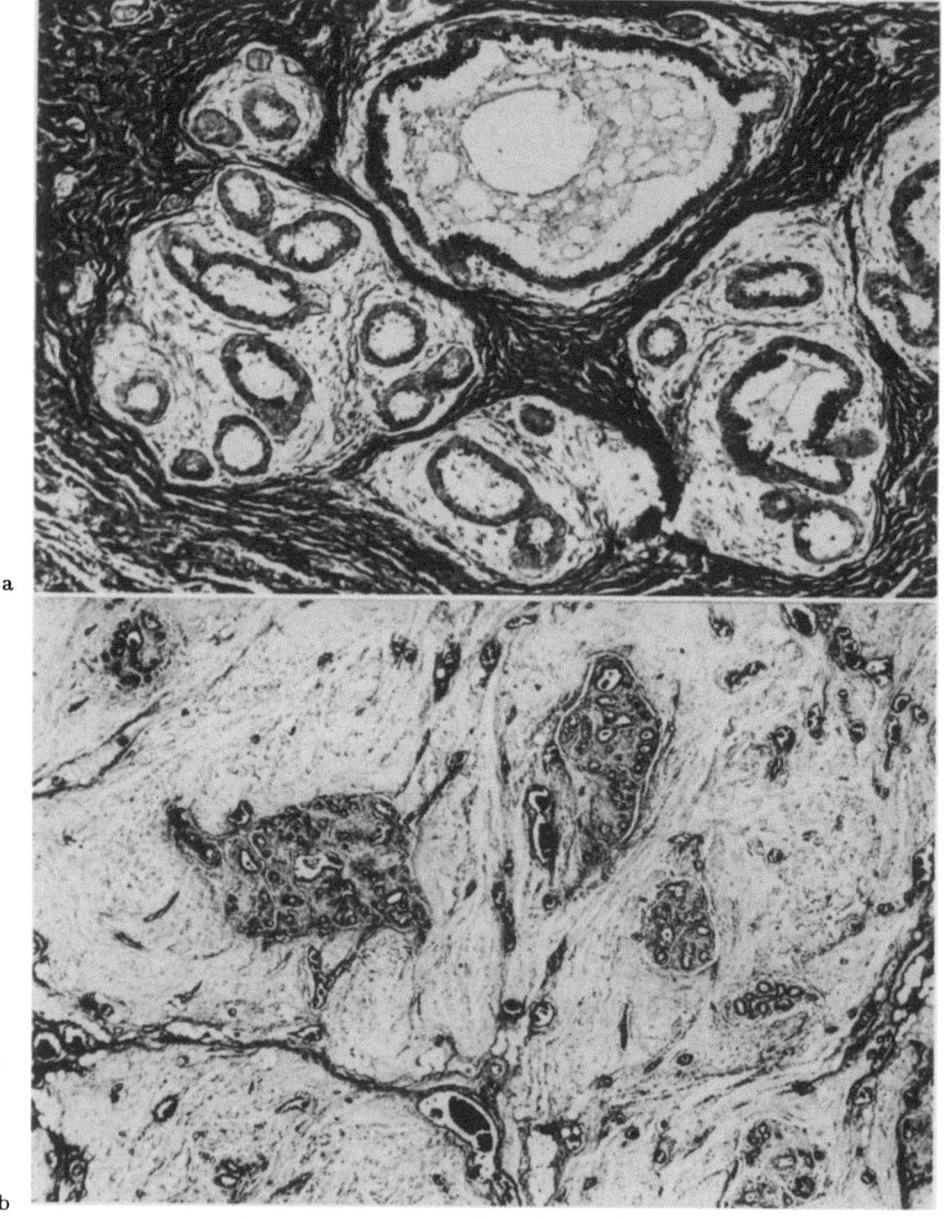

Fig. 26a and b. Two contrasting reaction types of the mesenchyma of the mammary gland. a Swelling and oedema of the mantle tissue during apocrine secretion of the glandular epithelium due to strong hormonal stimulation in macromastia. Formalin, paraffin, Azan., magnification 240 ×. b Oedematous loosening of supporting tissue with hyperemia and mantle tissue that is largely regular. Angiomesenchymal form of macromastia in Cushing's disease. Formalin, paraffin, HE, magnification 90 ×

Supporting tissue of the mammary gland. When the secretion of "witch's milk" has ceased, collagenous connective tissue appears between the tubules as interstitium. It directly envelops the epithelial components of the mammary gland and acts as supporting tissue until the onset of puberty. Before maturity the body of the gland consists mainly of a regular, dense stroma. Its isomorphism is subsequently maintained normally. With increasing age and in dysplasias focal and flat *hyalinoses* occur, which may be accompanied by *elastosis* (RIEDEL, 1925; BOHLE, 1951; VILLANI and ZANELLA, 1951) and atrophy of the parenchyma. The increase of supporting tissue is of particular importance in fibrocystic mastopathy. This increase is supposed to commence in the intralobular mantle tissue according to BÖHMIG (1964) and to observations by FOOTE and STEWART (1945) and COPELAND (1947).

Atrophy of the parenchyma and fibrosis are often accompanied by lipomatosis of the glandular body. My own observations have confirmed that even the stroma and residues of the intralobular connective tissue may be included in this, so that the epithelial portions of the lobuli are surrounded by fat cells only (stroma-free lobules).

Experimental work on fibrosing is based on the fact that the mammary gland of mature rodents has no mantle tissue in BERKA's sense. Under the influence of sex hormones neutral and acid mucopolysaccharides are deposited in the circumtubular and lobular stroma (CHAIN and DUTHIE, 1940; DURAN-REYNALS, BUNTING and VAN WAGENEN, 1950; VITRY, 1953; OZZELLO and SPEER, 1958). The retention and absorption of residual secretion from proliferating glands is the precondition of fibrosing. This last is stronger after lactation and galactostasis (SCHRIEVER, 1968). Reactions of the mesenchyme analogous to fibro-cystic mastopathy have not been observed, although after treatment of rats with oestrogen fibroadenomatous structures have occasionally been found in the circumtubular mesenchyme.

3. Aetiology and Pathogenesis of Benign Dysplasias

Structural changes of the mammary gland are due, on the whole, either to changes of the mechanisms of hormonal regulation or to tissue reactions being inadequate. The multitude of morphological and endocrinological symptoms makes classification difficult from a pathogenetic point of view, but to three large groups may be distinguished:

1. *Dysplasias and functional disorders due to changes of the quantity of mammotropic hormones.*

Accessory endogenous or exogenous compounds may stimulate development, secretion, and growth. They may cause hyperplasia (macromastia) of the mammary gland, when usually special tissue patterns are being developed.

a) *Secretion of "witch's milk"* is due to the joint action of hormones transferred through the placenta (choriogonadotropic hormones, follicular hormone) and of the mammotropin of the child (PHILIPP, 1938; LYONS, 1938; MERZ, 1946; DICZFALUSY, TILLINGER and WESTMAN, 1957).

b) *Macromastia of puberty* (virginal hypertrophy) at the beginning of sexual maturity through the influence of oestrogen (GESCHICKTER, 1948; BÄSSLER, 1966). Gynaecomastia of puberty [mastitis in adolescence, "early ripening"

(GESCHICKTER, 1948)]. This is usually transient, uni- or bilateral at the beginning of puberty. Morphologically corresponds to virginal hypertrophy.

c) *Gynaecomastia*, a polyaetiological syndrome due to increased growth impulses caused by hormones. Types: usually tubular gynaecomastia; more rarely true lobular gynaecomastia. Causes: endogenous or exogenous action of oestrogen, rarely other hormones or drugs (BREDT, 1932; KARSNER, 1946; NORDMANN, 1948; BOEMKE and BIRKLE, 1949; OVERZIER, 1949; KUNERT, 1951; SCHNURBUSCH, 1951; TREVES, 1958; BÄSSLER and SCHÄFER, 1968, 1969).

d) *Macromastia* due to hormone-active tumours of the ovary (granulosa-cell tumour: HABBE, 1931; carcinoma of the ovary: MÜLLERHEIM, 1928; together with disgerminoma and acromegaly: BÄSSLER, 1966), after administration of digitalis (CALOV and WHYTE, 1954; BLOCH, 1961); in endocrine disorders (CUSHING's disease: BÄSSLER, 1966).

e) *Hypoplasia and atrophy* in lack or deficiency of hormones.

f) *Atypical and papillary proliferation of epithelium* in harmless fibroadenomas of the mammary gland following the use of *oral contraceptives for several months* (GOLDENBERG, WIEGENSTEIN and MOTTET, 1968).

2. *Dysplasias due to changes of hormonal equilibrium*.

Preponderance of oestrogen and relative diminution of progesterone is a frequent cause of local and diffused disorders of the mammary gland.

a) *Mastodynia* (mazoplasia, CHEATLE and CUTLER, 1931; simple fibroadenomatosis, SEMB, 1928): Painful circumscribed swellings, increased consistency, usually in the upper outer quadrant, age 25—40 years. Menstrual cycle is shortened (GESCHICKTER, 1948; CUTLER, 1961). Irregular structure of the lobules, small cysts, multilayered epithelium, secretion, oedematous swelling of mantle tissue. Pregnandiol excretion in urine is only a third of normal, oestrogen remains unchanged (GESCHICKTER, 1948).

b) *Adenosis* (papillary cystadenoma, SCHIMMELBUSCH, 1892). Occurs at the ages of between 35 and 45 years, uni- or bilateral, prefers upper outer quadrant and middle of gland. Menstrual cycle is irregular. Microscopically strong proliferation of epithelium is seen in terminal tubuli with intracanalicular adenomas and papillomas and formation of cysts. Condition is to be understood as advanced stage of mastodynia. Hormone excretion as in mastodynia. According to GESCHICKTER (1948) it is due to relative hyperoestrogenism.

c) *Chronic cystic mastopathy.* (Morphology and symptomatology, KONJETZNY, 1942; GESCHICKTER, 1948; FRANTZ a.o., 1951; KONJETZNY, 1954; CUTLER, 1961; BÖHMIG, 1964, references, MÖBIUS a. NIZZE, 1966). Occurs between 40—50 years, prefers the upper and outer quadrant. — Excretion of pregnandiol greatly diminished, that of oestrogen sometimes greatly increased (GESCHICKTER, 1941, 1948). Numerous old and new investigations about aetiology and pathogenesis have shown that fibrocystic mastopathy is caused by persistent preponderance of oestrogen with relative diminution of progesterone. Although generally accepted, this concept has also been opposed (TAYLOR, 1936). It leaves a good many questions open, mainly those concerning quantity and quality of the pathogenetic factors.

The aetiological importance of hyperoestrogenism for fibrocystic mastopathy has been underscored by contrasting fibro-cystic mastopathy with the results of experimental research into hormonal action (BURROWS, 1935/36; HOFFMANN, 1939; TAYLOR and WALTMAN, 1940; INGLEBY, 1942; AVERBACH, 1956) and the happenings after administration of oestrogen for months, as described by GRUMBRECHT (1941) and EISEN (1942).

3. Dysplasias as inadequate reactions.

Physiological stimulation triggers off excess production. Example: macromastia of pregnancy.

4. Galactorrhoea in the Human Mammary Gland

Abnormal secretion is not only a guiding sign of disorders of the mammary gland, but is frequently due to increased formation of lactogenous hormones by tumours of the pituitary or to drugs. Apart from the sanguinous secretion of the mammary gland during excretion of "witch's milk", at the time of menstruation and in the case of tumours (SCHULTZ, 1933), only those kinds of galactorrhoea will be discussed where a *milk-like fluid is excreted from the mamilla outside the period of normal lactation*, in view of the importance of prolactin for secretion. Only this should be called galactorrhoea. It must be distinguished from common discontinuous excretions of the human mammary gland that accompany well-known syndromes and disorders of this organ and that may cause retention of secretion and lead to formation of cysts.

Causes and types of galactorrhoea:

1. *Chiari-Frommel syndrome.* The authors (1855 and 1881) called this a *post-partum abnormal lactation* in *post-partum amenorrhoea*, hypogenitalism, psychoses, and malnutrition. The review by DANOWSKI (1962) contains 13 case reports, four of which have been taken from a study by FORBES, HENNEMAN, GRISWOLD, and ALBRIGHT (1954). — The criticism may be voiced that intermediary forms of late lactation cannot be properly delineated from this syndrome, because morphological and endocrinological studies are lacking.

2. *Ahumada-del Castillo syndrome (1932).* Characterized by the triad: *galactorrhoea* with *amenorrhoea* in non-pregnant women, *lowered or lacking excretion of gonadotropin*, and signs of ovarian insufficiency. No pituitary tumour. In a subsequent study by ARGONZ and DEL CASTILLO (1953) and another by FORBES, HENNEMAN, GRISWOLD, and ALBRIGHT (1951, 1954) the assumption was made that the lowering of the blood oestrogen level caused an increase of lactogenic hormone and triggered off galactorrhoea. The acidophil cells of the adenohypophysis were proposed as site of production of the lactogenic hormone. Latest immunohistochemic investigations by KRACHT, HACHMEISTER, BREUSTEDT, and ZIMMERMANN (1967) have shown that prolactin and STH are produced by the acidophilic cell complex of the pituitary, although plurihormonal performance of individual cell types cannot be excluded. — Obesity, hirsutism, and hypoplasia of the genitals have been described as part of the syndrome. Galactorrhoea may persist for years (DANOWSKI, 1962). —

Observations of five cases with Ahumada-del Castillo syndrome by SPELLACY, CARLSON, and SCHADE (1968) showed normal values of growth hormone in blood. Symptoms presented that indicated a hypothalamic-hypophyseal disorder as cause of the galactorrhoea. — Whereas the asscociation of amenorrhoea and galactorrhoea is well recogniced, recently NYIRJESY (1968) has described *galactorrhoa in normal ovulatory women.*

3. Forbes-Albright syndrome. Galactorrhoea in tumours of the pituitary and brain disorders.

When the acidophilic cells of the adenohypophysis contain prolactin, it may be expected that adenomas of these cells may produce increased secretion. Galactorrhoea has been found in 4% of cases of *acromegaly* (LABHART, 1959; NEIMEIER, HAUSER, KELLER, LABHART, WENNER, STAMPFLI, 1959). Postpartum galactorrhoea in acromegaly is also called *Chiari-Frommel syndrome.* — In *Cushing's disease* abnormal secretion of the mammary gland is observed by SCHALTENBRAND (1951) and in a new case report with abnormal lactation, chromophobe adenoma of the pituitary and a marked elevated secretion rate of urinary steroids and cortisol by MAHESH, DALLA PRIA and GREENBLATT (1969). Finally, *chromophobic adenomas of the pituitary* have been thought to be causes of galactorrhoea. KRAUS (1935) reported two cases, FORBES, HENNEMAN, GRISWOLD and ALBRIGHT (1954) three cases, SUCHENWIRTH and BUES (1961) two cases, in which *galactorrhoea was the earliest endocrinological sign* of a tumour of the pituitary and where in one case it was accompanied by urinary excretion of prolactin corresponding to late pregnancy. For the aetiological clarification of galactorrhoea radiological and clinico-chemical examinations about the size of the sella and the function of the pituitary are absolutely necessary.

4. Galactorrhoea accompanied by disorders of thyroid function. Van Wyk-Grumbach syndrome: Galactorrhoea in hypothyroidism and premature menstruation. *Zondek-Bromberg-Rozin syndrome*: Galactorrhoea in hyperthyroidism. — An unusual coincidence of post-operative hypothyroidism, deficient function of the epithelial bodies, galactorrhoea, and undisturbed menstruation has been described by CLARK, SHAPIRO and MONROE (1956).

5. Further causes of galactorrhoea.

Disorders of the diencephalon in post-encephalitic Parkinsonism and administration of reserpine and chlorpromazine have been held responsible for galactorrhoea in rare cases (DANOWSKI, 1962). Individual cases of galactorrhoea in men may be due to angiosarcoma of the pituitary (HAENEL, 1928), be related to gynaecomastia (ZUM BUSCH, 1927; ALBORES CULEBRO, 1946; MCCULLAGH, ALIVISATOS, and SCHAFFENBURG, 1956), occur in tumours of the adrenals (BITTORF, 1919), tumours of the pineal gland (OESTREICH and SLAWYK, 1899) and chorion epithelioma (COOKE, 1915). *A familial nonpuerperal galactorrhoea* in three sisters is the first reported instance of galactorrhoea occuring either spontaneously or after oral contraceptive therapy (WIDER, MARSHALL and ROSS, 1969).

Further observations of *galactorrhoea subsequent to contraceptive hormones* are described by GREGG (1966), ROSEN and GAHRES (1967) and SCHACHNER (1966).

Galactorrhoea after castration and lowered excretion of FSH is studied by JAKOBOVITS (1960).

In a study of 5 cases of non-acromegalic persistent lactation by LEVINE, BERGENSTAL and THOMAS (1962) the analysis of milk secreted by 3 of these women revealed a consistently low lactose and a high protein content. — *Breast biopsies* demonstrated a pattern similar to subinvolution of a previously lactating mammary gland.— Secretion of milk due to tactile suckling stimulus of the nipple of men has been observed, so that fathers were able to suckle their children (HUMBOLDT, Journey into the Equinoctial Regions, 1889).

Much earlier it had been written: "Men who have a little milk may produce it in large quantities as soon as their breasts are suckled!" (ARISTOTELES, Historia animalium, Lib. III, c. 20).

I wish to thank Miss S. WALTER and Mrs. HANENBERGER for technical assistance and photographic work and Präparator Mr. W. MEYER for drawings and illustrations.

References

ADAIR, F. E.: Plasma cell mastitis. Arch. Surg. 26, 735—749 (1933).
AHRÉN, K.: (a) The effect of various doses of oestrone and progesterone on mammary glands of castrated hypophysectomized rats injected with insulin. Acta endocr. (Kbh.) 30, 435—458 (1959).
— (b) Mammary gland development in hypophysectomized rats injected with anterior pituitary hormones and testosterone. Acta endocr. (Kbh.) 31, 228—240 (1959).
— ETIENNE, M.: Stimulation of mammary glands in hypophysectomized male rats treated with ovarian hormones and insulin. Acta endocr. (Kbh.) 28, 89—102 (1958).
— — The effect of testosterone alone and combined with insulin on the mammary glands of castrated and hypophysectomized rats. Acta endocr. (Kbh.) 30, 109—136 (1959).
— HAMBERGER, L.: Direct action of testosterone propionate on the rat mammary gland. Acta endocr. (Kbh.) 40, 265—276 (1962).
— JACOBSOHN, D.: Mammary gland growth in hypophysectomized rats injected with ovarian hormones and insulin. Acta physiol. scand. 37, 190—203 (1956).
— — The action of cortison on the mammary glands of rats under various states of hormonal imbalance. Acta physiol. scand. 40, 254—274 (1957).
AHUMADA, I. C., DEL CASTILLO, E. B.: Amenorrea galactorrea. Biol. Soc. obstet. y Ginec. 11, 64—72 (1932).
ALBORES CULEBRO, C.: Un caso de ginecomastia o andro galactozemia. Toréon méd. 1, 80 (1946).
ALTMANN, H. W.: Der Zellersatz, insbesondere an den parenchymatösen Organen. Verh. dtsch. Ges. Path. 50, 15—51 (1966).
ANDERSON, R. R., BROOKRESON, A. D., TURNER, C. W.: Experimental growth of mammary gland in male and female mice. Proc. Soc. exp. Biol. (N. Y.) 106, 567—570 (1961).
ARGONZ, J., DEL CASTILLO, E. B.: A syndrome characterized by estrogenic insufficiency, galactorrhea and decreased urinary gonadotropin. J. clin. Endocr. 13, 79—87 (1953).

ARHELGER, ST. W., HUSELY, R. A.: Estrogen-Androgen antagonism: Histology of mammary glands and vaginal grafts of male mice receiving estrogens. Proc. Soc. exp. Biol. (N. Y.) 76, 811—817 (1951).

ARISTOTELES: Historia animalium. Lit. III. c. 20. Zit. nach Wenner.

ASBOE-HANSEN, G.: Hormonal effects on connective tissue. Physiol. Rev. (Baltimore) 38, 446—462 (1958).

— Endocrine control of connective tissue. Amer. J. Med. 26, 470—484 (1959).

ASTWOOD, E. B., GESCHICKTER, C. F.: Changes in mammary gland of rat produced by various glandular preparations. Arch. Surg. 36, 672—697 (1938).

— — RAUSCH, E. O.: Development of the mammary gland of the rat. A study of normal, experimental and pathologic changes and their endocrine relationships. Amer. J. Anat. 61, 373—405 (1937).

AVERBACH, M. M.: Über die Histogenese der Mastopathien und Fibroadenome der Mammae. Arch. Path. (Moskau) 18, H. 3, 65—71 (1956) [Russisch]. Ref. Ber. allg. spez. Path. 34, 186 (1957).

AVERILL, R. L. W.: The hypothalamus and lactation. Brit. med. Bull. 22, 261—265 (1966).

— RAY, E. W., LYONS, W. R.: Maintenance of pregnancy in hypophysectomized rats with placental implants. Proc. Soc. exp. Biol. (N. Y.) 75, 3—6 (1950).

BÄSSLER, R.: Zur Pathologie der kindlichen Brustdrüsen. Beitr. path. Anat. 118, 390—406 (1957).

— Beiträge zur Morphologie der kindlichen Brustdrüse. Frankfurt. Z. Path. 69, 37—52 (1958).

— Elektronenmikroskopische Beobachtungen bei experimenteller Milchstauung. Frankfurt. Z. Path. 71, 398—422 (1961).

— Formen der Makromastie. Beitr. path. Anat. 133, 430—460 (1966).

— Neuere Aspekte der normalen und pathologischen Feinstruktur der Mamma. Hippokrates (Stuttg.) 39, 237—244 (1968).

— Das sogenannte lobuläre Carcinom der Mamma. Dtsch. med. Wschr. 94, 108—113 (1968).

— BRETHFELD, V.: Enzymhistochemische Studien an der Milchdrüse. Gravidität-Laktation, Involution und experimentelle Stauung mit besonderer Berück, sichtigung myoepithelialer Zellen. Histochemie 15, 270—286 (1968).

— FLÖRCHINGER, J.: (a) Histometrische Studien an der laktierenden Milchdrüse. I. Mitteilung: Lactation und physiologische Involution. Arch. Gynäk. 203, 366—399 (1966).

— — (b) Histometrische Studien an der lactierenden Milchdrüse. II. Mitteilung: Experimentelle Milchstauung und vermehrtes Flüssigkeitsangebot durch Peristoninfusionen. Arch. Gynäk. 203, 400—422 (1966).

— FORSSMANN, W.: Experimenteller Strukturwandel der Drüsenzelle durch Hormonwirkung. Verh. dtsch. Ges. Path. 48, 240—244 (1964).

— PAEK, S.: Histochemisches Enzymmuster der Mamma unter dem experimentellen Einfluß von Geschlechtshormonen. Histochemie 13, 29—44 (1968).

— SCHÄFER, A.: Elektronenmikroskopische und experimentelle Untersuchungen zur Morphologie der Gynäkomastie. Verh. dtsch. Ges. Path. 52, 491—498 (1968).

— — (a) Elektronenmikroskopische Cytomorphologie der Gynäkomastie. Virchows Arch. Abt. A Path Anat. 348, 356—373 (1969).

— — (b) Elektronenmikroskopische Cytomorphologie der männlichen Brustdrüse. Z. Zellforsch. 101, 355—366 (1969).

— — PAEK, S.: Elektronenmikroskopische und histochemische Untersuchungen zur Morphologie und Funktion myoepithelialer Zellen. Verh. dtsch. Ges. Path. 51, 301—307 (1967).

Bässler, R., Schulze, G., Schriever, D.: Histochemische Untersuchungen am Bindegewebe der hormonal stimulierten Mamma. Experimentelle Beiträge zur Pathogenese von Fibrosierungen in der Brustdrüse. Beitr. path. Anat. (in press).

Baldwin, R. L., Martin, R. J.: Protein and nuclein acid synthesis in rat mammary glands during early lactation. Endocrinology 82, 1209—1216 (1968).

Balinsky, B. I.: (a) On the prenatal growth of the mammary gland rudiment in the mouse. J. Anat. (Lond.) 84, 227—235 (1950).

— (b) On the developmental processes in mammary glands and other epidermal structures. Trans. roy. Soc. Edinb. 62, 1—31 (1956).

Banerjee, M. R., Walker, R. J.: Variable duration of DNA-synthesis in mammary gland cells during pregnancy and lactation of C_3H/HE mouse. J. Cell Physiol. 69, 133—142 (1967).

Bardin, C. W., Liebelt, A. G., Liebelt, R. A.: The direct effect of pituitary isografts on mammary gland development in the mouse. Proc. Soc. exp. Biol. (N. Y.) 110, 716—718 (1962).

— — — Effect of hypophysial isografts on the mammary glands of intact and hypophysectomized mice. Endocrinology 74, 586—592 (1964).

Bargmann, W., Fleischhauer, K., Knoop, A.: Über die Morphologie der Milchsekretion. II. Zugleich eine Kritik am Schema der Sekretionsmorphologie. Z. Zellforsch. 53, 545—568 (1961).

Beato, M., Dienstbach, F.: Effect of estrogens and gestagens on the duration of DNA synthesis in the genital tract of ovariectomized mice. Virchows Arch. Abt. B. Zellpath. 1, 197—200 (1968).

Bengtsson, B., Norgren, A.: Interactions of oestrone and testosterone on mammary glands of male rabbit. Acta endocr. (Kbh.) 36, 141—156 (1961).

Benson, G. K., Cowie, A. T., Cox, C. P., Flux, D. S., Folley, S. J.: Studies on the hormonal induction of mammary growth and lactation in the goat. II. Functional and morphological studies of hormonally developed udders with special reference to the effect of "triggering" doses of oestrogen. J. Endocr. 13, 46—58 (1955).

— — — Folley, S. J., Hosking, Z. D.: Relative efficiency of hexoestrol and progesterone as oily solutions and as crystalline suspensions in inducing mammary growth and lactation in early and late ovariectomized goats. J. Endocr. 31, 157—164 (1965)

— — — Goldzweig, S. A.: Effects of oestrone and progesterone on mammary development in guinea-pig. J. Endocr. 15, 126—144 (1957).

— — Folley, S. J., Tindal, J. S.: Recent developments in endocrine studies on mammary growth and lactation. In: Recent progress in the endocrinology of reproduktion (C. W. Lloyd, ed.), p. 457—490. New York: Academic Press 1959.

— Folley, S. J.: (a) Oxytocin as stimulator for the release of prolactin from the anterior pituitary. Nature (Lond.) 177, 700 (1956).

— — (b) Retardation of mammary involution in the rat by oxytocin. J. Endocr. 14, 42 (1957).

— — (c) The effect of oxytocin on mammary gland involution in the rat. J. Endocr. 16, 189—201 (1957).

Berde, B.: Recent progress in oxytocin research. Amer. Lect. Series. Springfield, Ill.: C. C. Thomas Publ. 1959.

— Cerletti, A.: Über die Wirkung pharmakologischer Oxytocindosen auf die Milchdrüse. Acta endocr. (Kbh.) 34, 543—557 (1960).

Berger, H.: Beitrag zur elektronenoptischen Zelldifferenzierung des soliden Mammacarcinoms und der Mastopathia cystica des Menschen. Z. Krebsforsch. 66, 73—86 (1964).

Berk, F.: Beitrag zur Kenntnis der ersten Anlage der menschlichen Brustdrüse. Med. Inaug.-Diss. Greifswald 1913.

BERKA, F.: Die Brustdrüse verschiedener Altersstufen und während der Schwangerschaft. Frankfurt. Z. Path. **8**, 203—256 (1911).
BERSWORDT-WALLRABE, R. v.: (a) Die Hemmung der Galaktopoese der Albinomaus durch Dienöstroldiacetat und ihre Auswirkungen auf das inkretorische System. Arch. Gynäk. **190**, 549—618 (1958).
— (b) Versuch einer theoretischen Erklärung der Hemmung der Galaktopoese der Albinomaus durch Dienöstroldiacetat. Arch. Gynäk. **190**, 619—637 (1958).
— TURNER, C. W.: (a) Mammogenesis in ovary-thyro-parathyroidectomized rats. Proc. Soc. exp. Biol. (N. Y.) **103**, 536—537 (1960).
— — (b) Dihydrotachysterol (AT 10) and mammogenesis in ovary-thyro-parathyroidectomized rats. Proc. Soc. exp. Biol. (N. Y.) **104**, 599—602 (1960).
BIEDERMANN, K.: Das Verhalten des Genitalapparates weiblicher Ratten bei langdauernder Follikelhormonzufuhr. Arch. Gynäk. **167**, 465—476 (1938).
BITTORF, A.: Nebennierentumor und Geschlechtsdrüsenausfall beim Manne. Berl. klin. Wschr. **56**, 776 (1919).
BLOCH, K.: Zur Pathogenese der Mammahypertrophie bei der Digitalisapplikation. Z. Kreisl.-Forsch. **50**, 591—595 (1961).
BÖHMIG, R.: (a) Die Epithelproliferationen bei der Mastopathia fibrosa cystica. Zbl. allg. Path. path. Anat. **89**, 297—313 (1952).
— Mastopathia fibrosa cystica. Ergebn. allg. Path. path. Anat. **45**, 39—116 (1964).
BOEMKE, F., BIRKLE, K.: Zur Ätiologie der Fibrosis mammae virilis. Klin. Wschr. **1949**, 93—96.
BOHLE, A.: Beitrag zur Frage der Elastica-Vermehrung in Mammatumoren. Frankfurt. Z. Path. **62**, 167—183 (1951).
BOTTOMLEY, A. C., FOLLEY, S. J.: Effect of androgenic substances on growth of teat and mammary gland in immature male guinea pig. Proc. roy. Soc., London, Biol. Sci. **126**, 224—241 (1939).
BRADLEY, T. R., COWIE, A. T.: (a) The effects of hypophysectomy on the in vitro metabolism of mammary gland slices from lactating rats. J. Endocr. **14**, 8—15 (1956).
— CLARK, P. M.: (b) The response of rabbit mammary glands to locally administered prolactin. J. Endocr. **14**, 28—36 (1956).
BRANDES, D., ANTON, E., BARNARD, S.: Lysosomes and cellular regressive changes in rat mammary gland involution. Lab. Invest. **20**, 465—471 (1969).
BRANDT, G.: Die experimentelle Pathomorphogenese intramammärer Verkalkungen. Inaug.-Diss. Mainz, 1968.
— BÄSSLER, R.: Calciphylaktische Reaktionen der Mamma. Vortrag z. Tagg der nordwestdeutschen Pathologen, Bielefeld, 11.—13. Okt. 1968. Zbl. allg. Path. path. Anat. (in press).
— — Pathomorphogenese experimenteller Verkalkungen in der weiblichen Brustdrüse. Virchows Arch. Abt. A Path. Anat. **348**, 139—154 (1969).
BREDT, H.: Über Wesen und Formen der Gynäkomastie. Z. menschl. Vererb.- u. Konstit.-Lehre **17**, 29—54 (1932).
BRESCIANI, F.: DNA-synthesis in alveolar cells of the mammary gland: Acceleration by ovarian hormones. Science **146**, 653—655 (1964).
— Effect of ovarian hormones on duration of DNA synthesis in cells of the C_3H mouse mammary gland. Exp. Cell Res. **38**, 13—32 (1965).
BROMAN, J.: Die Entwicklung des Menschen vor der Geburt. München: J. F. Bergmann 1927.
BROUHA, H.: Recherches sur les diverses phases du developpement et de l'activité de la mamelle. Arch. Biol. (Liège) **21**, 459—605 (1905).
BROWNING, H. C., WHITE, W. D.: Local stimulation of mammary glands by pituitary or ovarian grafts in the mouse. Tex. Rep. Biol. Med. **23**, 26—37 (1965).

Browning, H. C., White, W. D., Gibbs, W.: Comparative stimulation of mammary gland by pituitary isografts with or without ovarian transplants. Tex. Rep. Biol. Med., 22, No. 1, Spring (1964).
Bunting, H.: The distribution of acid mucopolysaccharides in the mammalian tissues as revealed by histochemical methods. Ann. N. Y. Acad. Sci. 52, 977—982 (1950).
Burrows, H.: Pathological changes induced in the mamma by oestrogenic compounds. Brit. J. Surg. 23, 191—213 (1935/36).
Busch, J. P. zum: Gynäkomastie bei Hypernephrom. Dtsch. med. Wschr. 53, 323 (1927).
Busch, W., Merker, H.-J.: Elektronenmikroskopische Untersuchungen an menschlichen Mammacarcinomen. Virchows Arch. Abt. A Path. Anat. 344, 356—371 (1968).
Calov, W. L., Whyte, H. M.: Oedema and mammary hypertrophia: Toxic effect of digitalis leaf. Med. J. Aust. 41, 556—557 (1954).
Canivenc, R., Mayer, G.: Nature du facteur lutéotrophic de placenta de rat. C. R. Soc. Biol. (Paris) 147, 1067—1070 (1953).
Caspersson, T.: Cell growth and cell function. New York 1945.
Catchpole, H. R., Lyons, W. R.: The lactation hormone of the hypophysis. Anat. Rec. 55, 48—49 (1933).
— — Regan, W. M.: Induction of lactation in heifers with the hypophyseal lactogenic hormone. Proc. Soc. exp. Biol. (N. Y.) 31, 301—303 (1933).
Chain, E., Duthie, E. S.: Identity of hyaluronidase and opreading factor. Brit. J. exp. Path. 21, 324—338 (1940).
Chalkley, H. W.: Method for the quantitative morphologic analysis of tissues. J. nat. Cancer Inst. 4, 47—53 (1943).
Chamberlin, T. L., Gardner, W. U., Allen, E.: Local responses of the sexual skin and mammary glands monkeys to cutaneus applications of estrogen. Endocrinology 28, 753—757 (1941).
Chamorro, A.: Action de la progesteron seule sur la glande mammaire. C. R. Soc. Biol. (Paris) 138, 453—456 (1944).
Chaudhury, R. R., Walker, J. M.: Rate of disappearance of injected oxytocin from the blood. J. Physiol. (Lond.) 138, 50—61 (1957).
Cheatle, G. L., Cutler, M.: Tumors of the breast. London: Ed. Arnold & Co. 1931
Chen, Th. T., Johnson, R. E., Lyons, W. R., Li, C. H., Cole, D. R.: Hormonally induced mammary growth and lactation in the absence of the thyreoid. Endocrinology 57, 153—174 (1955).
Chentsov, Y., Chentsov, S.: Electron microscopy of rat mammary, glands on lactation, hormonal stimulation and in the case of postradiation fibroadenoma. Acta Un. int. Cancr. 20, 1377—1378 (1964).
Chiquoine, A. D.: The identification and electron microscopy of myoepithelial cells in the harderian gland. Anat. Rec. 132, 569—584 (1958).
Clark, B. G., Shapiro, S., Monroe, R. G.: Postthyroidectomie, hypothyroidism, hypoparathyroidism, exophthalamus and galactorrhoea with normal menstruation: metabolic response to propened. J. clin. Endocr. 16, 1245—1251 (1956).
Clifton, K. H., Furth, J.: Ducto-alveolar growth in mammary glands of adrenogonadectomized male rats bearing mammatropic pituitary tumors. Endocrinology 66, 893—897 (1960).
Cole, R., Hopkins, T. R.: Maintenance of the mammary gland in hypophysectomized — oophorectomized rats by injection of protein. Endocrinology 71, 395—398 (1962).
Consolandi, G.: La problema de cancero gelatinoso della mamella. Lav. Ist. Anat. Univ. Perugia 6, 35—76, 119—155 (1947).

COOKE, J. V.: Chorio-epithelioma of the testicle. Bull.-Johns Hopk. Hosp. 26, 215—221 (1915).
COPELAND, M. M.: New aspects of benign tumours of the breast. Arch. Surg. 55, 590—621 (1947).
CORNER, G. W.: The hormonal control of lactation. Amer. J. Physiol. 95, 43—55 (1930).
COWIE, A. T.: The relative growth of the mammary gland in normal, gonadectomized and adrenalectomized rats. J. Endocr. 6, 145—147 (1949).
— Recent studies on the endocrine control of the mammary development and milk secretion. Colloq. int. Cent. nat. Rech. sci., No. 32, p. 45—57 (1951).
— The hormonal control of milk secretion. In: Milk: The mammary gland and its secretion, ed. by S. K. Kon and A. T. Cowie, vol. I. New York and London: Academic Press 1961.
— FOLLEY, S. J.: Parathyreoidectomy and lactation in the rat. Nature (Lond.) 156, 719—721 (1945).
— — The mammary gland and lactation. In: Sex and internal secretions, ed. by W. C. Young and G. W. Corner, vol. II, p. 590—642. Baltimore: The Williams & Wilkins Co. 1961.
— — CROSS, B. A., HARRIS, G. W., JACOBSOHN, D., RICHARDSON, K. C.: Terminology for use in lactational physiology. Nature (Lond.) 168, 421 (1951).
— — MALPRESS, F. H., RICHARDSON, K. C.: Studies on the hormonal induction of mammary growth and lactation in the goat. J. Endocr. 8, 64—88 (1952).
— LYONS, W. R.: Mammogenesis and lactogenesis in hypophysectomized, ovarectomized, adrenalectomized rats. J. Endocr. 19, 29—32 (1959).
— TINDAL, J. S., YOKOYAMA, A.: The induction of mammary growth in the hypophysectomized goat. J. Endocr. 34, 185—195 (1966).
CURTISS, C.: Factors influencing lobulo-alveolar development and mammary secretion in the rat. Endocrinology 45, 284—295 (1949).
CUTLER, M.: Benign lesion of the female breast simulating cancer. J. Amer. med. Ass. 101, 1217—1222 (1933).
— Tumors of the breast. Philadelphia: Lippincott 1961.
DAANE, TH. A., LYONS, W. R.: Effect of estrone, progesterone and pituitary mammotropin on the mammary glands of castrated C_3H male mice. Endocrinology 55, 191—199 (1954).
DABELOW, A.: Der Entfaltungsmechanismus der Mamma. I. Das Verhalten von Gefäßsystem und Drüsenbaum während der Laktationsentwicklung der Mamma bei Maus, Ratte, Meerschweinchen und Kaninchen. Morph. Jb. 73, 69—99 (1934).
— Vergleichende Untersuchungen zur Entwicklung einiger Drüsen, ihrer Gefäßbäume und ihrem Verhalten zum umgebenden Gewebe. Verh. anat. Ges. (Jena), p. 165—188 (1934).
— Der Entfaltungsmechanismus der Mamma. II. Die postnatale Entwicklung der menschlichen Milchdrüse und ihre Korrelationen. Morph. Jb. 85, 361—416 (1941).
— Die Milchdrüse. In: Handbuch der mikroskopischen Anatomie des Menschen, hrsg. von W. v. Moellendorff u. W. Bargmann, Haut- und Sinnesorgane, Ergänz. zu Bd. 3/1, S. 277ff. Berlin-Göttingen-Heidelberg: Springer 1957.
DAMM, H. C., TURNER, C. W.: Effects of anterior pituitary preparations on mammary gland growth in mouse. Prox. Soc. exp. Biol. (N. Y.) 107, 893—895 (1961).
DANOWSKI, T. S.: Clinical endocrinology, vol. I. Baltimore: The Williams & Wilkins Comp. 1962.
DAWSON, E. K.: Carcinoma in the mammary lobule and its origin. Edinb. med. J. 40, 57—60 (1933).
DELLWEG, H.: Antibiotica und Hormone — ihre Wirkung auf die Biosynthese von Nucleinsäuren und Proteinen. In: Molekularbiologie, hrsg. von T. WIELAND und G. PFLEIDERER, S. 83—94. Frankfurt/M.: Umschau Verlag 1967.

DEMPSEY, E. A., BUNTING, H., WISLOCKI, G. B.: Observations on the chemical cytology of the mammary gland. Amer. J. Anat. 81, 309—341 (1947).
DESCLIN, L.: (a) L'ocytocine peut — elle déclencher la libération de lutéotrophine hypophysaire chez la rat? C. R. Soc. Biol. (Paris) 150, 1489—1491 (1956).
— (b) Hypothalamus et libération d'hormone lutéotrophique. Expériences de greffe hypophysaire chez la rat hypophysectomisée. Action lutéotrophique de l'ocytocine. Ann. Endocr. (Paris) 17, 586—595 (1956).
DICZFALUSY, E., TILLINGER, K. G., WESTMAN, A.: Studies on oestrogen metabolism in new born boys. I and II. Acta endocr. (Kbh.) 26, 303—312 and 313—321 (1957).
DIECKMANN, H.: Über die Histologie der Brustdrüse bei gestörtem und ungestörtem Menstruationsablauf. Virchows Arch. path. Anat. 256, 321—356 (1925).
DJOJOSOEBAGIO, S., TURNER, C. W.: (a) The effect of crystalline dihydrotachysterol on milk secretion in thyroparathyreoidectomized lactating rats. Proc. Soc. exp. Biol. (N. Y.) 116, 909—912 (1964).
— — (b) Effects of parathyreoid extract calciferol, hytakerol and crystalline dihydrotachysterol on feed consumption in normal lactating rats. Proc. Soc. exp. Biol. (N. Y.) 116, 646—648 (1964).
— — (c) Effects of parathyreoid extract, dihydrotachysterol (hytakerol) and calciferol on milk secretion in rats. Endocrinology 74, 554—558 (1964).
DONOVAN, B. T., JACOBSOHN, D.: Testosterone and the growth of mammary glands and other tissues of hypophysectomized rats treated with thyroxine, insulin and cortisone. Acta endocr. (Kbh.) 33, 214—229 (1960).
DORFMAN, R. I., SHIPLEY, R. A.: In: Androgens. New York: J. Wiley & Son 1956.
DUBOIS, J.: Méthode d'évolution quantitative du dévelopement de la glande mammaire chez la souris traitée par des corps oestrogènes. C. R. Soc. Biol. (Paris) 138, 149—151 (1944).
DUMONT, J. N.: Prolactin — induced cytologic changes in the mucosa of the pigeon crop during crop-"milk" formation. Z. Zellforsch. 68, 755—782 (1965).
DURAN-REYNALS, F., BUNTING, H., WAGENEN, G. VAN: Studies on the sex skin of Macaca mulatta. Ann. N. Y. Acad. Sci. 52, 1006—1014 (1950).
EGGELING, H. VON: Die Milchdrüse. In: Handbuch der mikroskopischen Anatomie des Menschen von v. MOELLENDORF, W. Bd. 1, Berlin: Springer 1927.
EISEN, M. J.: The occurence of benign and melignant mammary lesions in rats treated with crystalline estrogene. Cancer Res. 2, 632—644 (1942).
EISENFELD, A. J., AXELROD, J.: Selectivity of estrogen distribution in tissues. J. Pharmacol. exp. Ther. 150, 469—475 (1965).
ELGER, W., BERSWORDT-WALLRABE, R. VON, NEUMANN, F.: Der Einfluß von Antiandrogenen auf androgenabhängige Vorgänge im Organismus. Naturwissenschaften 54, 549—552 (1967).
— NEUMANN, F.: The role of androgens in differentiation of the mammary gland in male mouse fetuses. Proc. Soc. exp. Biol. (N.Y.) 123, 637—640 (1966).
ELLIS, R.: Fine structure of the myoepithelium of the eccrine sweat glands of man. J. Cell Biol. 27, 551—563 (1965).
EMGE, L. A.: Estrogenic hormones and carcinogenesis. Surg. Gynec. Obstet. 68, 472—479 (1939).
ESKIN, B. A., BARTUSKA, D. G., DUNN, M. R., JACOB, G., DRATMAN, M. D.: Mammary gland dysplasie in iodine deficiency studies in rats. J. Amer. med. Ass. 200, 691—695 (1967).
FAUVET, E.: Vergleichende Untersuchungen über die Entwicklung und Funktion der Milchdrüsen. V. Experimentelle Untersuchungen über den Einfluß der Ovarialhormone auf die Milchdrüsen der Ratten. Arch. Gynäk. 170, 244—262 (1940).
FERGUSON, D. J., VISSCHER, M. B.: The effects of androgen and estrogen in castrated and hypophysectomized C_3H mice. Endocrinology 52, 463—473 (1953).
— Endocrine control of mammary glands in C_3H mice. Surgery 39, 30—36 (1956).

Ferreri, F. L., Griffith, D. R.: Effect of hydrocortisone acetate on mammary gland nucleic content of pregnant rats. Proc. exp. Soc. Biol. (N.Y.) **130**, 1216—1218 (1969).

Fischer, R., Schaefer, H. E.: Geschlechtsdifferentes Vorkommen und östrogenabhängige Induktion der alkalischen Phosphatase in subkutanen Fibroblasten der Maus. Naturwissenschaften **54**, 342—343 (1967).

Fiske, S. W. C., Courtecuisse, V., Haguenau, F.: High resolution autoradiographic study of normal lactating mammary gland and mammary tumors of the mouse: Preliminary report. J. nat. Cancer Inst. **39**, 209—229 (1967).

Flux, D. S.: (a) Effect of 17-Vinyltestosterone on the mammae, uteri, thymus an adrenal glands of spayed female mice. Proc. Soc. exp. Biol. (N. Y.) **85**, 16—18 (1954).

— (b) The effect of adrenal steroids on the growth of the mammary glands, uteri, thymus and adrenal glands of intact, ovariectomized and oestrone-treated ovariectomized mice. J. Endocr. **11**, 238—254 (1954).

— Mammary gland growth in male mice of the CHI strain after hypophysectomy and castration. J. Endocr. **17**, 300—306 (1958).

— Munford, R. E.: The effect of adrenocorticotropin on the mammary glands of intact nature female mice of the Chi strain. J. Endocr. **14**, 343—347 (1957).

Folley, S. J.: Lactation. Biol. Rev. **15**, 421—458 (1940).

— The physiology and biochemistry of lactation. Edinburgh and London: Oliver & Boyd 1956.

— (a) Endocrine control of the mammary gland. Mammary development. Brit. med. Bull. **5**, 130—134 (1947).

— (b) Lactation. Brit. med. Bull. **5**, 135—141 (1947).

— Some effects of steroids on the mammary gland. In: Ciba foundation Colloquia on Endocrinology, ed. by G. E. W. Wolstenholme, vol. I, p. 69—86. London: J. & A. Churchill 1952.

— Hormones in mammary and function. Brit. med. Bull. **11**, 145—150 (1955).

— Greenbaum, A. L.: Changes in the arginase and alkaline phosphatase contents of the mammary gland and liver of the rat during pregnancy, lactation and mammary involution. Biochem. J. **41**, 261—269 (1947).

— Gutkelch, A. N., Zuckerman, S.: The mammary gland of the rhesus monkey and normal and experimental conditions. Proc. roy. Soc., London, Biol. Sci. **126**, 469—491 (1939).

— McNaught, M. L.: Biosynthesis of milkfat. In: Milk, the mammary gland and its secretion, ed. by S. K. Kon and A. T. Cowie, vol. 1, p. 441—479. New York and London: Academic Press 1961.

— Young, F. G.: Prolactin as a specific lactogenic hormone. Lancet **1941**, 380—381.

Foote, F. W., Stewart, F. W.: Lobular carcinoma in situ. A rare form of mammary cancer. Amer. J. Path. **17**, 491—496 (1941).

— — Comparative studies of cancerous versus noncancerous breasts. Ann. Surg. **121**, 197—222 (1945).

Forbes, A. P., Henneman, P. H., Griswold, G. C., Albright, F.: A syndrome, distinct from acromegaly, characterized by spontaneous lactation, amenorrhea, and low folliclestimulating hormone excretion. J. clin. Endocr. **11**, 749 (1951).

— — — — Syndrome characterized by galactorrhoea, amenorrhoea and low urinary FSH: Comparison with acromegaly and normal lactation. J. clin. Endocr. **14**, 265—271 (1954).

Forbes, Th. R.: Factor of age in the rate of absorption of, and in mammary stimulation by, testosterone monopropionate pellets in rats. Endocrinology **30**, 765—766 (1942).

Forssmann, W. G.: Elektronenmikroskopische Morphologie der Sekretion des Taubenkropfes unter dem Einfluß von Prolaktin. Frankfurt. Z. Path. **74**, 512—533 (1965).

Forsyth, J. A., Folley, S. J., Chadwick, A.: Lactogenic and pigeon crop-stimulating activities of human pituitary growth hormone preparations. J. Endocr. 31, 115—126 (1965).
Frantz, V. K., Pickren, J. W., Melcher, G. W., Auchincloss, H.: Incidence of chronic cystic disease in so called "normal breasts". Cancer (Philad.) 4, 762—783 (1951).
Frazier, C. N., Mu, J. W.: Development of female characteristics in adult male rabbits following prolonged administration of extrogenic substance. Proc. Soc. exp. Biol. (N. Y.) 32, 997—1001 (1935).
Gardner, W. U.: Growth of the mammary glands in hypophysectomized mice. Proc. Soc. exp. Biol. (N. Y.) 45, 835—837 (1940).
— Inhibition of mammary growth by large amounts of estrogen. Endocrinology 28, 53—61 (1941).
— Smith, G. M., Strong, L. C.: Stimulation of abnormal mammary growth by large amounts of estrogenic hormone. Proc. Soc. exp. Biol. (N. Y.) 33, 148—150 (1935).
— Strong, L. C.: The normal development of the mammary glands of virgin female mice of ten strains varying in susceptibility to spontaneous neoplasma. Amer. J. Cancer 25, 282—290 (1935).
— Turner, C. W.: The function, assay, and preparation of galactin, a lactation stimulating hormone of the anterior pituitary. Missouri Agr. Exp. Sta. Res. Bull. 190 (1933).
— White, A.: Mammary growth in hypophysectomized male mice receiving estrogen and prolactin. Proc. Soc. exp. Biol. (N. Y.) 48, 590—592 (1941).
Garrett, F. A., Talmage, R. V.: The influence of relaxin on mammary gland development in guinea-pigs and rabbits. J. Endocr. 8, 336—340 (1952).
Geschickter, C. F.: The endocrine aspects of chronic cystic mastitis. Sth. Surg. 10, 457—486 (1941).
— Diseases of the breast, 2nd ed. Philadelphia-London-Montreal: Lippincott 1948.
— Byrnes, E. W.: Factors influencing the development and time of appearance of mammary cancer in the rat in response to estrogen. Arch. Path. 33, 335—342 (1942).
— Hartman, C. G.: Mammary response to prolonged estrogenic stimulation in the monkey. Cancer (Philad.) 12, 767—781 (1959).
— Speert, H.: Zit. nach Speert, 1948.
Girardie, J., Wolff, E.: Localisation optique et ultrastructurale de l'activité phosphatasique alcaline dans l'epithélium mammaire. C. R. Acad. Sci. (Paris) 264, 2064—2067 (1967).
Glock, G. E., McLean, P.: Further studies on the properties and assays of glucose-6-phosphate-dehydrogenase and 6-phospho-gluconate-dehydrogenase of rat liver. Biochem. J. 55, 400—408 (1954).
— — Levels of enzymes of the direct oxydative pathway of carbohydrate metabolism in mammalian tissues and tumors. Biochem. J. 56, 171—175 (1954).
Gögl, H., Lang, F. J.: Brustdrüse. In: Lehrbuch der spez. pathologischen Anatomie von E. Kaufmann, hrsg. von M. Staemmler, 11./12. Aufl., II. Bd., 1. Teil. Berlin: W. D. Gruyter & Co. 1957.
Gössner, W.: Histochemischer Nachweis hydrolytischer Enzyme mit Hilfe der Azofarbstoffmethode. Histochemie 1, 48—96 (1959).
Goldenberg, V. E., Wiegenstein, L., Mottet, N. K.: Florid breast fibroadenomas in patients taking hormonal oral contraceptives. Amer. J. clin. Path. 49, 58—59 (1968).
Gomez, E. T., Turner, C. W.: Hypophysectomy and replacement therapy in relation to the growth and secretory activity of the mammary gland. Res. Bull. Mo. agric. Exp. Sta. Nr. 259 (1937).

Gorski, J., Noteboom, W. D., Nicolette, J. A.: Estrogen control of the synthesis of RNA and protein in the uterus. J. cell. comp. Physiol. **66**, 91—110 (1965).
Graumann, W.: (a) Entwicklung des Milchstreifens. Z. Anat. Entwickl.-Gesch. **114**, 500—510 (1950).
— (b) Mikroskopische Anatomie der männlichen Brustdrüse. 1. Kindheit und Pubertät. Z. mikr.-anat. Forsch. **59**, 358—380 (1952).
— (c) Mikroskopische Anatomie der männlichen Brustdrüse. 2. Mannesalter und Senium. Z. mikr.-anat. Forsch. **59**, 523—557 (1953).
Green, J. D., Harris, G. W.: The neurovascular link between the neurohypophysis and adenohypophysis. J. Endocr. **5**, 136—145 (1946/48).
Greenbaum, A. L., Slater, T. F.: Studies on the particulate components of rat mammary gland. II. Changes in the levels of the nucleic acids of the mammary glands of rats during pregnancy, lactation and mammary involution. Biochem. J. **66**, 155—161 (1957).
Gregg, W. I.: Galactorrhoea after contraceptive hormones. New Engl. J. Med. **274**, 1432—1434 (1966).
Griffith, D. R., Turner, C. W.: Desoxyribonucleic acid (DNA) content of mammary gland during pregnancy and lactation. Proc. Soc. exp. Biol. (N.Y.) **95**, 347—348 (1957).
— — Normal growth of rat mammary glands during pregnancy and lactation. Proc. Soc. exp. Biol. (N.Y.) **102**, 619—621 (1959).
— — (a) Normal growth of rat mammary glands during pregnancy and early lactation. Proc. Soc. exp. Biol. (N.Y.) **106**, 448—451 (1961).
— — (b) Thyroxine and mammary gland growth in rat. Proc. Soc. exp. Biol. (N.Y.) **106**, 873—874 (1961).
— — (c) Normal and experimental involution of rat mammary gland. Proc. Soc. exp. Biol. (N. Y.) **107**, 668—670 (1961).
Grosvenor, C. E., Turner, C. W.: (a) Evidence for adrenergic and cholinergic components in milk let down reflex in lactating rats. Proc. Soc. exp. Biol. (N. Y.) **95**, 719—722 (1957).
— — (b) Release and restoration of pituitary lactogen in response to nursing stimuli in lactating rats. Proc. Soc. exp. Biol. (N. Y.) **96**, 723—725 (1957).
Gruber, G. B.: Über die Milchdrüsenschwellung bei Neugeborenen. Z. Kinderheilk. **30**, 336—362 (1921).
Grumbrecht, P.: Pathologische Auswirkungen des Follikelhormones. Arch. Gynäk. **170**, 1—59 (1941).
Haagensen, C. D.: Diseases of the breast. Philadelphia: W. B. Saunders 1956.
Habbe, K.: Beitrag zur Frage über Granulosazelltumoren. Zbl. Gynäk. **55**, 1088 (1931).
Hadfield, D.: The nature and origin of the mammotrophic agent present in human female urine. Lancet **1957 I**, 1058—1061.
— Young, S.: The controlling influence of the pituitary on the growth of the normal breast. Brit. J. Surg. **46**, 265—273 (1958).
Haenel, H.: Ein Fall von dauernder Milchsekretion beim Manne. Münch. med. Wschr. **75**, 261—263 (1928).
Haguenau, F.: (a) Le cancer mammaire de la souris et de la femme étude comparative au microscope électronique. Path. et Biol. **7**, 989—1015 (1959).
— (b) Les myofilaments de la cellule myoepithelial. Etude au microscope électronique. C. R. Acad. Sci. (Paris) **249**, 182—184 (1959).
— Arnoult, J.: (c) Le cancer du sein chez la femme. Bull. Ass. franç. Cancer **46**, 177—211 (1959).
Hamada, H., Neumann, F., Junkmann, K.: Intrauterine antimaskuline Beeinflussung von Rattenfeten durch ein stark gestagen wirksames Steroid. Acta endocr. (Kbh.) **44**, 380—388 (1963).

Hamberger, L., Ahrén, K.: Influence of the adrenal cortex on growth processes in the rat mammary gland. J. Endocr. 30, 171—179 (1964).
Hamperl, H.: Über die Myothelien (myo-epitheliale Elemente) der Brustdrüse. Virchows Arch. path. Anat. 305, 171—215 (1940).
Hancock, J., Brumby, P. J., Turner, C. W.: Hormonal induction of lactation in identicaltwin dairy cattle. N. Z. J. Sci. Tech. A, 36, 111—116 (1954).
Hansen, R. G., Carlson, D. M.: General biochemistry of mammary tissue. In: Milk, the mammary gland and its secretion, ed. by S. K. Kon and A. T. Cowie, vol. 1, p. 371—388. New York and London: Academic Press 1961.
Hardy, M. H.: The Development in vitro of the Mammary Glands of the mouse. J. Anat. (Lond.) 84, 388—393 (1950).
Hartmann, M.: Einführung in die allgemeine Biologie. Sammlung Göschen, Sammlung Bd. 96, 1956.
Hayashida, T.: Further observations on the question of specificity of antihuman growth hormone rabbit serum. Endocrinology 70, 846—856 (1962).
Helminen, H. J., Ericsson, L. E., Orrenius, S.: Studies on the mammary gland involution. IV. Histochemical and biochemical observations on alterations in lysosomes and lysosomal enzymes. J. Ultrastruct. Res. 25, 240—252 (1968).
Herold, L., Effkemann, G.: Beziehungen des Follikelhormons zu patho-physiologischen Wachstumsvorgängen der Brustdrüse. Arch. Gynäk. 163, 85—93, 94—101, 309—315 (1936).
Heuverswyn, J. van, Folley, S. J., Gardner, W. U.: Mammary growth in male mice receiving androgens, estrogens and desoxycorticosterone acetate. Proc. Soc. exp. Biol. (N. Y.) 41, 389—392 (1939).
Hibbs, R. G.: The fine structure of the human eccrine sweat glands. Amer. J. Anat. 103, 201—218 (1958).
Higashi, K.: Studies on the prolactin-like substance in human placenta. Endocrin. Jap. 9, 1—11 (1962).
Higuchi, K.: Die Gewebsmastzellen in der Mamma. Fol. haemat. (Lpz.) 40, 401—414 (1930).
Höhn, E. O.: The effect of oestrone on the mammary gland of adrenalectomized guinea-pigs. J. Endocr. 16, 227—230 (1957).
Hoffmann, F.: Über die Wirkung des Follikelhormons auf den histologischen Aufbau der menschlichen Brustdrüse. Zbl. Gynäk. 63, 422—426 (1939).
Holmes, R.: Alkaline phosphatase in the rabbit mammary gland. Nature (Lond.) 178, 311 (1956).
Holzner, J. H., Kaufmann, F.: Histochemische Untersuchungen über das Verhalten der Phosphatasen bei der zyklischen Mastopathie, beim Fibroadenom und Karzinom der menschlichen Brustdrüse. Krebsarzt 20, 185—192 (1965).
Hoshino, K.: Development and growth of mammary glands of CBA mice prenatally exposed to progesterone. Anat. Rec. 154, 360 (1966).
Hughes, E. S. R.: The Development of the Mammary Gland. Ann. roy. Coll. Surg. Eng. 6, 99—119 (1950).
Humboldt, A. v.: Aus: Reise in die Aequinoktialgegenden. Ges. Werke, Stuttgart, Bd. 5, S. 230 (1889).
Humphrey, L. J., Swedlow, M.: The relationship of breast disease to thyroid disease. Cancer (Philad.) 17, 1170—1173 (1964).
Hunter, J.: Observation on certain parts of the animal occonomy, p. 191—198: On a secretion in the crop of breeding pigeons, for the nourishment of their young. London 1786.
Ihnen, M., Perez-Tamayo, R.: Breast stroma; morphological and histochemical study. Arch. Path. 56, 46—67 (1953).
Ingleby, H.: Normal and pathologic proliferation in the breast with special reference to cystic disease. Arch. Path. 33, 573—589 (1942).

JACOBSOHN, D.: Action of estradiol monobenzoate on the mammary glands of hypophysectomized rabbits. Acta physiol. scand. **32**, 304—313 (1954).
— Thyroxin and the reaction of the mammary glands to ovarian steroids in hypophysectomized rats. J. Physiol. (Proc. Physiol. Soc.) **148**, 10—11 (1959).
— Effects of thyroxine on growth of mammary glands, whole body, heart and liver in hypophysectomized rats treated with Insulin, Cortisone and ovarian steroids. Acta endocr. (Kbh.) **35**, 107—134 (1960).
— Hormonal Regulation of Mammary Gland growth. In: Milk: The mammary gland and its secretion by KON, S. K. and A. T. COWIE, vol. 1, p. 127—160. New York and London: Academic Press 1961.
— Modification by oestrogens of the reaction of the rat's mammary gland to androgens. Acta endocr. (Kbh.) **41**, 88—100 (1962).
— NORGREN, A.: Estrogens and corticoids in relation to mammary gland growth in male rats. Proc. Soc. exp. Biol. (N. Y.) **118**, 1106—1109 (1965).
JAKOBOVITS, A.: Extrapuerperale Milchabsonderung nach Kastration. Zbl. Gynäk. **82**, 438—441 (1960).
JEFFERS, K. R.: Cytology of the mammary gland of the albino rat. I. Pregnancy, lactation and involution. Amer. J. Anat. **56**, 257—277 (p 35).
JENSEN, E. V., JACOBSON, H. J.: Basii guides to the mechanism of oestrogen action. Recent Progr. Hormone Res. **18**, 387—414 (1962).
JERVELL, K. J., DINIZ, C. R., MUELLER, G. C.: Early effects of estradiol on nuclei acid metabolism in the rat uterus. J. biol. Chem. **231**, 945—948 (1958).
JOHNSON, R. M.: The effects of cortisone on lactation in rats. J. Anim. Sci. **15**, 1288 (1956).
— Effects of cortisone on lactation and involution of mammary glands in rats. J. Dairy Sci. **40**, 625 (1957).
— MEITES, J.: Effects of cortisone, hydrocortisone and ACTH on mammary growth and pituitary prolactin content of rats. Proc. Soc. exp. Biol. (N. Y.) **89**, 455—458 (1955).
JONES, D. B.: Florid papillomatosis of the nipple ducts. Cancer (Philad.) **8**, 315—319 (1955).
JOSIMOVICH, J. B., MCLAREN, J. A.: Presence in the human placenta and their serum of a highly lactogenic substance immunologically related to pituitary growth hormone. Endocrinology **71**, 209—220 (1952).
JUNKMANN, K.: Die physiologische Chemie der inneren Sekretion. In: FLASCHENTRÄGER-LEHNARTZ, Handbuch der physiologischen Chemie, Bd. II. Der Stoffwechsel, 2. Teil/Bandteil 6, S. 485—488. Berlin-Göttingen-Heidelberg: Springer 1957.
— NEUMANN, F.: Zum Wirkungsmechanismus von an Feten antimaskulin wirksamen Gestagenen. Acta endocr. (Kbh.) Suppl. **90**, 139—154 (1964).
KARLSON, P.: Biochemische Wirkungsweise der Hormone. Dtsch. med. Wschr. **86**, 668—674 (1961).
— Morphogenese und Metamorphose der Insekten. 13. Colloquium Ges. physiol. Chemie, S. 101—126 (1962).
— Chemie und Biochemie der Insektenhormone. Angew. Chemie **75**, 257—265 (1963).
KARSNER, H. T.: Gynecomastia. Amer. J. Path. **22**, 235—315 (1946).
KING, R. J. B., GORDON, J., INMAN, D. R.: The intracellular localization of oestrogen in rat tissues. J. Endocr. **32**, 9—15 (1965).
— GORDON, J., COWAN, D. M., INMAN, D. R.: The intranuclear localization of 6,7-^{3}H oestradiol-17-β in dimethyl-benzanthracen-induced. Rat mammary adenocarcinoma and other tissue. J. Endocr. **36**, 139—150 (1966).
KIRKHAM, W. R., TURNER, C. W.: Nucleic acids of the mammary glands of rats. Proc. Soc. exp. Biol. (N.Y.) **83**, 123—126 (1953).
— — Introduction of mammary growth in rats by estrogen and progesterone. Proc. Soc. exp. Biol. (N. Y.) **87**, 139—141 (1954).

KOCHAKIAN, C. D.: Regulation of libonucleic acid biosynthesis in the mouse kidney by androgens. Proc. 2nd Internat. Congr. on Hormonal Steroids, 1967, p. 794—802.

KOELLIKER, A.: Mikroskopische Anatomie oder Gewebelehre des Menschen, 2 Bd. Spezielle Gewebelehre. Leipzig. Engelmann 1852.

KON, S. K., COWIE, A. T.: Milk. The mammary gland and its secretion, vol. I. u. II. New York and London: Academic Press 1961.

KONJETZNY, G. E.: Pathologie, Klinik und Behandlung der Mastopathie. Stuttgart 1942.

— Mastopathie und Milchdrüsenkrebs. Stuttgart: Enke Verlag 1954.

KRACHT, J., HACHMEISTER, M., BREUSTEDT, H.-J., ZIMMERMANN, H.-D.: Immunhistologische Hormonlokalisation im Hypophysenvorderlappen des Menschen. Materia Medica Nordmark XIX/4, 224—238 (1967).

KRAUS, E. J.: Zur Pathogenese der Galaktorrhoe. Arch. Gynäk. **159**, 380—394 (1935).

KUECKENS, H.: Zur Frage der zyklischen Veränderungen der Mamma und des menschlichen Scheidenepithels. Z. Geburtsh. **96**, 55—76 (1929).

KUNERT, J.: Die Wirkung hoher Dosen örtlich verabreichten Follikelhormons auf die männliche Brustdrüse und das endokrine System. Experimentelle Studie zum Gynäkomastieproblem. Frankfurt. Z. Path. **62**, 373—383 (1951).

KURU, H.: Beiträge zur Geschwulstlehre. Dtsch. Z. Chir. **98**, 414—463 (1909).

KUZMA, J. F.: Myoepithelial proliferations in the human breast. Amer. J. Path. **19**, 473—489 (1943).

LABHART, A.: Klinik der inneren Sekretion. Berlin-Göttingen-Heidelberg: Springer 1957.

LANGER, E., HUHN, S.: Der submikroskopische Bau der Myoepithelzelle. Z. Zellforsch. **47**, 507—516 (1958).

LANI, K.: Enzymhistochemische und morphologische Untersuchungen über die Prolaktinwirkung auf die Mamma. Inaug.-Diss. Mainz 1967.

— BÄSSLER, R.: Tagg der nord- und westdeutschen Pathologen in Lüneburg 1967. Zbl. allg. Path. path. Anat. **111**, 473 (1968).

LAQUEUR, E., DE JONGH, S. E.: Zur Wirkung des weiblichen Sexualhormons Menformon, im besonderen auf die Mamma. Mschr. Geburtsh. **80**, 245 (1928).

LAQUEUR, G. L.: Effects of testosterone propionate on the mammary glands of female albino rats. Endocrinology **32**, 81—86 (1943).

— FLUHMANN, C. F.: Effects of testosterone propionate in immature and adult female rats. Endocrinology **30**, 93—101 (1942).

LAURITZEN, C.: Oestrogene und Gestagene beim Menschen. Naturw. Rdsch. **18**, 7—16 (1965).

LEESON, R.: (a) The histochemical identification of myoepithelium with particular reference to the Harderian and exorbital lacrimal glands. Acta anat. (Basel) **40**, 87—94 (1960).

— (b) The elctron microscopy of the myoepithelium in the rat exorbital lacrimal gland. Anat. Rec. **137**, 45—55 (1960).

LEONARD, S. L.: Stimulation of mammary glands in hypophysectomized rats by estrogen and testosterone. Endocrinology **32**, 229—237 (1943).

— REECE, R. P.: The relation of the thyroid to mammary gland growth in the rat. Endocrinology **28**, 65—69 (1941).

— — Failure of steroid hormones to induce mammary growth in hypophysectomized rats. Endocrinology **30**, 32—36 (1942).

LETTERER, E.: Die Morphologie der hormonalbedingten Veränderungen des Endometriums und der weiblichen Brustdrüse. Ärztl. Wschr. **1948**, 230—236.

LEUSCHNER, U.: Über die Lokalisation von Mucopolysacchariden und Mastzellen in scirrhösen Karzinomen der Mamma. Acta histochem. (Jena) **34**, 126—137 (1969).

LEVINE, H. J., BERGENSTAL, D. M., THOMAS, L. B.: Persistent lactation: Endocrine and histologic studies in 5 cases. Amer. J. med. Sci. 243, 118—128 (1962).
LEWIS, A. A., GOMEZ, E. T., TURNER, C. W.: Mammary gland development with mammogen in the castrate and the hypophysectomized rat. Endocrinology 30, 37—47 (1942).
— TURNER, C. W.: Effect of stilbestrol on the mammary gland of the mouse, rat, rabbit and goat. J. Dairy Sci. 24, 845—860 (1941).
— — (a) Growth of the male guinea pig mammary gland with diethylstilbestrol. Endocrinology 30, 585—590 (1942).
— — (b) Mammogen and unilateral mammary growth in the rabbit. Endocrinology 30, 985—989 (1942).
LIESER, H.: Beiträge zur Histologie und Feinstruktur der Mamma unter dem Einfluß von Geschlechtshormonen. Diss. Mainz 1964.
LINZELL, J. L.: The silver staining of myoepithelial cells, particulary in the mammary gland, and their relation of the ejection of milk. J. Anat. (Lond.) 86, 49—57 (1952).
— Some observations on the contractile tissue of the mammary glands. J. Physiol. (Lond.) 130, 257—267 (1955).
LITTEN, L.: Die histologischen Grundlagen der Sekretion nicht-gravider Mammae. Virchows Arch. path. Anat. 259, 126—146 (1926).
LITWER, G.: Die histologischen Veränderungen der Kropfwanderung bei Tauben zur Zeit der Bebrütung und Ausfütterung ihrer Jungen. Z. Zellforsch. 3, 695—722 (1926).
LUCHSINGER, Y., CENTENO, J.: Über die zyklischen Veränderungen der weiblichen Brustdrüse. Beitr. path. Anat. 78, 594—617 (1927).
LUSTIG, H.: Zur Entwicklungsgeschichte der menschlichen Brustdrüse. Arch. mikr. Anat. 87, 38—59 (1915).
LYONS, W. R.: The hormonal basis for "witches milk". Proc. Soc. exp. Biol. (N. Y.) 37, 207—209 (1938).
— The direct mammotrophic action of lactogenic hormone. Proc. Soc. exper. Biol. (N. Y.) 51, 308—311 (1942).
— Lobulo-alveolar mammary growth in the rat. Colloq. int. Cent. nat. Rech. sci. No. 32, 29—38 (1951).
— CATCHPOLE, H. R.: (a) "Assay with the guinea pig of the lactogenic hypophyseal hormone". Proc. Soc. exp. Biol. (N. Y.) 31, 299—301 (1933).
— — (b) "Availability of the rabbit for assay of the hypophyseal lactogenic hormone. Proc. Soc. exp. Biol. (N. Y.) 31, 305—309 (1933).
— JOHNSON, R. E., COLE, R. D., LI, C. H.: Mammary growth and lactation in male rats. In: The hypophyseal growth hormone, nature and actions (eds. R. W. SMITH, O. A. GAEBLER and C. N. H. LONG), p. 461—472. New York: The Blakiston Division 1955.
— LI, C. H., JOHNSON, R. E.: Localaction of pituitary and ovarian hormones on the mammary glands of hypophysectomized-oophorectomized rats. Anat. Rec. 127, 432—433 (1957).
— — — The hormonal control of mammary growth an lactation. Recent Progr. Hormone Res. 14, 219—254 (1958).
— McGINTY, D. A.: Effects of estrone and progesterone on male rabbit mammary gland. I. Varying doses of progesterone. Proc. Soc. exper. Biol. (N. Y.) 48, 83—86 (1941).
MAEDER, L. M. A.: Changes in the mammary gland of the albino rat (Mus norvegicus albus) during lactation and involution. Amer. J. Anat. 31, 1—26 (1922/23).
MAHESH, V. B., DALLA PRIA, S., GREENBLATT, R. B.: Abnormal lactation with Cushing's syndrom-a case report. J. clin. Endocr. 29, 978—981 (1969).
MASSHOFF, W.: Die physiologische Regeneration. In: Handbuch der allgemeinen Pathologie, Bd. VI/1, S. 489, von F. BÜCHNER, E. LETTERER und F. ROULET. Berlin-Göttingen-Heidelberg: Springer 1955.

Mayer, G., Klein, M.: Histology and cytology of the mammary gland. In: Milk: The mammary gland and its secretion, ed. by S. K. Kon and A. T. Cowie, vol. I, p. 47—126. New York and London: Academic Press 1961.

McCullagh, E., Alivisatos, J. G., Schaffenburg, C. A.: Pituitary tumor with gynecomastia and lactation. J. clin. Endocr. **16**, 397—405 (1956).

McDonald, G. J., Reece, R. P.: Quantitative response of rat mammary glands to mammogens. I. Estrogen alone with progesterone. Proc. Soc. exp. Biol. (N. Y.) **110**, 647—649 (1962).

McEuen, C. S.: Some effects of prolonged administration of oestrin in rats. Lancet **1936 I**, 775—776.

— Role of pituitary in effect of testosterone on the mammary gland. Proc. Soc. exp. Biol. (N. Y.) **36**, 213—215 (1937).

— Selye, H., Collip, J. B.: Effect of the testis on the mammary gland. Proc. Soc. exp. Biol. (N. Y.) **35**, 56—58 (1936).

Meier-Ruge, W.: Die diagnostische Bedeutung des Sexchromatingehaltes in Relation von Enzymhistochemie, DNS-Gehalt und Mitoseindex beim Mammacarcinom. Verh. dtsch. Ges. Path. **50**, 330—335 (1966).

Meites, J.: (a) Mammary growth and lactation. In: Reproduction in domestic animals, ed. by H. H. Cole and P. T. Cupps, vol. I, p. 539—593. New York and London: Academic Press 1959.

— (b) Induction and maintenance of mammary growth and lactation in rats with acetylcholin or epinephrine. Proc. Soc. exp. Biol. (N. Y.) **100**, 750—754 (1959).

— Farm animals: hormonal induction of lactation and galactopoesis. In: Milk: The mammary gland and its Secretion, ed. by S. K. Kon and A. T. Cowie. New York: Academic Press 1961.

— Maintenance of the mammary lobuloalveolar system in rats after adrenoorchidectomy by prolactin and growth hormone. Endocrinology **76**, 1220—1223 (1965).

— Effects of altering the balance between prolactin and ovarian hormones on initiation of lactation in rabbits. Endocrinology **55**, 530—534 (1954).

— Sgouris, J. T.: Can the ovarian hormones inhibit the mammary response to the prolactin? Endocrinology **53**, 17—23 (1953).

— Turner, C. W.: The induction of lactation during pregnancy in rabbits on the specifity of the lactogenic hormone. Amer. J. Physiol. **150**, 394—399 (1947).

Merz, W.: Brustdrüsenschwellung bei Neugeborenen. Schweiz. med. Wschr. **11**, 213—217 (1946).

Meyer, H.: Experimentelle Pathomorphogenese der Mamma unter dem Einfluß männlicher Geschlechtshormone. Inaug.-Diss. Mainz, 1967.

Mixner, J. P.: Influence of environmental temperature on growth of mammary lobule-alveolar system. Proc. Soc. exp. Biol. (N. Y.) **48**, 443—445 (1941).

— (a) Role of estrogen in the stimulation of mammary lobule-alveolar growth by progesterone and by the mammogenic lobule-alveolar growth factor of the anterior pituitary. Endocrinology **30**, 591—597 (1942).

— (b) Progesterone like-activity of some steroid compounds and of diethylstilbestrol in stimulating mammary lobule-alveolar growth. Endocrinology **30**, 706—710 (1942).

— (c) Influence of thyroxine upon mammary lobule-alveolar growth. Endocrinology **31**, 345—348 (1942).

— The mammogenic hormones of the anterior pituitary. II. The lobulo-alveolar growth factor. Res. Bull. Mo. agric. Exp. Sta. **378** (1943).

— Strain differences in response of mice to mammary gland stimulating hormones. Proc. Soc. exp. Biol. (N. Y.) **95**, 87—89 (1957).

— Turner, C. W.: Growth of the lobule-alveolar system of the mammary gland with pregneninolone. Proc. Soc. exp. Biol. (N. Y.) **47**, 453—456 (1941).

Möbius, G., Nizze, H.: Mastopathia fibrosa cystica und Epithelproliferationen in der weiblichen Brustdrüse des Sektionsgutes. Frankfurt. Z. Path. **75**, 297—305 (1966).
Moon, R. C.: Mammary gland cell content during various phases of lactating. Amer. J. Physiol. **203**, 939—941 (1962).
— Influence of graded thyroxin levels on mammary gland growth. Amer. J. Physiol. **203**, 942—946 (1962).
— Griffith, D. R., Turner, C. W.: Normal and experimental growth of rat mammary gland. Proc. Soc. exp. Biol. (N. Y.) **101**, 788—790 (1959).
— Turner, C. W.: Thyroid hormone and mammary growth in the rat. Proc. Soc. exp. Biol. (N. Y.) **103**, 149—151 (1960).
Mosimann, W.: Vergrößerung der Kernvolumina in der Parathyreoidea und vermehrte Kalziumausscheidung in der Milch bei Ziegen nach künstlicher Auslösung der Laktation durch Oestrogen. Schweiz. Arch. Tierheilk. **97**, 178—187 (1955).
— Das Volumen der Zellkerne im Epithel der Milchdrüse in Abhängigkeit vom Funktionszustand und bei Stilboestrol-Zufuhr. Z. mikr.-anat. Forsch. **63**, 303—316 (1957).
Mühlbrock, O.: The oestrone-sensitivity of the mammary gland in female mice of various strains. Acta brev. neerl. physiol. **16**, 22—27 (1948).
Müllerheim, R.: Ovarialtumoren bei Greisinnen mit Hypertrophie der Mammae und des Uterus und mit uterinen Blutungen. Zbl. Gynäk. **52**, 689 (1928).
Munford, R. E.: The effect of cortisol acetate on oestrone-induced mammary growth in immature ovariectomized albino mice. J. Endocr. **16**, 72—79 (1957).
— A review of anatomical and biochemical changes in the mammary gland with particular reference to quantitative methods of assessing mammary development. Dairy Sci., Abstr. **26**, 293—304 (1964).
Munger, B. L.: The ultrastructure and histophysiology of human eccrine sweat glands. J. biophys. biochem. Cytol. **11**, 385—402 (1961).
Munson, P. L.: Studies on the role of the parathyreoids in calcium and phosphorus metabolism. Ann. N. Y. Acad. Sci. **60**, 776—795 (1955).
Murad, T. M., Haam, E. v.: Ultrastructure of myoepithelial cells in human mammary gland tumors. Cancer (Philad.) **21**, 1137—1149 (1968).
Mylius, E. A.: The identification and the role of the myoepithelial cell in salivary gland tumors. Acta path. microbiol. scand., Suppl. **139**, 50 (1960).
Nandi, S.: (a) Role of somatotropin in mammogenesis and lactogenesis in C₃H/He CRGL mice. Science **128**, 772—774 (1958).
— (b) Endocrine control of mammary gland development and function in the C₃H/He CRGL mouse. J. nat. Cancer Inst. **21**, 1939—1963 (1958).
— (c) Hormonal control of mammogenesis and lactogenesis in the C₃H-He crgl. mouse. Univ. Calif. Publ. Zool. **65**, 1—128 (1959).
Needham, D. M., Shoenberg, C. F.: Proteins of the contractile mechanismen of mammalian an smooth muscle and their possible location in the cell. Proc. roy. Soc., Ser. B (London) **160**, 517—522 (1964).
Neimeier, R., Hauser, G. A., Keller, M., Labhardt, F., Wenner, R., Stampfli, V.: Die pathologische Lactation. Schweiz. med. Wschr. **89**, 442—445 (1959).
Nelson, W. O.: Endocrine control of the mammary gland. Physiol. Rev. **16**, 488—526 (1936).
— Studies on the physiology of lactation. VI. The endocrine influences concerned in the development and function of the mammary gland in the guinea pig. Amer. J. Anat. **60**, 341—365 (1937).
— (a) Growth of mammary gland following local application of estrogenic hormone. Amer. J. Physiol. **133**, 397—398 (1941).
— (b) Production of sex hormones in the adrenals. Anat. Rec., Suppl. **1**, **81**, 97 (1941).

Nelson, W. O., Heytler, P. G., Ciacco, E. I.: Guinea pig mammary gland growth changes in weight, nitrogen and nucleic acids. Proc. Soc. exp. Biol. (N. Y.) **109**, 373—375 (1962).
— Merckel, C. G.: Effects of androgenic substances in the female rat. Proc. Soc. exp. Biol. (N. Y.) **36**, 823—825 (1937).
Neumann, F., Elger, W.: The effect of the anti-androgen 1,2 α-methylene-6-chloro-Δ 4,6 pregnandiene-17 α-ol-3,20-dione-17 α-acetate (cyproterone-acetate) on the development of the mammary glands of male foetal rats. J. Endocr. **36**, 347—352 (1966).
— — Steroid stimulation of mammary glands in prenatally feminized male rats. Europ. J. Pharmacol. **1**, 120—123 (1967).
— — Berswordt-Wallrabe, R. von: The structure of the mammary glands and lactogenesis in feminized male rats. J. Endocr. (Lond.) **36**, 353—356 (1966).
Neumann, H. O., Oing, M.: Polymastie und Polythelie. Eine klinische Studie mit einem entwicklungsgeschichtlich-historischen Beitrag. Arch. Gynäk. **13**, 494—542 (1929).
Newman, W.: In situ lobular carcinoma of the breast. Report of 26 woman with 32 cases. Ann. Surg. **157**, 591—599 (1963).
— Lobular carcinoma of the female breast. Report of 73 cases. Ann. Surg. **164**, 305—314 (1966).
Nicoll, C. S.: Growth autoregulation and the mammary gland. J. nat. Cancer Inst. **34**, 131—140 (1965).
— Meites, J.: Prolactin secretion in vitro: effects of thyreoid hormones and insulin. Endocrinology **72**, 544—551 (1963).
Noble, R. L., McEuen, C. S., Collip, J. B.: Mammary tumors produced in rats by the action of estrone tablets. Canad. med. Ass. J. **42**, 412—417 (1940).
Nordmann, M.: Fibrosis mammae virilis. Klin. Wschr. **26**, 220—221 (1948).
Norgren, A.: Effects of different doses of oestrogen and progesterone on mammary glands of gonadectomized rabbits. Acta Univ. Lund. Sectio II, No. 31 (1966).
Nyirjesy, I.: Galactorrhoea without amenorrhoea. J. Obstet, Gynec. **32**, 52—57 (1968).
Oestereich, R., Slawyk: Riesenwuchs und Zirbeldrüsen-Geschwulst. Virchows Arch. path. Anat. **157**, 475—484 (1899).
Olivi, M., Barbieri, G.: La mastopathia fibrocistica. Lav. Ist. Anat. Univ. Perugia **12**, 311—323 (1952).
Overzier, C.: Gynäkomastie bei paradoxer Fettsucht — ein Beitrag zum Gynäkomastieproblem. Ärztl. Wschr. **4**, 4—10 (1949).
Ozzello, L., Speer, F. D.: The mucopolysaccharides in the normal and diseased breast. Their distribution and significance. Amer. J. Path. **34**, 993—1009 (1958).
Paek, S.: Histochemisches Enzymmuster der Mamma unter dem experimentellen Einfluß von Geschlechtshormonen. Inaug.-Diss. Mainz, 1967.
Perrini, F.: Action of stilboestrol and progesterone on the mammary gland. G. Ostet. Ginec. **17**, 59—74 (1953).
Philipp, E.: Schwangerschaftsveränderungen beim Neugeborenen. Klin. Wschr. **17**, 797—800 (1938).
Price, D., Williams-Ashman, H. G.: The accessory reproductive glands of mammals. In: Sex and internalse cretions, 3d, ed. by Young, W. C., p. 366—448. Williams & Wilkins 1961.
Rapoport, S. M.: Medizinische Biochemie, Berlin 1962.
Ratzenhofer, M.: Zum Verhalten des Mesenchyms bei chronischer Mastopathie und Mammacarcinom. Wien. med. Wschr. **101**, 681—686 (1951).
— Schauenstein, E.: (a) Weitere biophysikalische Untersuchungen des Gewebssaftes bei Mammacarcinom. Z. Krebsforsch. **58**, 707—710 (1952).

Ratzenhofer, M., Schauenstein, E.: (b) Über den Nachweis von Albuminen im Gewebssaft bei krebsig entarteter Mastopathie. Z. Krebsforsch. **58**, 198—200 (1952).

Ray, E. W., Averill, S. C., Lyons, W. R., Johnson, R. E.: Rat placental hormone activities corresponding to those of pituitary mammotropin. Endocrinology **56**, 359—373 (1955).

Raynaud, A.: (a) Effet des injections d' hormones sexuelles à la souris gravide, sur le développement des ébauches de la glande mammaire des embryous. I. Action des substances androgènes. Ann. Endocr. (Paris) **8**, 248—253 (1947).

— (b) Action de fortes doses des substances oestrogènes. Ann. Endocr. (Paris) **8**, 318—329 (1947).

— (c) Inhibition du développement des ébauches mammaires de l'émbryon de souris sous l'effet d'une hormone oestrogène injectée directement á l'embryon. C. R. Soc. Biol. (Paris) **146**, 544—549 (1952).

— (d) Morphogenesis of the mammary gland. In: Milk: The mammary gland and its secretion, ed. by S. K. Kon, and A. T. Cowie, vol. I, p. 1—46. New York and London: Academic Press 1961.

— (f) Le développement embryonnaire de la glande mammaire de la souris après déstruction au moyen des rayons X des glandes génitales de l'embryon. Bull. Soc. zool. France, **74**, 156—159 (1949).

— (h) La production expérimental de malformations mammaires chez les foetus de souris par l'action des hormones sexuelles. Ann. Inst. Pasteur **90**, 39—219 (1956).

— Frilley, M.: (e) Etat de développement des ébauches mammaires et du cordon vaginal chez le foetus mâles et femelles de souris, dout les ébauches des glandes génitales ont été détruites par une irradiation au moyen des rayon X, a l'âge de treize jours. C. R. Acad. Sci. (Paris) **225**, 1380—1382 (1947).

— Raynaud, J.: (g) Les diverses malformations mammaires produites chez les foetus de souris, par l'action des hormonelles sexuelles. C. R. Soc. Biol. (Paris) **148**, 963—968 (1954).

Reece, R. P., Mixner, J. P.: Effect of testosterone on pituitary and mammary gland. Proc. Soc. exp. Biol. (N. Y.) **40**, 66—67 (1939).

— Leathem, J. H.: Growth of mammary glands of hypophysectomized rats following estrogen and lactogen administration. Proc. Soc. exp. Biol. (N. Y.) **59**, 122—124 (1945).

— Leonard, S. L.: Lobule-alveolar growth of mammary glands of hypophysectomized female rats. Proc. Soc. exp. Biol. (N. Y.) **49**, 660—662 (1942).

Rein, G.: Untersuchungen über die embryonale Entwicklungsgeschichte der Milchdrüse. Arch. mikr. Anat. **20**, 431—501 (1882); **21**, 678—694 (1882).

Reinecke, E. P., Meites, J., Cairy, C. F., Huffman, D. F.: Hormonal induction for lactation in sterile cows. In: Proceedings annual meeting American Veterinary Medical Association, 1952, p. 325—328, Atlantic City. Amer. Veterinary Med. Ass.

Richardson, K. C.: (a) Some structural features of the mammary tissues. Brit. med. Bull. **5**, 123—129 (1947).

— (b) Contractile tissues in the mammary gland with special reference to myoepithelium in the goat. Proc. roy. Soc. B **136**, 30—45 (1949).

— (c) Measurement of the total area of secretory epithelium with lactatin mammary gland of the goat. J. Endocr. **9**, 170—184 (1953).

— (d) Mammary tumors and mammary gland development in normal and oestrogen-treated F_1 hybrids of strains C_3H/J and R III/An mice. J. nat. Cancer Inst. **36**, 1167—1187 (1966).

— (e) The acinar pattern in the mammary glandes of virgin mice at different ages. J. nat. Cancer Inst. **38**, 305—315 (1967).

Riddle, O.: Prolactin invertebrate function and organization. J. nat. Cancer Inst. 31, 1039—1110 (1963).
— The preparation, identification and assay of prolactin — a hormone of the anterior pituitary. Amer. J. Physiol. 105, 191—216 (1933).
— Bates, R. W., Dykshorn, S. W.: A new hormone of the anterior pituitary. Proc. Soc. exp. Biol. (N. Y.) 29, 1211—1212 (1932).
— Braucher, P. F.: Studies on the physiology of reproduction in birds. XXX. Control of the special secretion of the crop-gland in pigeons by an anterior pituitary hormone. Amer. J. Physiol. 97, 617—625 (1931).
Riedel, G.: Die Entwicklung und Entartung des elastischen Gewebes in der senilen Mamma. Virchows Arch. path. Anat. 256, 242—267 (1925).
Rosen, S. W., Gahres, E. E.: Nonpuerperal galactorrhoea and the contraceptive pill. J. Obstet. Gynec. 29, 730—731 (1967).
Rosenburg, A.: Über menstruelle, durch das Corpus luteum bedingte Mammaveränderungen. Frankfurt. Z. Path. 27, 466—506 (1922).
Ross, R., Klebanoff, S.: Fine structural changes in uterine smooth muscle and fibroblasts in response to estrogen. J. Cell Biol. 32, 155—167 (1967).
Saameli, K.: Untersuchungen über den Blutspiegel und die Abbaugeschwindigkeit von Oxytocin. Gynaecologia (Basel) 152, 329—332 (1961).
Salter, J., Best, C. H.: Insulin as a growth hormon. Brit. med. J. 1953 II, 353—359.
Sandritter, W., Federlin, K., Pfeiffer, E. F.: Quantitative histochemical studies on islet cells. In: The structure and metabolismen of the pancreatic islets. Proc. 3rd. Internat. Symp. Stockholm, 1963. Oxford-London-Edinburgh-New York-Paris-Frankfurt: Pergamon Press 1964.
Schachner, S. H.: Galactorrhoea subsequent to contraceptive hormones. New Engl. Med. J. 275, 1138—1141 (1966).
Schäfer, A., Bässler, R.: Vergleichende elektronenoptische Untersuchungen am Drüsenepithel und am sog. lobulären Carcinom der Mamma. Virchows Arch. Abt. A Path. Anat. 346, 269—286 (1969).
Schaefer, H. E., Fischer, R.: Östrogenbedingte Induktion alkalischer Phosphatase in Fibroblasten des subkutanen Bindegewebes der Maus. Acta endocr. (Kbh.) 57, 261—273 (1968).
Schairer, E.: Kernmessungen und Chromosomenzählungen an menschlichen Geschwülsten. Z. Krebsforsch. 43, 1—38 (1936).
Schaltenbrand, G.: Die Nervenkrankheiten. Stuttgart: Thieme 1951.
Scharf, G., Lyons, W. R.: Effects of estrone and progesterone on male rabbit mammary glands. II. Varying doses of estrone. Proc. Soc. exp. Biol. (N. Y.) 48, 86—89 (1941).
Schimmelbusch, C.: Das Cystadenom der Mamma. Arch. klin. Chir. 44, 117—134 (1892).
Schipp, R.: Der Feinbau filamentärer Strukturen im Endothel peripherer Lymphgefäße. Acta anat. (Basel) 71, 341—351 (1968).
Schmidt, Hugo: Über normale Hyperthelie menschlicher Embryonen und über die erste Anlage der menschlichen Milchdrüsen überhaupt. Schwalbes morphol. Arb. 7, 157—199 (1897).
Schmitt, Heinrich: Über die Entwicklung der Milchdrüse und die Hyperthelie menschlicher Embryonen. Schwalbes morphol. Arb. 8, 236—303 (1898).
Schnurbusch, F.: Untersuchungen über die Morphologie der männlichen Brustdrüse während des Lebensablaufes als Grundlage für ein Studium der Gynäkomastie. Frankfurt. Z. Path. 62, 402—418 (1951).
Schriever, D.: Histochemische Untersuchungen am Bindegewebe der Mamma in physiologischen Funktionsphasen. Inaug.-Diss. Mainz, 1968.
Schultz, A.: Pathologische Anatomie der Brustdrüse. In: Handbuch der speziellen pathologischen Anatomie und Histologie von O. Lubarsch und F. Henke, Weibliche Geschlechtsorgane, 7. Bd., 2. Teil. Berlin: Springer 1933.

Schulze, G.: Histochemische Untersuchungen am Bindegewebe der hormonal stimulierten Mamma. Inaug.-Diss. Mainz, 1968.
Segal, S. J., Scher, W.: Estrogenes, nuclei acids and protein synthesis in uterine metabolism. In: R. M. Wynn, Cellular biology of the uterus, p. 114—150. Amsterdam: North Holland publ. 1967.
Seifert, G.: Über Gewebsreaktionen der menschlichen Brustdrüse bei Leukämien. Virchows Arch. path. Anat. 322, 336—357 (1952).
Selye, H.: On the nervous control of lactation. Amer. J. Physiol. 107, 535—538 (1934).
— Activity of progesterone in spayed female not pretreated with estrin. Proc. Soc. exp. Biol. (N. Y.) 43, 343—344 (1940).
— (a) Stress and lactation. Rev. canad. Biol. 13, 377—384 (1954).
— (b) The effect of cortisol upon the mammary glands. Acta endocr. (Kbh.) 17, 394—401 (1954).
— Browne, J. S. L., Collip, J. B.: The effect of large doses of progesterone in the female rat. Proc. Soc. exp. Biol. (N. Y.) 34, 472—474 (1936).
— McEuen, C. S., Collip, J. B.: Effect of testosterone on mammary gland. Proc. Soc. exp. Biol. (N. Y.) 34, 201—203 (1936).
Semb, C.: Fibroadenomatosis cystica mammae. Acta chir. scand. 64, Suppl. X, 1—483 (1928).
Short, R. H. D.: Alveolar epithelium in relation to growth of the lung. Phil. Trans. B 235, 35—86 (1951).
Silver, I. A.: Myoepithelial cells in the mammary and parotid glands. J. Physiol. (Lond.) 125, 8—9 (1954).
Smith, Th. C.: The action of relaxin on mammary gland growth in the rat. Endocrinology 54, 59—70 (1954).
— The effect of estrogen and progesterone on mammary gland growth in the rat. Endocrinology 57, 33—43 (1955).
— Action of estrogen and progesterone on mammary nucleic acids and enzymes in rats. Endocrinology 65, 51—55 (1959).
— Braverman, L. B.: The action of desoxycorticosterone acetate on the mammary gland of the immature ovariectomized rat. Endocrinology 52, 311—317 (1953).
— Richterich, B.: Synergism of estrogen and progesterone on mammary growth in guinea pigs. Endocrinology 63, 89—98 (1958).
Smithcors, J. F., Leonard, S. L.: Limited effects of certain steroid hormones on mammary glands of hypophysectomized rats. Proc. Soc. exp. Biol. (N. Y.) 54, 109—111 (1943).
Soemarwoto, J. N., Bern, H. A.: The effect of hormones on the vascular pattern of the mouse mammary gland. Amer. J. Anat. 103, 403—435 (1958).
Speert, H.: The normal and experimental development of the mammary gland of the rhesus monkey with some pathological correlations. Contr. Embryol. Carneg. Inst. 32, 9—65 (1948).
Spellacy, W. N., Carlson, K. L., Schade, S. L.: Human growth hormone studies in patients with galactorrhea (Ahumada-del-Castillo-Syndrome). Amer. J. Obstet. Gynec. 100, 84—89 (1968).
Spuler, A.: Abriß der Entwicklungsgeschichte der Milchdrüse. In: Handbuch der Gynäkologie, hrsg. von W. Stoeckel, Bd. 1, S. 490—510. Berlin: Bergmann 1930.
Stein, O., Stein, Y.: Formation of milk glycerides in lactating mice studied by electronmicroscopic autoradiography. Israel J. med. Sci. 2, 773—778 (1966).
Steinbeck, H.: Die Wirkung der verschiedenen Gestagene auf Morphologie und Funktion der Milchdrüse. In: Handbuch der experimentellen Pharmakologie, hrsg. von O. Eichler, A. Farah, H. Herken und A. D. Welch, Bd. 22/2, S. 341—425. Berlin-Heidelberg-New York: Springer 1969.

Stöcker, E.: (a) Autoradiographische Untersuchungen zur Deutung der funktionellen Kernschwellung am exokrinen Pankreas. Z. Zellforsch. **57**, 47—62 (1962).
— (b) Autoradiographische Untersuchungen mit 12 H³ und 5 C¹⁴ markierten Aminosäuren zur Größe des nukleolären und zytoplasmatischen Eiweißstoffwechsels bei verschiedenen Zellarten von Maus und Ratte. Z. Zellforsch. **70**, 419—448 (1966).
Stricker, P.: Recherches expérimentales sur les fonctions du lobe antérieur de l'hypophyse: influence des extraits du lobe antérieur sur l'appareil génital de la lapine et sur la montée laiteuse. Presse méd. **37**, 1268—1271 (1929).
— Grueter, F.: Action du lobe antérieur de hypophyse sur la montée laiteuse. C. R. Soc. Biol. (Paris) **99**, 1978—1980 (1928).
Suchenwirth, R., Bues, F.: Galaktorrhoe als Leitsymptom bei Hypophysenadenomen. Endokrinologie **41**, 66—75 (1961).
Suetina, J. A., Chentsov, S., Chentsov, Y., Smirnova, J. O., Samoilov, W. J.: Action mechanism of estrogens and progesteron on the mammary glands. Arh. Patol. (Moskva) **28**, 16—22 (1966).
Sykes, J. F.: Hormonal development of mammary tissue in dairy heifers. J. Dairy Sci. **34**, 1174—1179 (1951).
— Wrenn, T. R.: Hormonal development of the mammary gland of dairy heifers. J. Dairy Sci. **33**, 194—204 (1950).
Sylven, B.: Über die Elektivität und Fehlerquellen der Schleimfärbung mit Mucicarmin im Vergleich mit metachromatischer Färbung. Virchows Arch. path. Anat. **303**, 280—394 (1938).
Takahashi, N.: Electron microscopic studies on the ectodermal secretory glands in man. The fine structure of the apocrine sweat glands with special reference to the myoepithelium. Bull. Tokyo med. dent. Univ. **4**, 259—269 (1957).
— Electron microscopic studies on the extodermal secretory glands in man. II. The fine structures of the myoepithelium in the human mammary and salivary glands. Bull. Tokyo med. dent. Univ. **5**, 177—192 (1958).
Talwalker, P. K.: Mammary lobulo-alveolar growth in adreno-ovariectomized rats following transplantation of "mammotropic" pituitary tumor. Proc. Soc. exp. Biol. (N. Y.) **117**, 121—124 (1964).
— Meites, J.: Mammary lobulo-alveolar growth induced by anterior pituitary hormones in adreno-ovariectomized and adreno-ovariectomized-hypophysectomized rats. Proc. Soc. exp. Biol. (N. Y.) **107**, 880—883 (1961).
— Nicoll, C. S., Meites, J.: Induction of mammary secretion in pregnant rats and rabbits by hydrocortisone acetate. Endocrinology, **69**, 802—808 (1961).
Tamarin, A.: Myoepithelium of rat submaxillary gland. J. Ultrastruct. Res. **16**, 320—338 (1966).
Tandler, B.: Ultrastructure of the human submaxillary gland. Z. Zellforsch. **68**, 852—863 (1965).
Taylor, H. C.: (a) The relation of chronic mastitis to certain hormones of the ovary and pituitary and to coincident gynecological lesions. Surg. Gynec. Ostet. **62**, 129—148 (1936).
— (b) The relation of chronic mastitis to certain hormones of the ovary and pituitary and to coincident gynecological lesions. Surg. Gynec. Obstet. **62**, 562—584 (1936).
— Waltman, C. A.: Hyperplasias of the mammary gland in the human being and in the mouse. Arch. Surg. **40**, 733—820 (1940).
Terzakis, I. A.: The ultrastructure of monkey eccrine sweat glands. Z. Zellforsch. **64**, 493—509 (1964).
Thölen, H.: Das embryonale und postnatale Verhalten der männlichen Brustdrüse beim Menschen. I. Das Mammaorgan beim Embryo und Säugling. Acta anat. (Basel) **8**, 201—235 (1949).
Thoenes, W.: Mikromorphologie des Nephron nach temporärer Ischämie. Stuttgart: Thieme 1964.

TRAURIG, H.: (a) Cell proliferation in the mammary gland during late pregnancy and lactation. Anat. Rec. **157**, 489—504 (1967).
— (b) A radioautographic study of all proliferation in the mammary gland of the pregnant mouse. Anat. Rec. **159**, 239—248 (1967).
TRENTIN, J. J.: The experimental development of the mammary gland with special reference to the interaction of the pituitary and ovarian hormones. Mo. agric. Exp. Sta. Res. Bull Nr. 418 (1948).
— TURNER, C. W.: Effect of adrenalectomy on the mammary gland of the castrated and estrogen treated male rat. Endocrinology **41**, 127—134 (1947).
TREVES, N.: Gynecomastia. The origins of mammary swelling in the male: an analysis of 406 patients with breast hypertrophy, 525 with testicular tumors and 13 with adrenal neoplasma. Cancer (Philad.) **11**, 1082—1102 (1958).
TUCKER, H. A.: (b) Nuclei acid content of mammary glands of lactating rats. Proc. Soc. exp. Biol. (N. Y.) **112**, 409—412 (1963).
— (d) Nuclei acid of rat mammary glands during post-lactational involution. Proc. Soc. exp. Biol. (N. Y.) **112**, 1002—1004 (1963).
— REECE, R. P.: (a) Nuclei acid content of mammary glands of pregnant rats. Proc. Soc. exp. Biol. (N. Y.) **112**, 370—372 (1963).
— — (c) Nuclei acid content of mammary gland of rats lactating 41 and 61 days. Proc. Soc. exp. Biol. (N.Y.) **112**, 688—690 (1963).
TURNER, C. W.: The mammary gland. I. The anatomy of the udder of cattle and domestic animals. Columbia: Lucas Brothers 1952.
— GOMEZ, E. T.: The experimental development of the mammary gland. I. The male and female albino mouse. II. The male and female guinea pig. Mo. agric. Exp. Sta. Res. Bull. Nr. 206 (1934).
— YAMAMOTO, H., RUPPERT, H. L.: The experimental induction of growth of the cow's udder and the initiation of milk secretion. J. Dairy Sci. **39**, 1717—1729 (1956).
URBAN, J. A., ADAIR, F. E.: Sklerosing adenosis. Cancer (Philad.) **2**, 625—634 (1949).
VERLEY, J. M., HOLLMANN, K. H.: Synthese et réabsorption des proteines dans la glande mammaire en stase étude autoradiographique au microscope électronique. Z. Zellforsch. **75**, 605—610 (1966).
VERNE, J.: État actuell de la cytochimie de la glande mammaire. Cell. int. Cent. nat. Rech. sci. **32**, 59—66 (1951).
VERONESI, U., CANDIANI, M. A.: La glandola mammaria muliebre nella senescenca. Biol. lat. (Milano) **8**, 7—100 (1955).
VIGNEAUD, P. G. DU, RESSLER, C., SWAN, J. M., ROBERTS, C. W., KATSOYAMIS, P. G., GORDON, S.: The synthesis of an octapeptide amide with the hormonal activity of oxytocin. J. Amer. chem. Soc. **75**, 4879—4880 (1953).
VIGNEAUD, V. DU, LAWLER, H. C., POPENOE, E. A.: Enzymatic clearage of glycinamide from vasopressin and a proposed structure for this pressor-antidiuretic hormone of the posterior pituitary. J. Amer. chem. Soc. **75**, 4880—4881 (1953).
VILLANI, G., ZANELLA, E.: Il tissue elastico nei tumori e in altre forme patologiche della mammella. Arch. De Vecchi Anat. pat. **17**, 537—552 (1951).
VITRY, G.: Modification histochimique de la substance fondamentale du tissu conjonctif, de la tetine du cobaye sans l'action de diverse hormones sexuelles. C. R. Soc. Biol. (Paris) **147**, 124—126 (1953).
VOGLER, E.: Über das basilare Helle-Zellen-Organ der menschlichen Brustdrüse. Klin. Med. (Wien) **2**, 159—167 (1947).
VOLKMANN, H.: Zahlen und Daten zur Funktion der Milchdrüsen. Zusammenstellung und Tabelle (Beilage). Med. Klin. **39** (1951).
VOSS, H. E.: Die hormonale Regelung der Laktation. Dtsch. med. Wschr. **83**, 288—291, 328—331 (1958).

WAGENEN, G. VAN, FOLLEY, S. J.: Effect of androgens on mammary gland of female rhesus monkey. J. Endocr. 1, 367—372 (1939).
WATTENWYL, H. V.: Tierexperimentelle Untersuchungen über die Wirkung langdauernder Follikelhormonapplikation und die hormonale Tumorentstehung. Inaug.-Diss. Basel, 1944.
WATZKA, M.: Zellen mit spezialen Funktionen. In: Handbuch der allgemeinen Pathologie, hrsgg. von F. BÜCHNER, E. LETTERER und R. ROULET, Bd. II/1. Berlin-Göttingen-Heidelberg: Springer 1955.
WAUGH, D., HOEVEN, E. VAN DER: Fine structure of the human adult female breast. Lab. Invest. 11, 220—228 (1962).
WEBER, A. T., KITCHELL, R. L., SAUTTER, I. H.: Mammary gland studies. I. The identity and characterization of the smallert lobule unit in the udder of the dairy cow. Amer. J. vet. Res. 16, 255—263 (1955).
WEBER, W.: Zur Histologie und Cytologie der Kropfmilchbildung der Taube. Z. Zellforsch. 56, 247—276 (1962).
WEICHERT, C. K., BOYD, R. W., COHEN, R. S.: A study of certain endocrine effects in the mammary glands of female rats. Anat. Rec. 61, 21 (1934).
WELLINGS, S. R., NANDI, S.: Electron microscopy of induced secretion in mammary epithelial cells of hypophysectomized-ovarectomized-adrenalectomized BALB/c Crgl mice. J. nat. Cancer Inst. 40, 1245—1258 (1968).
— PHILP, J. R.: The function of the Golgi apparatus in lactating cells of the BALB/c Crgl mouse. An electron microscopic and autoradiographic study. Z. Zellforsch. 61, 871—882 (1964).
WENNER, R.: Physiologische und pathologische Lactation. Arch. Gynäk. 204, 171—206 (1966).
WERNER, K. H.: Über die Wirkung des Follikelhormons auf die Milchdrüsen kastrierter Ratten. Diss. Leipzig 1938.
WIDER, J. A., MARSHALL, J. R., ROSS, G. T.: Familial galactorrhoea in three sisters with oligo-ovulation. J. Amer. med. Ass. 209, 669—671 (1969).
WILLIAMS-ASHMAN, H. G.: Androgenic control of nucleic acid and protein synthesis in male accenory genital organs. J. cell. comp. Physiol. 66, 111—124 (1965).
WYK, J. J. V., GRUMBACH, M. M.: Syndrom of precocious menstruation and galactorrhea in juvenil hypothyreoidism: an example of hormonal overlap in pituitary feedback. J. Pediat. 57, 416—435 (1960).
YAMAMOTO, H., TURNER, C. W.: Experimental mammary gland growth in rabbits by estrogen and progesterone. Proc. Soc. exp. Biol. (N. Y.) 92, 130—132 (1956).
ZAKS, M. G.: The motor apparatus of the mammary gland, ed. by A. T. COWIE. Edinburgh and London: Oliver and Boyd 1962.
ZARZYCKI, L., PERYT, A., KLUBINSKA, B., HJAC, T., ZAK, K.: Histochemische Untersuchungen über den Involutionsmechanismus der Milchdrüse. Histochemie 18, 314—320 (1969).
ZONDEK, B., BROMBERG, Y. M., ROZIN, S.: An anterior pituitary hyperhormotrophic syndrome. J. Obstet. Gynaec. Brit. Emp. 58, 525—537 (1951).

Neurological Institute of University of Vienna
(Director: Prof. Dr. F. SEITELBERGER)

Spongy Degeneration of the Central Nervous System in Infancy

KURT JELLINGER and FRANZ SEITELBERGER

With 15 Figures

Table of Contents

I. Introduction	91
A. The Problem of "Status Spongiosus"	92
B. Classification of Spongy Dystrophies	97
II. Historical Aspects	98
III. Genetic and Geographic Aspects	99
IV. Clinical Aspects	105
A. Pre- and Paranatal Histories	105
B. Clinical Course	105
C. Clinical Symptomatology	106
D. Personal Observations	108
1. Infantile Cases	108
2. Late Infantile Cases	108
3. Juvenile Cases	108
V. Clinical Laboratory Findings	109
VI. Pathological Aspects	110
A. General Necropsy	110
B. Brain Autopsy	110
C. Histological Findings	111
1. Quality of the CNS Lesions	111
2. Topography of the Lesions	119
3. Peripheral Nerves and Muscle	123
D. Ultrastructural Findings	124
VII. Biochemical Aspects	127
A. Histochemical Findings	127
B. Water Content of Brain Tissue	127
C. Electrolytes	127
D. Brain Lipids	127
VIII. Differential Diagnosis	128
IX. Nosological Aspects	130
A. Atypical Cases	130
1. Transition to Progressive Poliodystrophy	130
2. Transition to Sudanophilic Leukodystrophies	131
3. Spongy Degeneration and Axonal Dystrophy	132
B. Relationship to other Spongy Encephalopathies	132
1. Hepatic Encephalopathies	133

2. Inborn Errors of Amino Acid Metabolism 133
   3. Encephalopathy in Infantile Dystrophy 134
   4. Presenile Spongiform Encephalopathy 135
   5. Border Disease of Sheep 135
   6. Experimental Spongy Encephalopathies 135
 X. Pathogenetic Aspects 138
   A. Chronic Edema 139
   1. Myelin Swelling 139
   2. Astroglial Reactions 141
   B. Pathogenesis of Myelin Destruction 143
   C. Myelin Deficit in Other Spongy Encephalopathies 144
   D. Localization Problems 146
 XI. Etiological Problems 147
References 148

Eponyma. Progressive degenerative subcortical encephalopathy; Early infantile familial cerebral sclerosis; Early infantile "diffuse sclerosis" of the brain; Idiotie familiale avec dégénérescence spongieuse du névraxe; Familial idiocy with spongy degeneration of the neuraxis; Spongy degeneration of the cerebral white matter; Spongy type of diffuse sclerosis; Familial idiocy with spongy degeneration of the CNS; Spongy degeneration of the CNS in infancy; Spongy degeneration of the nervous system; dégénérescence spongieuse familiale; Ödemkrankheit des ZNS im frühen Kindesalter; Maladie oedémateuse progressive cérébrale de la première enfance; Idiotie amaurotique atypique; CANAVAN's sclerosis (disease); Familial spongy degeneration of the brain; CANAVAN's spongy degeneration; Diffuse Form der spongiösen Dystrophien des Nervensystems — Typ CANAVAN; Spongy degeneration of the CNS (VAN BOGAERT-BERTRAND type).

I. Introduction

Among the large variety of encephalopathies of obscure origin in infancy and childhood, a group of progressive diseases is morphologically characterized by striking vacuolation of the neuraxis. Although spongy changes of the CNS are present in a wide range of disorders of different origin, several nosological entities have been recognized among these "spongy encephalopathies" in infancy and childhood. On the basis of their clinical and particularly pathological features, these rare diseases can be separated from other deteriorating disorders of early age which usually take the form of one of the varieties of leukodystrophy or lipidosis or result from other metabolic disorders.

Considering the pathological features and pattern of the CNS lesions, three principal groups of "spongy encephalopathies in infancy and childhood" can be distinguished which are believed to represent separate clinico-pathological entities (VAN BOGAERT, 1960):

1. Diffuse forms referred to as *"Spongy degeneration of the CNS in Infancy"* (VAN BOGAERT-BERTRAND type), also known under various eponymous designations[1], which will be reviewed here.

---
[1] Vide supra.

2. Focally disseminated forms with predilective affection of the brain stem, commonly called *"Subacute necrotizing encephalomyelopathy"* (LEIGH) or referred to as "infantile Wernicke's syndrome". A review of this and related conditions has been given recently by JELLINGER and SEITELBERGER (1970b).

3. Progressive cerebral degeneration with spongy necrosis limited almost exclusively to the cerebral gray matter. Since these changes are nonspecific in nature, the nosological entity of this group, usually called *"Progressive infantile poliodystrophy"* (CHRISTENSEN-KRABBE) or ALPERS' disease is still controversial (DREIFUSS and NETSKY, 1964; GREENHOUSE and NEUBUERGER, 1964). Whereas a number of cases described under this term apparently belong to conditions with different causes, e.g. anoxic and toxic disorders, a group of cases shows a distinctly familial tendency of the disease suggesting a genetically determined metabolic abnormality (BLACKWOOD et al., 1963; LAURENCE and CAVANAGH, 1968; KLEIN and DICHGANS, 1969; JELLINGER, 1970).

Although recent ultrastructural and biochemical studies have made valuable contributions towards a better morphogenic understanding of these conditions and their basic disorders, the pathogenesis and etiology of the "spongy encephalopathies" in infancy and childhood still remain obscure.

In the following report the currently available data on the first type of infantile spongy encephalopathies, the "Spongy Degeneration of the CNS in Infancy" (SDI) are reviewed. First of all, the problem of "spongy degeneration" of the nervous tissue will be critically discussed with special reference to its characteristic type of lesion commonly called "status spongiosus".

A. The Problem of "Status Spongiosus"

The term "spongy degeneration of the nervous tissue" has been applied to conditions which by light microscopy are characterized by striking vacuolar changes in the gray and/or white matter of the neuraxis resulting in a sponge- or sieve-like appearance. This type of transformation usually referred to as "spongy state" appears characteristic for the central nervous tissue as it is not seen in other organs. This is due to the ultrastructural architecture of the CNS, its functional compartmentation, and the peculiarities of the intracerebral transport mechanism. The spongy state, however, does *not* represent a specific CNS lesion. In practice, this term has been applied with considerable frequency to CNS tissues altered in a large variety of circumstances, apparently by pathogenic factors of varying character.

FISCHER (1911) was the first to describe the "status spongiosus" resulting from neuronal loss in progressive degenerative diseases. BIELSCHOWSKY (1919) and STRÄUSSLER and KOSKINAS (1926) interpreted spongy changes found in general paralysis of the insane as the result of serous inbibition of the cerebral tissue. According to SPIELMEYER (1922), this condition represents the effect of a rapid disintegration of the neuropil associated with insufficient substitution by reactive glia. This interpretation was deduced from the cribriform appearance of lesions in subacute combined degeneration of the spinal cord and in hepato-cerebral disease. Later, these disorders were summarized as "spongy neurodystrophies" (ERBSLÖH, 1958).

BRAUNMÜHL (1957) distinguished two types of spongy state. The first, as seen in Wilson's disease, funicular myelosis or amaurotic idiocy, was considered to result from fulminant disintegration of the nervous tissue with lack of reparative capacity of the astroglia. The second, rather frequent type was suggested to be the consequence of serous inbibition of the ground substance. Conversely, according to LÜERS and SPATZ (1957) and CROMPTON (1969), the spongy state is not an expression of edema but probably represents the compensatory effect of a rapid disintegration of the neuropil, in which there is not time for cortical shrinkage or enlargement of the ventricles and perivascular spaces, the usual and slower mechanism by which destruction or disappearance of brain tissue is compensated.

SEITELBERGER (1967) interpreted the status spongiosus as a consequence of selective partial necrosis of single components of the nervous tissue. From light microscopical analysis, he theoretically distinguished a neurogenic type, a gliogenic type and a — non-existing — mesenchymogenic form.

1. The *neurogenic type* of spongy state originates in severe selective neuronal loss due to atrophic or degenerative processes, e.g. in Pick's disease, neuroaxonal dystrophy, special types of cerebral lipidoses or anoxic parenchymal necrosis, if the outfall of the neuronal component of the neuropil (neurons and axons) is not sufficiently substituted by reparative gliosis. This change can also occur in the white matter due to intense loss of nerve fibers in neuroaxonal dystrophies, leukodystrophies or leukoencephalitides.

2. The *gliogenic type* of spongy state is suggested to be caused by selective affection and loss of the astroglial element of the neuropil, in the sequence of which three stages can be distinguished:

a) Hypertrophic-proliferative phase with increase in volume and hypertrophic proliferation of the cell processes. Aggregates of intensely swollen astrocytes can cause a "status prespongiosus".

b) Regressive phase characterized by disintegration of the luxuriant processes ("clasmatodendrosis") and hydropic ballooning of the astroglia progressing to microcystic vacuolation of the tissue.

c) Defective stage associated with disintegration of the glial cells with slight but insufficient fibrillary proliferation, formation of vacuoles and their secondary confluence to form large spaces.

This latter type of spongy change is seen in conditions for which SEITELBERGER (1965) proposed the term "dystrophies of transport structures" because the primary lesion apparently affects the compartments which play an important role in cerebral transport mechanisms.

According to ISHINO et al. (1968), the spongy state of the neuropil occurs in various forms ranging from grumelous to polycystic states. Sieve-like transformation of the gray matter can be caused by neuronal loss in the final stage of necrosis or can be associated with relative preservation of the nervous parenchyma.

Reviewing the light optical features of cavitating change of the CNS tissue referred to as the spongy state, it becomes evident that this term has been synonymously used for two different types of lesion:

1. Spongy transformation resulting from severe *loss of nervous tissue components*. This type of spongy state represents a terminal stage of disintegration of the nervous parenchyma with deficient glial response as seen in selective parenchymal necrosis and atrophic neuronal processes of various origin. It is akin to FISCHER's and SPIELMEYER's original descriptions and to SEITELBERGER's neurogenic type.

2. Spongy change of the nervous tissue *without primary loss of neural elements*. This type is characterized by the occurrence of rounded, empty spaces or cavities of various extent separated by fibers or bands of more or less *intact* neural tissue. Although, at the light microscopic level, it is similar in appearance among various disorders, it differs considerably at the ultrastructural level. Here, a spongy appearance of the tissue may predominantly correspond to:

a) severely *swollen astrocytes* or astrocytic processes, as seen in most types of human and experimental brain edema, especially in the gray matter (LONG et al., 1966; KLATZO, 1967; ULE, 1967; SCHEINBERG et al., 1969), in Jakob-Creutzfeldt disease (MARIN and VIAL, 1964; TORACK, 1969), and in various toxic and deficiency states (ROBERTSON et al., 1968);

b) vacuolation or *swelling of oligodendroglia* (HARRIS, 1964; HIRANO et al., 1965; MAXWELL and KRUGER, 1966; SLUGA, 1967; O'LEARY et al., 1965);

c) large *intramyelinic vacuoles* as the outstanding findings in SDI (ADACHI et al., 1966), TET intoxication (ALEU et al., 1963; LEE and BAKAY, 1965; KOLKMANN and ULE, 1967; HIRANO et al., 1968), and INH-induced encephalopathy (LAMPERT and SCHOCHET, 1968; REIN et al., 1968);

d) *intra-axonal vacuoles*, as seen in experimental cyanide encephalopathy (HIRANO et al., 1967) or as initial lesion in subacute combined degeneration of the spinal cord (PANT et al., 1968);

e) *distended extracellular spaces* in human and experimental forms of white matter edema (GONATAS et al., 1963; HIRANO et al., 1967; LONG et al., 1966; SCHRÖDER and WECHSLER, 1965; LAMPERT et al., 1966; SCHEINBERG et al., 1969);

f) *Swelling of postsynaptic dendrites* as reversible findings in experimentally induced respiratory acidosis (SCHLOTE et al., 1969).

g) *combined affection of several compartments* of the CNS, such as

α) *swelling of astrocytes and neuronal processes*, e.g. in Jakob-Creutzfeldt disease (GONATAS et al., 1964; SLUGA and SEITELBERGER, 1967; KIDD, 1967; FONCIN, 1967), in SDI (ULE, 1968), thiamine deficiency (ULE et al., 1968), after injection of ouabain (CORNOG et al., 1967), methionine sulfoximine (DE ROBERTIS et al., 1967; ULE, 1968) or sodium acide (KOLKMANN, 1970);

β) *vacuolation* of neuronal perikarya, axons and dendrites in experimental Kuru (LAMPERT et al., 1969); and Jakob-Creutzfeldt-disease (RIBADEAU-DUMAS et al., 1969).

γ) *swelling of astroglia and intramyelinic vacuolation*, as seen in SDI (ADACHI et al., 1966; GAMBETTI et al., 1969);

δ) *intramyelinic vacuolation associated* with swelling of the inner and outer oligodendrocytic covering of the myelin sheath in experimental cyanide poisoning (HIRNER, 1969), vacuolation of astroglia and oligodendroglia in

Cuprizone intoxication (SUZUKI and KIKKAWA, 1969) or with swelling of astroglia and postsynaptic dendrites in SDI (ULE, 1968).

It should be emphasized that some of these lesions are inconstant findings and that there exist considerable species differences with regard to the affected tissue component (ULE, 1968).

In all these conditions the spongy transformation is primarily caused by intense *dilatation of various tissue elements*. It usually results from accumulation of excess fluid associated with changes in ion distribution between the various compartments which is consistent with the common definition of "*cerebral edema*" (cf. BAKAY and LEE, 1965; KLATZO and SEITELBERGER, 1967). This type of spongy loosening of the CNS tissue is seen in the initial stages of anoxic necrobiosis (VAN HARREVELD and KHATTAB, 1967; HAGER, 1968; BAKAY and LEE, 1968), in perifocal and histotoxic edema (ULE and KOLKMANN, 1962; HIRANO et al., 1965, 1967; SCHRÖDER and WECHSLER, 1965) and in various toxic and metabolic disorders of different origin. One of the basic pathogenic mechanisms appears to be a selective disorders of the active, energy-bound ion and water transport systems at the cell membranes.

Evidence accumulated in recent years suggests that a membrane-bound ATPase activated by Na^+ and K^+ is closely associated with the active transport of ions and water across cell membranes (SKOU, 1965; VAN HARREVELD, 1966). This enzyme system is present in a wide variety of tissues and is especially active in the brain (BONTING, 1964; SAMAHA, 1967). ATPase activity has been demonstrated in the endothelial cells, in the basement membrane, in myelinated axons, and in the interspace between the plasma membranes of neurons and glial processes as well as in synaptic terminals (TORACK and BARNETT, 1963, 1964; TORACK, 1965). Na^+-K^+-activated ATPase has been localized primarily in cholinergic nerve endings (ALBERS et al., 1965; RODRIGUEZ DE LOPEZ ARNAIZ et al., 1967; FAHN et al., 1968; LING et al., 1968). A large increase in this enzyme during neonatal maturation suggests that it has a major role in synaptic function (SAMSON et al., 1967; ABDEL-LATIF et al., 1967). Electrolyte study in the rat brain during maturation has revealed that total brain Na^+ and Cl^- concentration decreases progressively while there is evidence of a large increase in Na^+-K^+-stimulated ATPase (VERNADAKIS et al., 1963). Recent data further indicate a close relationship between the sodium localization and the distribution of this enzyme in normal brain tissue (TANI et al., 1969).

Inhibition of this membrane-bound enzyme system has been observed in various experimental forms of brain edema (TORACK, 1965; ZADUNAISKY et al., 1965; TORACK et al., 1967; REULEN and BAETHMANN, 1967; DE ROBERTIS et al., 1969). These changes are not combined with increased permeability of the BBB for macromolecules, and thus are consistent with the "*cytotoxic*" type of brain edema (KLATZO, 1967). Increased vascular permeability, however, may occur in advanced stages of these conditions (LAMPERT and SCHOCHET, 1968). Another type of cerebral edema results from primarily increased permeability of the BBB, including leakage of plasma constituents into the surrounding tissue. This form, referred to as the "*vasogenic*" type, is associated with tumors, injuries, radiation damage, inflammation and chemical lesions. The conditions referred to as "spongy degenerations" are usually more akin to the "intracellular" type of edema than to the latter form which is characterized by enlargement of the extracellular spaces in the white matter.

A strict and definite separation of these two principal types of cerebral edema is, however, impossible, since perifocal "vasogenic" edema has an almost exclusive intracellular location in the gray matter, whereas TET-edema, a special form of "toxic" edema, occupies the embryonal extracellular space.

The precise mechanism by which swelling and vacuolation of various tissue components develop, producing spongy loosening of the CNS tissue in any of the aforementioned conditions, is unknown. The variable affection of the different compartments very probably depends (a) on the fundamental biochemical mechanism which give rise to these changes and (b) on the local mechanic, ultrastructural and metabolic peculiarities of the affected CNS tissue.

Spongy loosening of the CNS tissue due to increased water content can be reversible or may progressively increase and give rise to secondary lesions up to the point of frank necrosis (ALEU et al., 1966; HIRANO et al., 1964, 1967; SCHRÖDER and WECHSLER, 1965; LONG et al., 1966). This can result from progressive enlargement of swollen cells and subsequent cell membrane rupture with formation of "pseudoextracellular spaces" and progressive extracellular fluid accumulation with separation and simultaneous affection of cellular tissue components. The neuronal perikarya which often do not appear significantly changed in early stages of edema are compressed by large vacuoles or undergo other damage. In advanced stages, increased vascular permeability may give rise to transition of protein-rich fluid which promotes further tissue damage. Comparatively early, the astroglia undergo progressive and regressive changes, and microglial cells also proliferate. Myelin sheaths undergo disintegration due to primary toxic "myelinolysis" or due to secondary damage and are removed by phagocytes. Progressive astroglial fibrillary proliferation is associated with mesodermal and vascular reactions. After intense loss of neural elements, a residual glio-mesenchymal network persists. Vacuolation and spongy loosening of the nervous tissue ultimately may result in the first type of status spongiosus.

In summary, two types of sieve-like transformation of the CNS tissue are to be distinguished. Although of different origin, they are often closely related because the first type can ultimately result from lesions seen in the second type of spongy change.

1. The *"spongy state"* in its original meaning which represents the final stage of severe disintegration of the nervous parenchyma with intense loss of nervous tissue components, especially neurons. The deficiency of glial response is believed to be an important factor in the formation of the vacuolation so commonly termed status spongiosus.

2. *"Spongy alterations"* resulting from swelling and vacuolation of various tissue elements associated with accumulation of excess fluid in corresponding tissue compartments. This type of cavitating transformation appears to be in close relationship to the "cytotoxic" type of brain edema. It is associated with relative preservation of the neural tissue components, at least in the initial stage of the lesion. The identification of cerebral "edema" with "spongy change" of various origin, however, appears conjectural. Although the exact

ultrastructural and pathophysiological backgrounds of either state are not yet fully elucidated, in the future one should attempt to separate the "ordinary" edema from other forms of spongy loosening of the CNS tissue of different origin.

B. Classification of Spongy Dystrophies

The term "spongy degeneration of the neuraxis" primarily refers to disorders which are characterized by "spongy alterations" of various types. As in other conditions, however, this vacuolation can represent only the initial stage of the lesion which, by secondary disintegration and loss of nervous tissue components, may give rise to a real "spongy state". In other instances, simple spongy change without secondary necrosis may represent a permanent kind of lesion.

As the pathogenesis of spongy change of this kind appears closely connected with disorders of cerebral transport mechanisms, the conditions referred to as "spongy degenerations" are consistent with the *"dystrophies of the cerebral transport structures"* as proposed by SEITELBERGER (1965, 1968). According to the suggested basically affected functional compartment or unit, one can distinguish three principal types:

1. *Glial* dystrophies or "spongy dystrophies" *sensu strictiori* in which the primary pathologic defect is believed to affect the *astroglia*. This type is represented by SDI, where astroglial involvement is usually associated with intramyelinic vacuolation. In TET-edema and INH-induced encephalopathy which, from their ultrastructural features, are considered as experimental models of this human condition, similar disorders of the *glio-myelinic* unit are apparent. They probably result from primary affection of the *oligodendroglia* as was demonstrated in experimental cyanide poisoning (HIRNER, 1969).

2. In *glio-neuronal* dystrophies, the astroglial lesion is associated with neuronal changes of a type corresponding to NISSL's acute cell disease or vacuolation of neuronal perikarya and processes. This affection of the glio-neuronal unit (HYDEN, 1962) is present e.g. in Jakob-Creutzfeldt disease which is considered a primary disorder of the neuropil (FRIEDE and DE JONG, 1964; ULE, 1967; ROBINSON, 1969). Ouabain intoxication was believed to be an experimental model but, at the ultrastructural level, the changes differ from those in the human condition. "Progressive infantile poliodystrophy" is thought to be another type of glio-neuronal disorder (JELLINGER, 1970).

3. In *glio-vasal* dystrophies, the primary astroglial disorder is associated with secondarily increased permeability of the BBB which later gives rise to a mesodermal reaction and hypervascularity. Representatives of this type are hepato-cerebral diseases, many toxic-metabolic disorders of various origin including conditions referred to as the "Wernicke tissue syndrome". Hence, subacute necrotizing encephalopathy (LEIGH) appears to belong to this type of disorders (JELLINGER and SEITELBERGER, 1970).

II. Historical Aspects

Spongy Degeneration of the CNS in Infancy (SDI) is a rare neurological disorder. The first reported instance of this disease was described in 1928 by GLOBUS and STRAUSS under the designation of "progressive degenerative subcortical encephalopathy" or Schilder's disease. Their case IV, a 6,5 month old girl who died within 4 days from apathy, seizures and general rigidity, pathologically differs from their other cases by the existence of "status spongiosus" of the subcortical white matter with myelin destruction and diffuse astroglial reaction, the cortex and basal ganglia remaining intact.

CANAVAN (1931) reported the case of a 16,5 month old boy whose illness was marked by progressive enlargement of the head, blindness and optic atrophy, mental retardation, spasticity and signs of increased intracranial pressure. The neuropathological changes were that of macrocephalus with normal-sized ventricles and white matter "resembling mucoid degeneration". A "mass of lacy edema" and lacunae were noted in the subcortical white matter, cerebellum and white matter of the medulla. The changes were thought to represent Schilder's disease. The peculiarity of the spongiform lesions was not specifically recognized. For this reason, the eponym, "Canavan's disease", often used in the Anglo-American literature, does not seem justified. Restudy of the material by E. P. RICHARDSON disclosed severe glial changes which were not originally described.

EISELSBERG (1937) was the first to draw attention to the familial incidence of this condition, although she considered her cases to be examples of Krabbe's type of diffuse sclerosis. Examination of the brain of the first child who at 4 months developed hypertonicity, seizures, generalized rigidity, tonic fits and optic atrophy, and died at 7,5 months, showed spongy degeneration without "globoid cells". An older brother had died of a similar illness.

Two similar cases were published by JERVIS (1942) under the title of Krabbe's disease. In his case II, who was the product of a consanguineous marriage and suffered from apathy, spasticity, tonic fits and decerebrate posture, vacuolation of the CNS was not mentioned, but the photographs suggest such a change at the junction of the cerebral cortex and white matter.

In 1949, VAN BOGAERT and BERTRAND clearly defined SDI as a nosological entity on the basis of certain clinical and pathological features. Their report concerned 3 children of Polish-Jewish stock. Two girls were born to the family "Rot" whose genetic data later elaborated by VAN BOGAERT (1963) indicated the affection of four out of 5 children. Like the third case of the original report, they were products of a consanguineous marriage. The clinical symptoms becoming evident in the first months of life included apathy, limb flaccidity, inability to control the head, and involuntary movements. The course was progressive with failure of mental and motor development, blindness, optic atrophy, and spasticity terminating in decerebrate rigidity. The histological features were diffuse demyelination and sponginess, especially in the subcortical white matter, associated with marked proliferation of the astroglia in gray and white matter, with "bare" nuclei. A degenerative disorder was postulated, probably "abiotrophic" and morphologically characterized by "chronic edema of the gray and white matter" based on an abnormality of metabolism. In a recent review, VAN BOGAERT and BERTRAND (1967) discussed the nosologic position of this disorder.

Thus far 84 cases[2] of this disease entity have been reported in the literature, 56 of which were verified at necropsy, and 9 by cerebral biopsies. Clinically similar but not pathologically examined neurological disorders have been recognized in 18 siblings of confirmed cases. The sufficiently reported instances are listed in Table 1[3].

Two additional biopsy cases examined biochemically were mentioned by CUMINGS (1965), one of which was confirmed at necropsy. Three familial cases, two of them confirmed and one living, were mentioned by DONOHUE (1967), and one autopsy case by COLMANT (1968). Recently ANDERSON (1969) described spongy degeneration of the CNS white matter of unknown etiology in two premature infants without clinical neurological abnormality who died from apnoea on the 6th and 24th day of life respectively. In summary, more than 100 cases of this condition appear to have been observed up to date.

III. Genetic and Geographic Aspects

Sex incidence shows slight prevalence for the male children, the ratio of the affected boys and girls being 41:37. It is often observed in patients of *Jewish* origin, particularly of Polish-Russian stock. Of the 78 acceptable cases at least 37 are of Jewish descent (5—10, 14—21, 25, 26, 29—37, 40, 41, 49—52, 63, 64, 68, 73, 74), whereas 21 patients are not (22—24, 25 A, 26 A, 39, 48, 53—62, 65—67, 72, 75, 76). Among the latter, two were Puerto Rican colored infants (65, 66). In the rest, the racial origin is not stated.

Familial occurrence is stated in at least 60% of all reported cases. 22 pairs of siblings either of the same sex — 8 boys and 5 girls — or of different sex (9 sibs) and one girl twin (27, 28) are mentioned. In family "Rot" (8, 9, 29, 30), 4 out of 5 children succumbed to the disease, 3 of which were girls and one a boy. In family "H" (19—21), 3 sons of one generation were affected, whereas 3 daughters remained free of it. In some families, 2 out of three (33—34, 36—37, 5—6, 49—50) or 2 out of 4 children (25 A—26 A, 46—47) were afflicted in one generation; in another, 3 out of 5 daughters were affected (22—24). In some families, both of the two children suffered from SDI (3—4, 17—18, 40—41, 31—32, 57—58), whereas in others only one of two siblings succumbed to the disease (1, 13, 39, 48, 55, 60). Thus the number of the children attacked per family is usually high. In one exceptional family only one out of 6 children, including a healthy fraternal twin, was afflicted (62). In addition, some apparently sporadic cases were reported both in Jewish (7, 10, 51, 52, 64) and Aryan families (24 A, 39, 48, 55, 59—62, 72). In some families, affected

---
2 Including 7 personal observations presented in this paper.
3 In the following we shall refer to these cases by the numbers indicated in Table 1.

Table 1. *Pathologically confirmed cases of Spongy Degeneration in Infancy. Normal brain by other authors).*

Nr.	Author	Case		Sex	Age onset	Age death (Last Exam.)
1	Globus-Strauss (1928)		IV.	F	6.50 mo	6.50 mo
2+	Canavan (1931)			M	2.50 mo	16.50 mo
3	Eiselsberg (1937)	S.K.	1	M	4.00 mo	7.50 mo
4	Eiselsberg (1937)	S.L.	2	M	2.00 mo	5.50 mo
5	Jervis (1942)	fam. C.: A.C.	1	M	4.00 mo	17.00 mo
6	Jervis (1942)		2	F	5.00 mo	24.00 mo
7	Jervis (1942)	H.S.	3	M	4.00 mo	34.00 mo
8	Bogaert-Bertrand (1949)	P. Rot	1	M	3.00 mo	8.50 mo
9	Bogaert-Bertrand (1949)	M. Rot	2	F	4.00 mo	56.00 mo
10	Bogaert-Bertrand (1949)	J. Me	3	F	6.00 mo	34.00 mo
11	Meyer (1950)			F	6.00 mo	9.00 mo
12	Meyer (1950)			F	?	24.00 mo
13	Blackwood-Cumings (1954)	C. M.	1	M	2.00 mo	23.00 mo
14	Jervis (1954)		1	M	4.00 mo	16.00 mo
15	Jervis (1954)		2	F	4.00 mo	14.00 mo
16	Wolman (1958)			M	birth	16.75 mo
17	de Vries et al. (1958)	THi.	1	F	birth	24.00 mo
18	de Vries et al. (1958)	THi	2	M	3.00 mo	12.00 mo
19	de Vries et al. (1958)	H. Ja	3	M	4.00 mo	14.00 mo
20	de Vries et al. (1958)	H. Ar	4	M	6.00 mo	26.00 mo
21	de Vries et al. (1958)	H. Is	5	M	5.00 mo	12.00 mo
22	zu Rhein et al. (1960)	fam. S.S.	1	F	2.00 mo	99.00 mo
23	zu Rhein et al. (1960)		2	F	birth	7.00 mo
24	zu Rhein et al. (1960)		3	F	2.00 mo	21.00 mo
24A	Nakai et al. (1960)	K. B.		M	101.00 mo	114.00 mo
25A	Seitelberger (1961)	C. McF	1	F	12.00 mo	70.00 mo
26A	Seitelberger (1961)	L. McF	2	M	28.00 mo	34.00 mo
25	Tariska (1961)		1	M	?	42.00 mo
26	Tariska (1961)		2	M	?	24.00 mo
27	Verhaart (1962)		1	F	?	22.00 mo
28	Verhaart (1962)		2	F	?	?
29	van Bogaert (1963)	A. Rot	3	F	10.00 mo	42.00 mo
30	van Bogaert (1963)	H. Rot	4	F	2.00 mo	37.00 mo
31	Banker et al. (1964)	fam. A	1	M	5.00 mo	105.00 mo
32	Banker et al. (1964)		2	F	2(?) mo	39.00 mo
33	Banker et al. (1964)	fam. B: H.S.	3	F	5.00	114.00 mo
34	Banker et al. (1964)	fam. B.: R.S.	4	M	6.00 mo	40.00 mo
(2)+	Banker et al. (1964)	fam. C	5			
35	Banker et al. (1964)		6	M	5.00 mo	13.00 mo
36	Banker et al. (1964)	fam. D	7	M	0.50 mo	9.00 mo
37++	Banker et al. (1964)	I. G.	8	M	1.25 mo	17.00 mo
38	Jervis (1964, unpubl.)			F	3.00 mo	36.00 mo
39	Hogan-Richardson (1965)	E.R.	1	F	2.00 mo	38.50 mo

yrs = years; mo = months; ds = days, hr = hours.

weights according to ARONSON et al.: Arch. Neurol. Psychiat. 79, 151, 1958 (data given
A = atypical cases.

Duration illness	Jewish descent	Affected siblings	Normal siblings	Consang. parents	Histologic. exam.	Brain weight g	Normal brain weight g
4.00 ds	?	—	1	?	+	?	
14.50 mo	?	?	?	?	+	1,890	1,020
3.50 mo	?	sibs	—	?	+	?	
3.50 mo	?	sibs	—	?	+	?	
13.00 mo	+	sibs	1	—	+	1,350	1,042
alive	+	sibs	1	—	—	—	
31.00 mo	+	—	—	+	+	960	1,140
5.50 mo	+	sibs	1	+	+	820	489 (714)
51.00 mo	+	sibs	1	+	—	—	
28.00 mo	+	—	—	1st.cous.	+	?	
3.00 mo	?	—	—	?	+	?	
?	?	—	—	?	+	?	
21.00 mo	?	—	1 M	?	+	1,595	1,062 (1,059)
12.00 mo	+	sibs	1	?	—	—	
10.00 mo	+	sibs	1	?	+	1,210	750
16.75 mo	+	—	1 M	?	+	1,350	1,026
24.00 mo	+	sibs	—	—	—	—	
9.00 mo	+	sibs	—	—	+	1,720	925
10.00 mo	+	sibs	3 F	—	+	?	
20.00 mo	+	sibs	3 F	—	+	?	
7.00 mo	+	sibs	3 F	—	+	1,085	925 (965)
92.00 mo	—	sibs	2 F	—	+	biopsy	
7.00 mo	—	sibs	2 F	—	—	—	
19.00 mo	—	sibs	2 F	—	—	—	
13.00 mo	—	—	—	—	+	1,250	1,280
58.00 mo	—	sibs	1 M, 1 F	—	+	—	
4.00 mo	—	sibs	1 M, 1 F	—	+	—	
?	+	sibs	—	?	+	1,380	1,141
?	+	sibs	—	?	—	—	
?	?	twins	—	?	+	?	
alive	?	twins	—	?	—	—	
32.00 mo	+	sibs of Nr. 8, 9	1 M	+	—	—	
35.00 mo	+	sibs of Nr. 8, 9	1 M	+	+	?	
100.00 mo	+	sibs	—	—	+	1,340	1,275
37.00 mo	+	sibs	—	—	—	—	
alive	+	sibs	1	—	+	biopsy	
36.00 mo	+	sibs	1	—	+	1,480	1,145
8.00 mo	+	sibs	1	—	—	—	
8.50 mo	+	sibs	3 F	?	—	—	
17.75 mo	+	sibs	3 F	?	+	1,540	1,026
33.00 mo	?	?	?	?	+	?	
36.50 mo	—	—	1	?	+	850	1,141

Table 1

Nr.	Author	Case	Sex	Age onset	Age death (Last Exam.)
(37)++	Hogan-Richardson (1965)	I. G.	2		
(33)	Hogan-Richardson (1965)	R.S.	3		
(34)	Hogan-Richardson (1965)	H.S.	4		
40	Buchanan-Davis (1965)	1	M	3.00 mo	16.00 mo
41	Buchanan-Davis (1965)	2	M	5.50 mo	?
42	Buchanan-Davis (1965)	3	F	3.00 mo	30.00 mo
43	Buchanan-Davis (1965)	4	M	4.00 mo	84.00 mo
44	Sacks et al. (1965)	1	M	2.00 ds	80.00 hr
45	Sacks et al. (1965)	2	M	birth	19.00 hr
46	Gaburro et al. (1965)	Mi. N. 1	F	birth	3.00 ds
47	Gaburro et al. (1965)	2	F	birth	8.00 ds
48	Henn et al. (1965)		F	birth	5.00 mo
49	Adachi-Aronson (1966)	RIS 1	F	3.00 mo	26.00 mo
50	Aronson-Aronson (1967)		F	?	15.00 mo
51	Aronson-Aronson (1967)	2	F	birth	57.00 mo
52	Adachi et al. (1966)		M	4.00 mo	12.00 mo
53	Kolkmann-Völzke (1966)	W.S. 1	M	2.50 mo	6.50 mo
54	Kolkmann-Völzke (1966)	K.S. 2	M	2.00 mo	7.00 mo
55	Kolkmann-Völzke (1966)	I. H. 3	F	birth	2.50 mo
56	Nelson-Aurebeck (1966)		?		6.50 mo
57	Jellinger-Seitelberger (1967)	A. Hö. 1	F	birth	3.00 mo
58	Jellinger-Seitelberger (1967)	J. Hö. 2	M	?	10.00 mo
59	Jellinger-Seitelberger (1967)	J. Sch. 3	M	<24.00 mo	56.00 mo
60	Jellinger-Seitelberger (1967/69)	B. K. 4	M	60.00 mo	20.50 yrs
61	Jellinger-Seitelberger (1967/69)	Sch. A. 5	F	60.00 mo	17.00 yrs
62	Kamoshita et al. (1967)	HPJ	M	3.00 mo	48.00 mo
63	Kamoshita et al. (1968)	2	F	<6.00 mo	48.00 mo
64	Kamoshita et al. (1968)	1	F	5.00 mo	20.00 mo
65	Feigin et al. (1968)	4	M	10.50 mo	13.00 mo
66	Feigin et al. (1968)	5	F	birth	14.00 mo
67	Feigin et al. (1968)	6	M	2.50 mo	5.50 mo
68	Gambetti et al. (1969)	1	M	1.00 mo	6.00 yrs
69	Gambetti et al. (1969)	2	M	?	13.00 mo
70	Ule (1968)	1	M	1.25 mo	5.00 mo
71	Ule (1968)	2	M	3.00 mo	8.00 mo
72	Brucher et al. (1968)	M.S.	F	72.00 mo	12.00 yrs
73	Adachi-Volk (1968)	1	M	4.00 mo	11.15 yrs
74	Adachi-Volk (1968)	2	F	?	2.00 yrs
75	Morcaldi et al. (1969)	S.D.C. 1	F	0.75 mo	10.00 mo
76	Morcaldi et al. (1969)	M.M.D.C. 2	F	birth (?)	18.00 mo

yrs = years; mo = months; ds = days; hr = hours.

Spongy Degeneration of the Central Nervous System in Infancy

(continued)

Duration illness	Jewish descent	Affected siblings	Normal siblings	Consang. parents	Histologic. exam.	Brain weight g	Normal brain weight g
13.00 mo	+	sibs	—	—	+	?	
?	+	sibs	—	—	+	950	?
27.00 mo	?	1	1	—	+	1,400	1,064
80.00 mo	?	?	?	—	+	1,250	1,263
32.00 hr	?	sibs	—	?	+	450	335
19.00 hr	?	sibs	—	?	+	445	335
3.00 ds	?	sibs	1 M, F	—	+	?	
8.00 ds	?	sibs	1 M, F	—	—	—	
5.00 mo	—	—	1	1st.cous.	+	?	
23.00 mo	+	sibs	1 M	—	+	1,080	1,064
?	+	sibs	1 M	—	—	—	
57.00 mo	+	—	—	—	+	1,500	1,237
alive	+	—	—	—	+	biopsy	
4.00 mo	—	sibs	—	—	+	685	
3.00 mo	—	sibs	—	—	+	840	
2.50 mo	—	—	1 M	—	+	610	
alive	?	?	?	?	+	biopsy	
3.00 mo	—	sibs	—	—	+	680	
?	—	sibs	—	—	—	—	
32.00 mo	—	—	—	—	+	?	
15.50 yrs	—	—	1	—	+	?	
12.00 yrs	—	—	—	—	+	?	
45.00 mo	—	—	4F, 1 M	—	+	875	1,191
43.00 mo	+	1 F	2	—	+	?	
15.00 mo	+	—	2F	—	+	1,300	
2.50 mo	—	?	?	—	+	1,040	944
14.00 mo	—	?	2	—	+	840	944
3.00 mo	—	?	?	—	+	610	656
alive	+	sibs	?	—	+	biopsy	
alive	+	sibs	?	—	—	—	
alive	?	?	?	?	+	biopsy	
alive	?	+	?	?	+	biopsy	
18.00 yrs	—	—	—	?	+	?	
10.65 yrs	+	sibs	—	+	+	1,420	1,320
?	+	sibs	—	+	—	—	
9.25 mo	—	sibs	1 F	—	—	—	
18.00 mo	—	sibs	1 F	—	+	biopsy	

cases appeared in more than one generation (BANKER et al., 1964): in the pedigree of family "B" (33—34) a first cousin of the patient's father very likely succumbed with SDI and in 2 paternal uncles the diagnosis was highly suspect, whereas 2 other members suffered from amaurotic idiocy. In the pedigree of family "C" (2, 35), the sons of 2 paternal uncles were suspected to have died from the same illness, while in family "D" (36, 37) a first cousin of the patient's mother and a firstborn sister of their father probably died from SDI.

The hitherto reported genetic features appear to indicate an *autosomal recessive* mode of inheritance with a variable penetration tendency. However, the large number of sibling cases would seem an unusually high incidence for a disease based on a recessive form of inheritance (BUCHANAN and DAVIS, 1965). *Sex-linkage* was seen in five families (19—21, 22—24, 2—35, 36—37, 75—76).

Consanguinity was known to be a feature in both Jewish (7, 10, 73—74) and non-Jewish families (48). The study of the family "Rot" even showed double consanguinity (VAN BOGAERT, 1963). Intermarriage of the grandparents was described (73—74).

The *geographical factors* are of interest since the progenitors of many affected Jewish families came from Eastern Europe, particularly from Poland and the Western Ukraine: Family "Rot" and part of family "S" (49—50) originated from Warsaw. Other families were of Polish (10, 16, 64) or Russian descent (14—15). The 4 families reported by BANKER et al. (1964), the paternal ancesters of a protracted case (73) and of another patient (63) derived from two restricted regions in Eastern Europe, the one being Vilna-Kovno (presently Lithuania) and adjacent Byalistock (Eastern Poland) and the other Volhynia (Western Ukraine). Although these regions are separated by the Pinsk marshes, the Jews of these counties form a single ethnical group, since they migrated in the second quarter of the 18th century from the Vilna-Kovno region via Byalistock to the Western Ukraine (BANKER et al., 1964). In addition to SDI, it appears that the Jewish strains of these regions are rich in Tay-Sachs disease (ARONSON and VOLK, 1962), Niemann-Pick and Gaucher's disease (KNUDSON and KAPLAN, 1962).

SDI also has been reported in Jewish-Maltese families partly of Arabian blood (19—21) and in families of part Jewish and part Aryan origin (17—18), while in other families there is no evidence of Jewish ancestry: for example it occurs also in German (22—24, 48, 53—54, 71), Tyrolian (57—58), Irish-American (25 A, 26 A, 39, 62), Italian (46—47, 75—76) and in Puerto Rican families (65, 66).

With regard to general condition, BANKER et al. (1964) pointed out that none of the children with SDI had black hair or a pigmented skin, although these were dominant characteristics in the unaffected members of all 4 families reported. Six afflicted children had blond hair, 4 had red hair, and all had a fair complexion. Blue eyes were more common than brown. Conversely, two children in family "B" whose disease proved to be amaurotic idiocy, had black hair. Other cases of SDI were also blond (9,39), whereas another had dark hair (48).

IV. Clinical Aspects

A. Pre- and Paranatal Histories

The maternal histories, in terms of pregnancy and delivery, were normal except for nephropathy with albuminuria (11), prolonged labor with toxemia gravidarum (3—4), premature birth (22, 76), Caesarian section (31) and respiratory distress at birth (34). Often, however, there was no record of the pregnancy and birth available. Undescended testicles were noted (2, 31). The neonatal period usually was free of abnormalities except for two instances with obvious neurologic defects at birth, quadriplegia with tremor (16) and spasticity of the lower limbs (23). In one infant, a fit was reported on the second postnatal day (9).

B. Clinical Course

The *date of onset* of the illness is often difficult to establish with precision. In several cases, the disease was said to be apparent at birth (16, 17, 23, 45—48, 51, 55, 57, 66) or within the very first weeks of life (36, 44, 75, 76), but usually the first symptoms were recognized in the second or third month of life (23 cases) or between the age of 3 to 6 months (21 cases). Rarely the symptoms have first appeared in the second half of the first year (1, 29, 65), in the second year (59) or later (26 A). In 3 patients the initial manifestations became evident at the age of 5 years (60, 61) or even later (72). Occasionally, the age of onset is not stated.

With regard to the onset of symptoms, a "congenital", an infantile and a rare late infantile form of the disease can be distinguished.

Although the *age at death* ranged between 19 hours and 20,5 years, the majority of the patients died in infancy. Of 66 fatal cases, only 23 survived beyond the second year, whereas 21 children died in the first year and a further 22 in the second year of life. This group can be referred to as the *infantile* form. Of the remaining patients, 18 died at age 2—5 years and 3 others between 5 and 10 years of age, thus representing the *late infantile* group. It further includes 5 patients who were still alive between 5 and 49 months of age (6, 50, 56, 69, 70), while two others were still alive at age 6 and $9^1/_2$ years respectively (33, 68). Only 4 patients survived beyond the age of 10. One was a protracted infantile case with early onset dying at age 11 (73); the others were *juvenile* cases in which death supervened at the age of 17 to 20,5 years (60, 61, 72).

The *duration of the illness* ranged from 19 hours to 15,5 years, but two-thirds of the reported cases died within 2 years. In some patients death occurred within several days or weeks (1, 44—47), 12 infants died after 2—6 months and 15 children after one to two years' illness. 24 patients had a longer survival, but only 7 of them showed a protracted course of more than 5 years. Five of them showed early infantile onset (31, 33, 43, 68, 73), and three belonged to the juvenile group (60, 61, 72).

With regard to the onset of symptoms, SDI usually is a disease of early infancy and childhood with rapidly progressive and fatal course. Only a few patients had a prolonged course and even survived to late adolescence. Thus, an *infantile* and a *juvenile* form of the disease might be distinguished, the latter presenting a different clinical course. Whereas the majority of the infantile cases were of Jewish extraction of Ashkenazic background and often showed familial incidence of the disorder, the rare juvenile patients with SDI appeared to be sporadic cases and were of non-Jewish stock. As the infantile form of SDI, however, is not confined to Jewish families, there is no evidence, as yet, to speculate on a possible genetic basis for these age varieties.

C. Clinical Symptomatology

The *initial symptoms* becoming evident in the early postnatal period usually consist of a lack in psychomotor maturation (25—27, 50, 59) with poor head control (2, 38, 49, 72), listlessness and apathy (5, 7, 32, 50, 51) and feeding difficulties (23, 55, 66, 75, 76).

Progressive limb *flaccidity* and generalized muscle *atonia* (16, 18, 30, 46, 47) with inability to support the head (8, 10, 21, 22, 35, 45) and retarded psychomotor development (14, 20, 67, 76) have been noted as prominent early signs of the disease. Some children certainly had normal muscle tone in the first months of life (21, 30, 33). In others increased muscle tone has been recognized at the onset of the illness. Rigidity with lack of development (15) or spastic quadriplegia present from birth (2, 16) or in the early postnatal period (37) and a decerebrate posture with opisthotonus were noted immediately after delivery (23).

An *increase in the size of the head* was evident very early in the course of the disease (11, 22, 31, 36, 43, 62, 63, 73), representing the first symptom or being associated with psychomotor retardation and poor head control (22, 34).

Occasionally, *convulsions* or tonic and clonic *spasms* and jerky movements heralded the onset of the illness (3, 9, 13, 26A, 29, 40, 53, 54, 56, 57, 67, 75, 76). Seizures were accompanied by apathy (1, 4), retarded development (40), rigidity (1, 3, 36, 37), spasticity with floppy head (17, 39, 44) or generalized hypotonia (75, 76) and sucking difficulties (33).

Among the rare symptoms indicating the onset of the disorder are suspected blindness (24, 64, 68), tremor (41) and hemiparesis (65).

In summary, reduced motor activity and impairment of muscle tone with atonia rather than hypertonia as well as arrest of normal psychomotor development or loss of acquired developmental attributes are frequently recognized early manifestation of this disorder except in rare cases in which it apparently begins with seizures.

The initial flaccid state is almost invariably followed by increased muscle tone including *spasticity* (5, 8, 11, 16, 22, 23, 31, 36—39, 48—53, 55, 59, 65, 68, 73) and/or generalized *rigidity* (3, 4, 6, 7, 13, 15, 22, 29, 55, 66), although the time of occurrence varies considerably. The spastic changes usually occur within a few months of the onset of the disease but occasionally spasticity is not recognized until comparatively late stages (10, 13, 31, 34, 35). Increased tendon reflexes (2, 5, 13, 15, 18, 22, 25, 36—40, 42, 48, 49, 53, 62, 64, 66, 72), clonus and Babinski signs (5, 7, 13, 25, 33, 40, 49, 62, 65, 72) are common. Although some patients remain flaccid until their death (17, 25A, 29, 76), the majority of the cases ultimately show generalized spasticity and/or rigidity usually leading to a decerebrate (or decorticate) state with tonic tendon reflexes (3—5, 10, 16, 18, 32, 34, 37, 40, 57, 58, 64, 72) and cervical and labyrinthine tonic reflex movements (10). Tonic extensor spasms usually precipitated by some external stimulus, e.g. noise or manipulation of the limbs, are often superimposed on the initial atonia (3, 5, 7, 9, 10, 13, 19—21, 36, 75). Opisthotonus may occur in these attacks (3—7, 10, 15, 18, 30, 33, 43, 73). Tonic attacks or "cerebellar" fits with periodic exaggeration of decerebrate posture also occur in the later stages of the disease (10, 21, 22, 25, 33, 36). In some cases, there is hyperacusis without reflexes of decerebration (17, 63).

Seizures of some type occurred in almost half of the patients. Although focal and generalized convulsions are not uncommon, their recognition may be difficult because the seizure activity may be obscured by involuntary movements or irregular myoclonic twitches that occur in the interseizure periods (35, 40). In two sibs (25 A, 26 A) myoclonic seizures were prominent. In the state of permanent rigidity small involuntary movements involving all limbs (18, 21), rhythmical buccal, lingual and facial automatisms (9), trembling of the limbs (11, 16, 29, 39, 55), choreiform (29, 30) and athetoid movements (34) may be superimposed.

Enlargement of the head is frequent with megalencephaly being described in almost half of the patients. In some cases, however, it was definitely absent (25 A, 26 A, 57, 58). Increase in the cranial circumference is occasionally recognized as an initial symptom (11, 22, 31, 36, 43, 62, 63), but it usually becomes conspicuous after the onset of other neurological signs. Often it is already marked between the fourth and sixth month of life (31, 34, 36, 73). In most cases, however, head circumference shows a slowly progressive increase with age and the course of the disease. There was a maximum increase of 5,25 cm in one month (2) and of 11 cm in 4 months in a patient who reached a head circumference of 58,8 cm at the age of 11 months (37), while the most marked case attained 60 cm at the age of 8 years (31).

Internal strabismus (2, 9, 31, 34, 35, 38, 42, 48), nystagmus (2, 3, 5—8, 10, 11, 21, 33, 38, 42, 52, 76), roving or rolling eye movements (18, 21) and episodic rapid ocular oscillations (52, 62) are rather common. They were first noted between the age 5 months (39) and 33 months (15). Bilateral ptosis is rare (13, 15, 60, 61).

Visual impairment was noted in almost half of the cases and may be either early (8, 11, 18, 19, 21—24, 33, 40, 48, 64, 68, 73) or late in the course of the disease (9, 20, 25, 25 A, 35, 36, 60, 61, 67). Pupillary light reflex may be present, though often sluggish, or may be absent (13). *Optic atrophy* was noted in at least 32 patients, sometimes appearing early at age 2 to 9 month (8, 9, 13, 17, 20—23, 29, 33, 36, 48, 52, 72) or rather late (2, 5, 7, 10, 25, 25 A, 26 A, 32, 35, 60, 61, 63, 68, 76). Occasionally, pallor of the optic discs was absent (14, 15, 32, 42, 53, 54, 62, 67, 75). Rarely there was a suggestion of tapetoretinal degeneration or chorioretinal atrophy (17, 25 A, 39, 40, 60). Cherry-red spots and pigmentary degeneration were not present in any of the reported cases.

Deafness may have been present in some cases (11, 25, 40, 67) but its diagnosis is quite difficult in sick infants in this age group.

Ultimately most children are completely apathetic and unresponsive. Usually they develop pseudobulbar palsy and decerebrate or decorticate states with or without tonic attacks and convulsions of other types. Occasionally, autonomic dysfunction appears in the terminal state characterized by episodes of profuse sweating, pallor, vomiting with a tendency to collapse, excessive vasomotor reaction and dermographia or an upset of thermostasis with hyperthermia or hypothermia (17, 18, 33, 38, 39). Death may supervene in hyperthermia, collapse or coma, but most children succumb to intercurrent disorders, bronchopneumonia, inanition or respiratory failure.

D. Personal Observations

Among 7 cases — 6 confirmed at autopsy, 3 infantile and 2 late infantile cases showed typical clinical features, whereas 2 juvenile cases exhibited some deviations of the otherwise uniform course.

1. Infantile Cases

In two siblings of a Tyrolian family of pure Aryan stock, originating from healthy, non-consanguineous parents, seizures were the first signs of illness reported. The girl (57) appeared normal at birth and had generalized convulsions at the age of 2 months. Motor development was retarded without enlargement of the head. At 3 months of age, she died in a decerebrate state. The history of her elder brother (58) who died at 10 months of age, was virtually the same but no necropsy was performed. In a further sporadic non-Jewish case with non-contributory family history (59), the exact date of onset of clinical symptoms is unknown. At 2 years, mental development was retarded. This boy had lack of head control, spastic quadriplegia and frequent seizures. He died at 56 months of age.

2. Late Infantile Cases

Two out of 4 children in a non-Jewish American family were mentioned by SEITELBERGER (1961). The elder sib, a girl (25A), appeared mentally retarded and showed clumsy gait at the end of the first year. Stiffness and coordination disorders developed, and at age 4, myoclonic twitches started, later associated with clonic seizures and status epilepticus. At age 6, there were flaccid quadriparesis with absence of all deep tendon reflexes, muscle atrophies, roving eye movements and frequent myoclonic jerks. Death supervened in coma at the age of 70 months. Her brother's (26A) symptoms began at 28 months of age with an initial general convulsion, mental retardation, slurred speech, progressive stiffness of the limbs and frequent myoclonic movements. Trephination for suspected subdural hematoma was negative. There was pallor of the optic discs and retinal degeneration. Myoclonic seizures increased, and he died at the age of 34 months.

3. Juvenile Cases

Cases of later onset and survival up to late adolescence are very rare. BRUCHER et al. (1968) reported the case of an 18 year-old girl (72) whose brain showed a protracted form of SDI combined with pallidonigral neuro-axonal dystrophy. Two apparently sporadic cases with late infantile onset and protracted course in different non-Jewish families have been reported by JELLINGER and SEITELBERGER (1969):

A boy (60) was the second child of healthy, non-consanguineous parents; one sister was healthy. Pregnancy, delivery and early infantile development were unremarkable. The initial symptoms became evident at the age of 5 years and consisted of ataxic gait, tremor of the hands, vacant look and mental retardation. At age 12, bilateral ptosis, loss of vision and dysarthria became manifest. Bilateral optic atrophy and retinal pigmentation were noted. At age 15, a spastic-ataxic syndrome with slurring bulbar language and intense tremor was prominent. After progressive deterioration with blindness and deafness, the ultimately unresponsive patient died at the age of $20^1/_2$ years. A girl (61) had healthy parents and an unremarkable family history. Her symptoms started at about 5 years of age and included progressive mental deterioration, tremor and ataxia, followed by loss of vision, optic atrophy and terminal spasticity of all limbs. She died after 12 years of illness. In both cases neither megalencephaly nor convulsions were reported.

V. Clinical Laboratory Findings

Cerebrospinal fluid has usually been reported normal (7, 9, 13, 18, 21, 22, 26A, 53, 55, 60—62, 65, 67, 75) except for an elevation in pressure ranging from 120 to 350 mm H_2O (1—3, 35, 37, 39). Moderately elevated albumin content has been noted (3, 25A, 33, 36, 71) and was as high as 168 and 249 mg-% (44, 45). Enzyme determinations were normal (49).

Skull radiographs show a symmetrically enlarged and thin calvarium.

Pneumoencephalography is normal or shows slight and, later, marked ventricular dilatation (3, 9, 21, 22, 29, 35, 49, 53, 54, 62, 63, 67, 72, 73, 75).

Electroencephalography is normal (13, 17, 40, 42, 63) or discloses various abnormalities, such as fast activity (25 c/s) or low and moderate voltage with bursts of 3—4 c/s high voltage slow waves in the occipital leads (33). It may be diffusely abnormal (34, 53, 61, 62, 67, 71, 75, 76) or shows some spike activity (25A, 26, 54), diffuse high voltage rhythmic activity of 4—7 c/s without focal lesions (49, 73) or numerous waves of 1—2 c/s of high amplitude in the temporal area (24). There may be marked asymmetry in activities between the two hemispheres (39). Continuous phasic groups of motor-unit potential synchronous with myoclonies were seen (25A, 26A).

Electroretinogram has shown lowered photoptic components with normal scotopic reaction indicating a retinal disorder (25 A).

Increased vestibular *chronaxies* and neuromuscular chronaxies in the upper and lower limbs were present in one case (10), and prolonged conduction velocity of the peripheral nerves in another (63), but no conduction defect was noted in a third (64).

Electromyogram was normal or disclosed fibrillations (63, 64).

Blood counts, *urinary analysis* and the usual blood chemical examinations failed to disclose any distinctive abnormalities except for an elevation in the urine levels of copper and zinc in one infant (22). Random examination of urine for phenylpyruvic acid, other abnormal amino acids (DONOHUE, 1967), and metachromatic bodies were negative, as were chromatographs for abnormal amino acids.

Analysis of *serum enzymes* showed no significant changes (46, 49, 73) except for slight increase of malic dehydrogenase. Enzyme analysis of skeletal muscle disclosed marked increase of acetylcholine activity and slight reduction of aldolase, phosphatase and malic dehydrogenase activities (46).

VI. Pathological Aspects
A. General Necropsy

Postmortem examination is often unremarkable except for occasional fatty degeneration of the liver (8, 11, 13, 17, 21, 44, 45, 54) and intercurrent disorders, e.g. bronchopneumonia (2, 21, 49, 53, 64, 66, 73), otitis media (2, 3), enteritis, myocarditis, hepatitis and lymphadenitis (53) or ductus Botalli persistens (55). Cachexia was rarely reported (4, 31).

B. Brain Autopsy

Enlargement of the brain in weight and volume has been one of the most constantly noted features in this disorder, especially in the younger children.

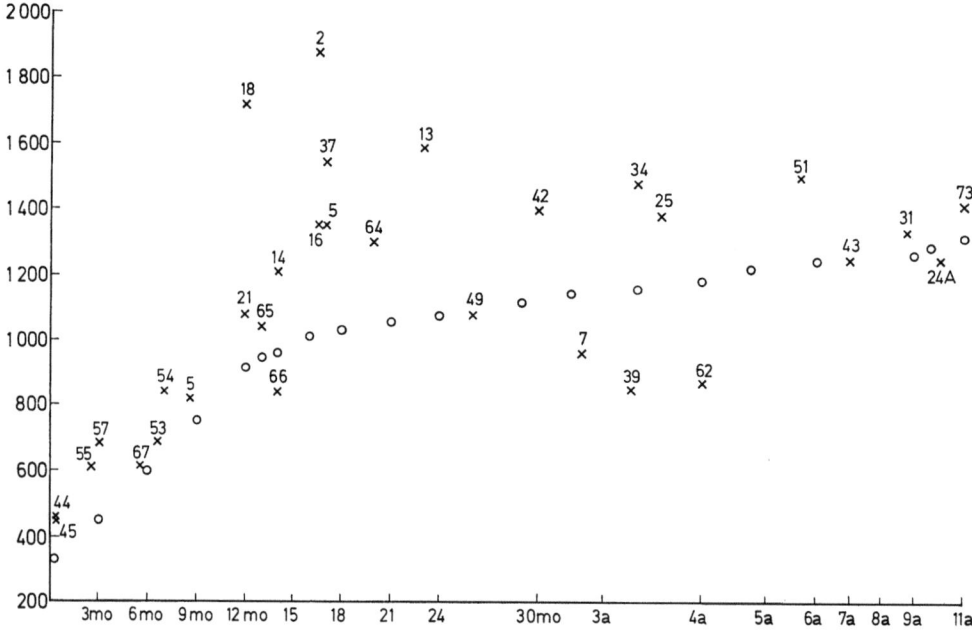

Fig. 1. Brain weights of Spongy Degeneration of C.N.S. in Infancy compared with normal brain weight. Numbers refer to cases in Table 1. × Spongy degeneration of CNS; ○ normal brain

In the cases available for analysis there are 31 published reports which list both brain weight and age at death. A graph showing the relationship of age at death and brain weight in SDI compared with the average brain weight indicates that in many instances the brain was considerably heavier than normal (Fig. 1). This is particularly true for those patients who died in the second year of life, whereas this difference is less conspicuous in the first year.

In some older children brain weight was considerably above normal (25, 31, 34, 42, 51, 73); in others it was much below average, thus indicating brain atrophy which was confirmed at necropsy (7, 39, 62).

ADACHI et al. (1966, 1968) emphasized that the increasing megalencephaly and the weight of the brain in this disease do not parallel the progress of the cerebral disorder. In those lethal cases which terminate within the first two years of life, the ratio of brain weight to normal ranges from 1,87 to 1,12 and averages 1,38 (cf. ADACHI and ARONSON, 1966). In two neonatal cases (44, 45), the ratios of brain weight were 1,32 and 1,34 respectively. In children older than 2 years at death, the ratio of brain weight to normal shows minor differences and approaches unity. The values

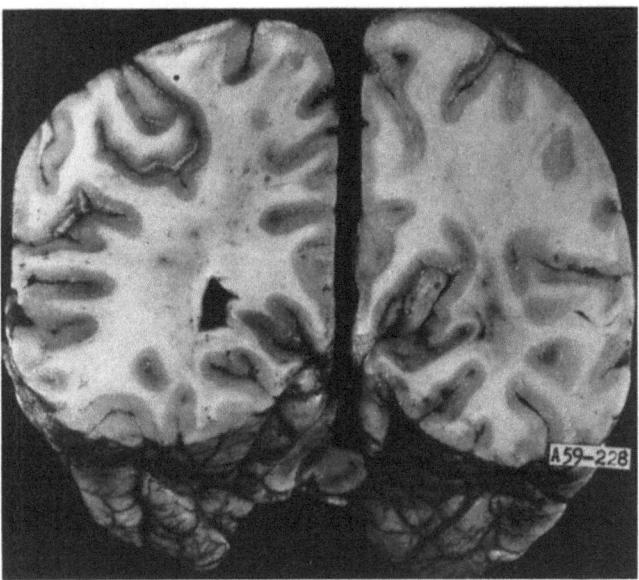

Fig. 2. Coronal section of occipito-parietal hemispheres showing flattening of convolutions and marked uncal herniation. (NA 6-59; case 25A)

ranged from 0,83 to 1,31 and the average was 1,04. The brain weight ratios are comparable to those based on age at death if they are calculated on the basis of the duration of illness being either less than or greater than 24 months. In cases where the age at death is over 3 years or the duration of illness is greater than 36 months, the ratios of the brain weight were between 0,87 and 1,29 with an average of 1,00. Thus, after 2 years of illness, the weight of the brain declines and approaches the average weight or is even below normal. It was considered that this phenomenon might be related to progressive degeneration and loss of cerebral white matter.

Grossly, the brain may be normal (65, 66). Often the cerebral hemispheres are diffusely enlarged (4, 18, 39, 47, 51) and soft (4, 8, 27, 25A, 39, 47) with flattening of the gyri (Fig. 2), but in cases of long duration moderate to marked brain atrophy is noted (39, 59, 60, 62, 73). Localized frontal atrophy is rare (3). The leptomeninges show no gross changes. The ventricles are either normal (16, 18, 48, 60, 67) or smaller than normal (2, 4, 25A), while in other instances slight to moderate (3, 21, 26A, 39, 43, 49, 51, 10) or even marked enlargement (31, 60, 61, 72) is noted. The ventricular enlargement may be greater in the parieto-occipital regions (39, 49, 51). In one case severe hydrocephalus was related to a deformity of the occipital bone and complicating meningitis (31). The enlarged white matter of the cerebral hemispheres is often soft and presents a mucoid (2, 49) or gray gelatinous appearance (11, 15, 31, 39, 40, 65) or is of grayish tan (31) or pinkish, translucent color (39). In the prolonged type including the juvenile cases, however, it shows increased consistency and large areas of patchy discoloration (Fig. 3A) or gray opacity (72). Occasionally,

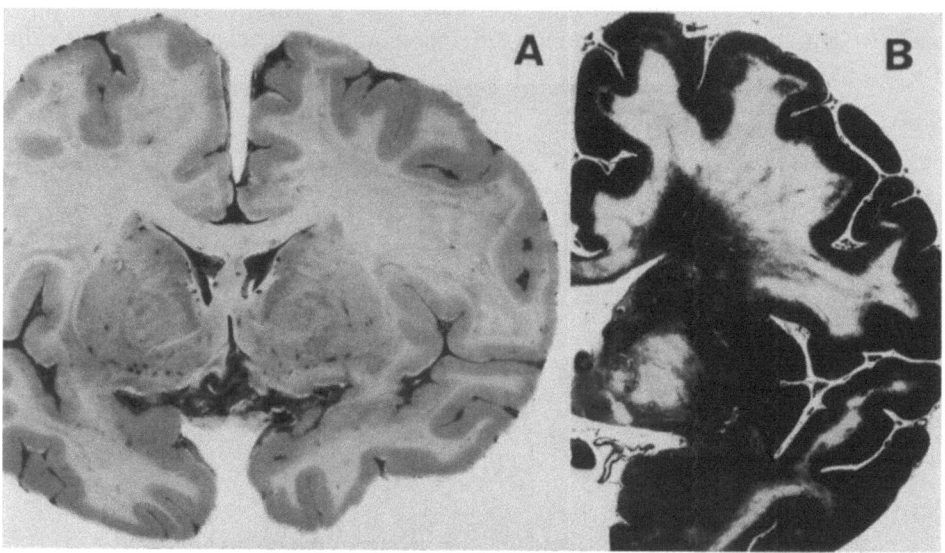

Fig. 3A and B. Juvenile form of SDI (NI 86-63 — case 60). A Coronal section of brain, illustrating diffuse and gray patchy gray discoloration of the convolutional white matter and increased volume of globus pallidus. B Coronal section of brain, demonstrating diffuse demyelination of the white matter and corpus callosum with sparing of the most central portions of the centrum ovale. Severe spongy lesion of globus pallidus. Heidenhain's myelin stain

numerous small cystic cavities are obvious to the naked eye at the junction of the cortex and white matter (31, 48) or in the deep centrum ovale (25). The cerebellum may show increased consistency of the translucent or grayish white matter (38, 48, 60, 61) and atrophic folia (13, 26A, 31, 49, 60, 61). The spinal cord is grossly normal or shows a gray appearance of the dorsal and lateral tracts (31, 60).

C. Histological Findings

1. Quality of the CNS Lesions

The microscopic findings are remarkably stereotyped in most of the reported cases although of variable intensity and extent. The essential features as seen by the light microscope are as follows:

a) spongy changes in both the white and gray matter of the neuraxis;
b) reduction of myelin uniformly associated with spongy degeneration;

c) relative absence of myelin breakdown products;
d) relative preservation of axons, nerve cells and oligodendroglia;
e) diffuse increase of astroglia in both the white and gray matter with abundant occurrence of Alzheimer type II cells;
f) scarcity of fibrillary gliosis;
g) lack of vascular reaction, microglial and inflammatory response.

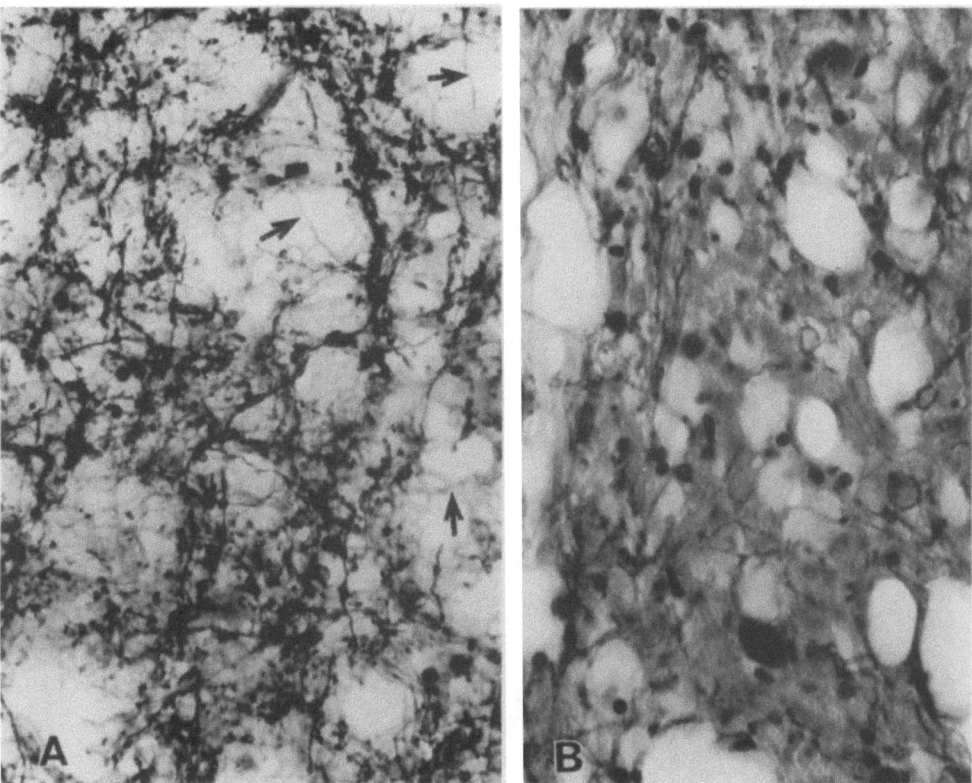

Fig. 4. A Sieve-like vacuolation of subcortical white matter (case 25 A). Small myelin-stained septa within the vacuoles (arrows) indicate splitting of the myelin. Heidenhain's myelin stain × 265. B Spongy vacuolation of the globus pallidus with swelling and disintegration of myelin sheath and preserved nerve cell (NI 149-63 — case 57). Heidenhain's myelin stain × 440

Ad a). The most striking change is an intense and widespread *vacuolation of tissue* affecting both the white and gray matter. This sponginess is manifested by independent cavities 15—200 μ in diameter, round or oval, which may also be clustered around neurons and glial elements. These cystic spaces may be bordered by small bands of cytoplasm in the wall of which one observes swollen astrocytic nuclei or oligodendrocytes (Figs. 4 B, 7 A, 8 A, B). Others are defined at their perimeter by astrocytic fibers, distorted axonal fibers or thin myelin lamellae (Figs. 4 A, B). The spongy cavities often appear empty, and no material is demonstrated within the vacuoles by any of the routine and histochemical staining techniques (13, 48, 49). Occasionally, however, within these cystic spaces, one can discern small islets of granular material staining palely with hematoxylin, or small bridges of an amorphous, slightly PAS-positive material (Fig. 12A). With myelin-staining methods, small septa can be demonstrated within the vacuoles (Fig. 4A). These findings along with the bending of the axis cylinders around these spaces indicate that the vacuoles probably arise within the lamellae of the myelin sheath (SACKS *et al.*, 1965; KOLKMANN and VÖLZKE, 1966). In the white matter, the vacuoles have their long axis in the direction of the nerve fibers. Frequently they appear to

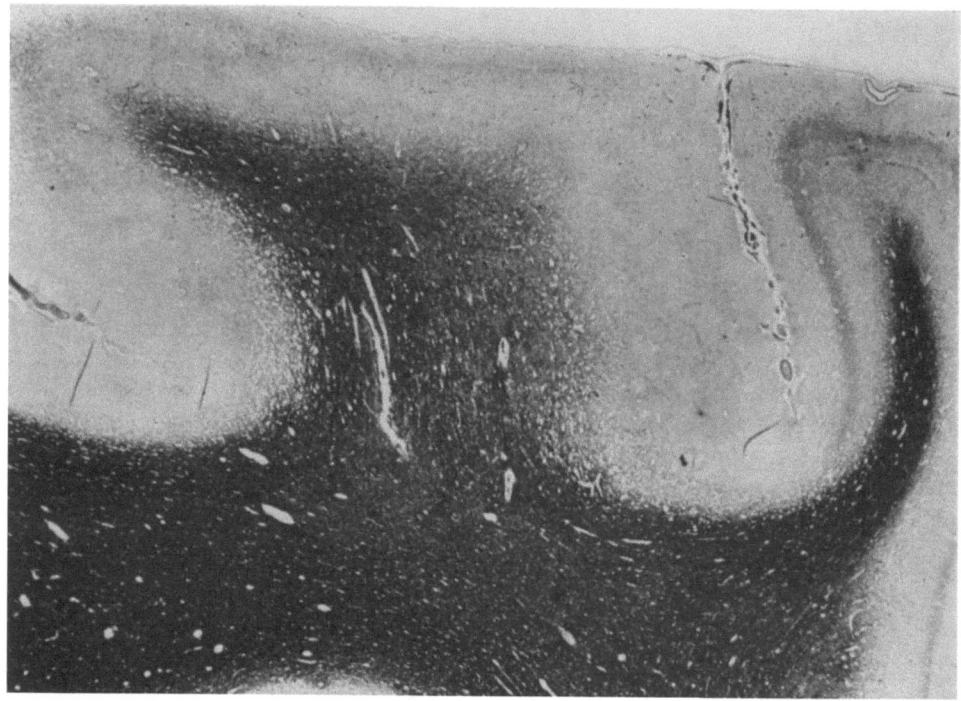

Fig. 5. Spongy vacuolation in the deep occipital cortex and at the cortico-subcortical Junction (case 25A). Weil's myelin stain × 12

displace the nerve cells (Fig. 4B) and to surround vessels. Usually the cavities are independent of vascular elements, and the perivascular spaces are not enlarged (Fig. 7B). Conversely, some vacuoles are related to small blood vessels and capillaries (11, 12). The latter may have an apparently empty space around them (8) representing the distended space of Held.

Ad b). There is widespread and marked *disintegration of myelin* which involves the areas of spongy degeneration but may even extend far beyond them. The pattern of myelin loss usually follows closely that of the spongy change but its intensity and extent vary considerably, often in accordance with the duration of the illness. Reduction of myelin content is conspicuous in the peripheral white matter with constant involvement of the subcortical U-fibers and of the radiating fibers of the cerebral cortex (Fig. 5) but relative sparing of the corpus callosum, internal capsule and the large fiber tracts. In cases of short duration relative preservation of myelin sheaths in the deep white matter is a constant feature, but in protracted cases, both infantile and juvenile (Fig. 3 B), diffuse demyelination is distinctly noticeable (31, 42, 60 61, 72, 73).

Ad c). Despite of the considerable myelin change, fatty products of myelin breakdown usually are *not* conspicuous. Though sudanophilic degradation

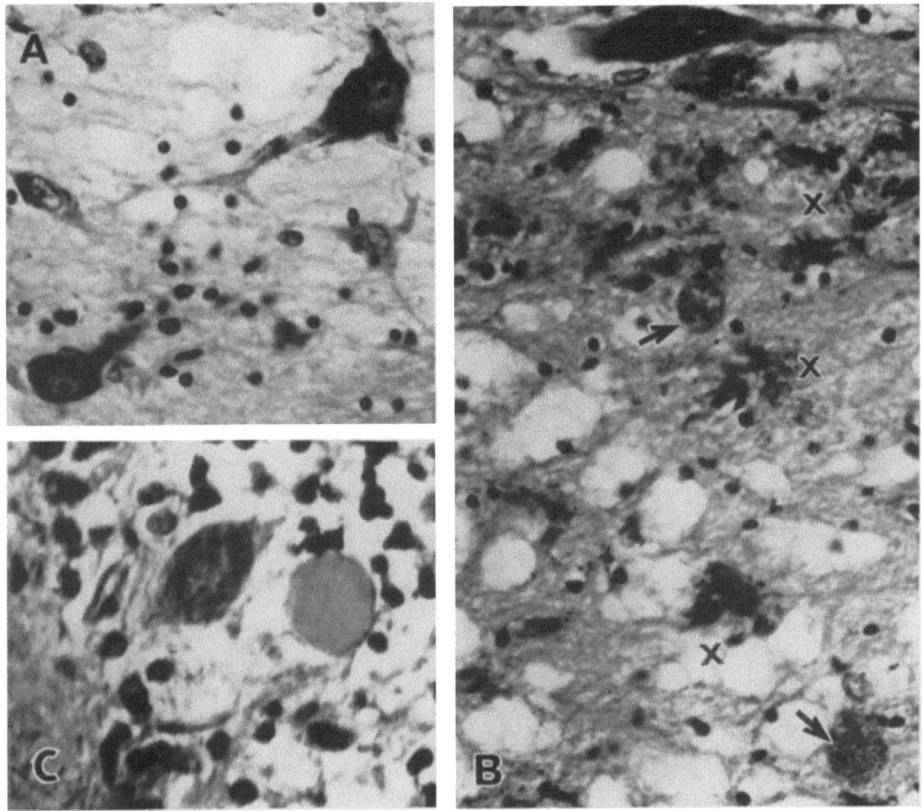

Fig. 6. A and B Juvenile form of SDI (NI 15-65 — case 61). A Well preserved nerve cells in severely vacuolated substantia nigra. K. V. × 560. B Granular lipid pigment (×) and spheroids (arrows) in markedly vacuolated internal pallidal segment. Kresylviolett × 560. C Axonal spheroid ("torpedo") in spongy granular layer of cerebellar cortex (case 24A); H&E × 560

material and macrophages are seen in the vacuolated interstices or are clustered within the perivascular spaces, they are never present in significant amounts. No metachromatic material can be demonstrated.

Ad d). In the areas of spongy degeneration and in the demyelinated zones, *oligodendroglia* are often *preserved* (Fig. 7) or only appear slightly decreased (73). Occasionally, oligos even seem to be increased in number within the affected areas, perhaps due to condensation of the tissue (31). They may contain fine sudanophilic granules (18, 21). In rare cases, complete loss of oligos is noted (16).

Axis cylinders, in general, are relatively better preserved than myelin sheaths, but, nevertheless, are decreased in number or may be completely absent in some severely affected areas. Often considerable destruction of axons with uneveness of color and caliber, varicosities and fragmentation (5, 16, 22, 31, 62, 73) in the gray and less in the white matter is present (8).

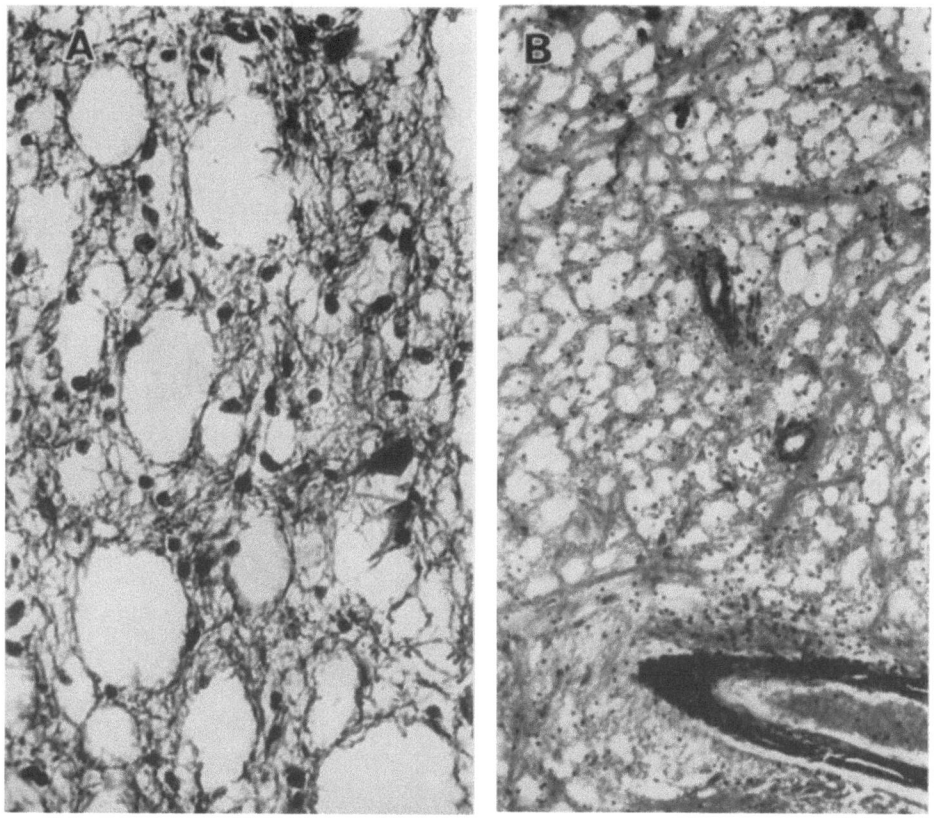

Fig. 7. A Severe spongy lesion of medial thalamus with incomplete lose of nerve cells (case 25A). H.&E. ×300. B Intense spongy lesion of globus pallidus with complete loss of nerve cells oligodendrocytes being preserved (case 61). H.&E. ×60

Axonal dystrophy was reported in some cases of SDI, where numerous eosinophilic ovoid bodies with marked argyrophilia were present in the demyelinated spongy lesions. Silver impregnations demonstrated that they arose in the course of axons indicating the axonal origin of these spheroids (60, 62, 72). Axonal dystrophy in the pallidonigral system (Fig. 6B) was conspicuous in juvenile cases (60, 61, 72) but axonal spheroids were also seen in the spongy white matter in both infantile and juvenile cases (60—62).

Neuronal changes are relatively mild when compared to the degree of the spongy transformation of tissue, but may be evident to a variable extent in the cerebral and cerebellar cortices and gray matter nuclei. Whereas in some cases neither neuronal degeneration nor evident neuronal loss were demonstrable

(8, 11, 12, 18, 21, 49, 62) (Figs. 6A, 8B), the protracted cases showed moderate to noticeable loss of cortical and subcortical nerve cells (10, 31, 33, 43, 72, 26A) (Figs. 7A and B). In rare cases, severe neuronal loss up to the point of subtotal necrosis is conspicuous (Fig. 9).

Ad e). Throughout both the white and gray matter of the neuraxis, there is a considerable *increase in the number and size of astrocytes*. Often this is the

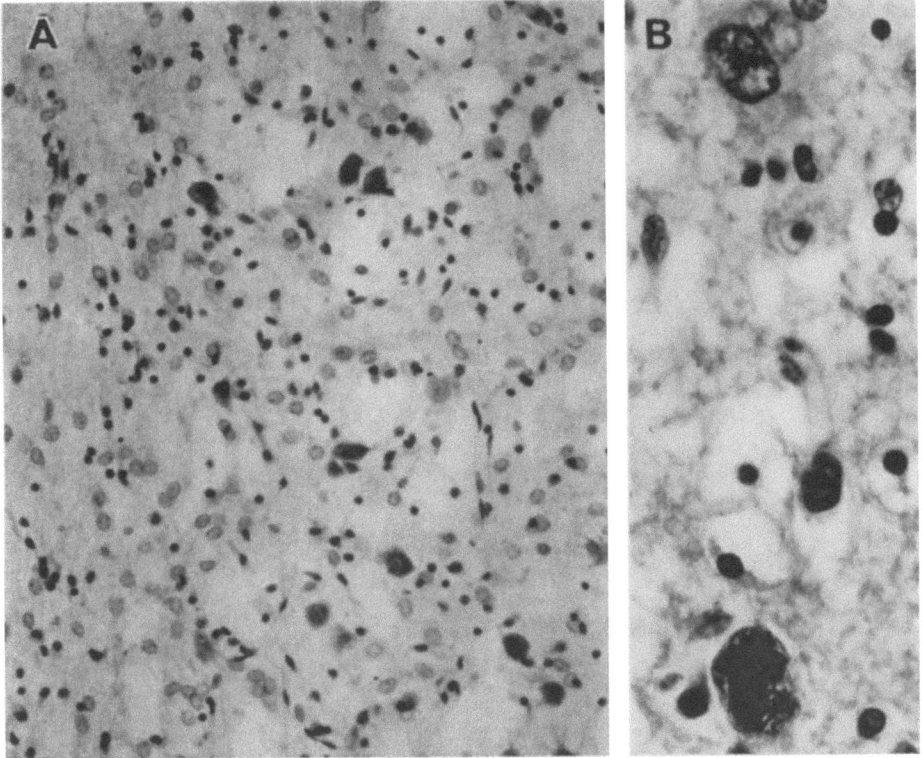

Fig. 8. A Spongy vacuolation of the dentate nucleus with numerous large "naked" pale nuclei (Alzheimer type II glial cells) and intact nerve cells (SN 262-61 — case 48). Nissl × 280. B Occasional bizarre naked giant nucleus (bottom), and large, multinucleated astrocyte of gemistocytic type (top) in the deep cerebral cortex (case 25A). H. & E. × 1056

first alteration seen under the light microscope. Many of the astrocytes show enlarged, oval or lobated, clear nuclei of 20—30 μ diameter. They have a very definite nuclear membrane and a small, often excentrically placed nucleolus. Cytoplasm is often absent. These "naked" nuclei referred to as Alzheimer type II cells are abundant within the affected zones and outside the spongy areas (Fig. 8A). Such cells have been found in almost all cases of this malady. Some naked giant nuclei measuring 45—75 μ (Fig. 8B) were seen (25A, 73). In a few cases bizarre giant cells resembling the Alzheimer type I cell have been noted (10, 30), but these usually are absent. Large astrocytes of the gemistocytic type may occur (Fig. 9) and are prominent in rare cases (25A, 26a). Their cytoplasm may contain granular lipid material.

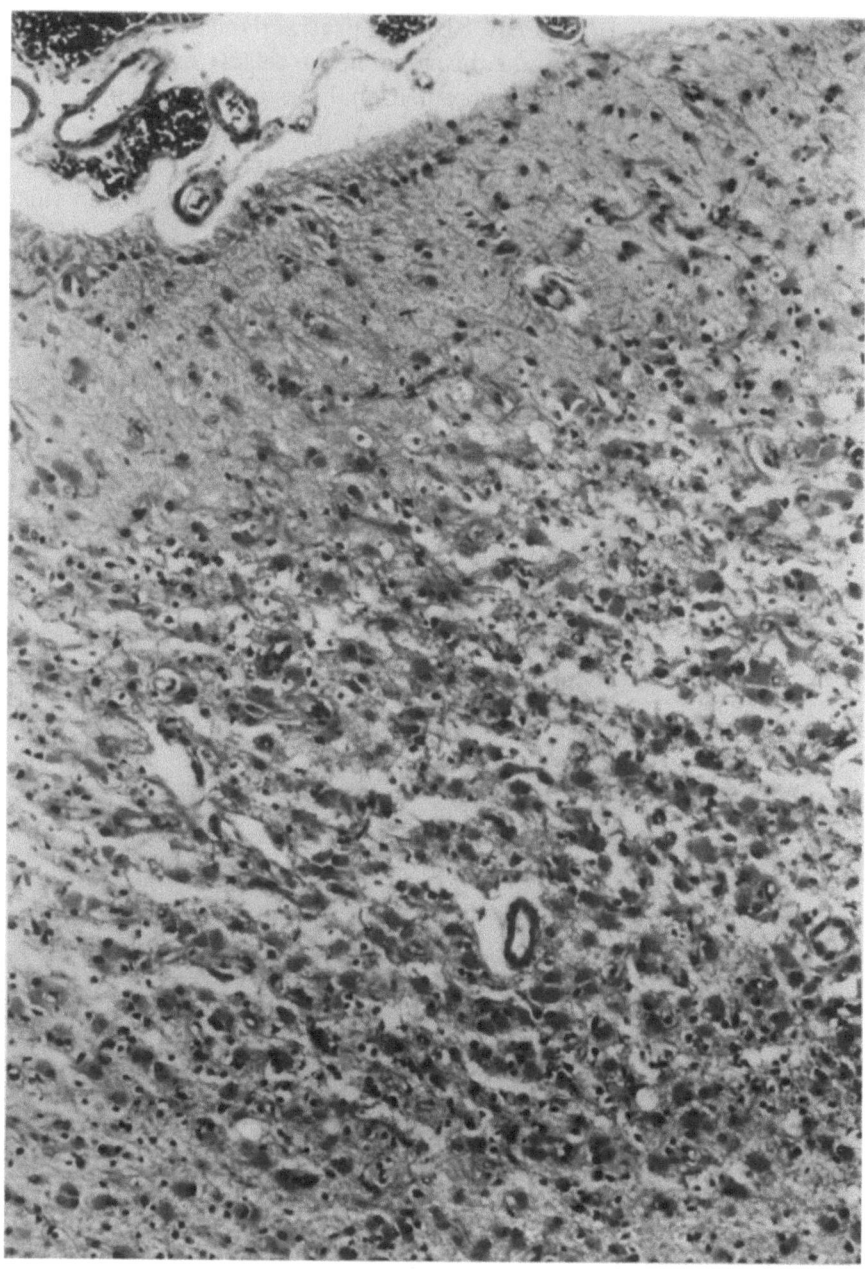

Fig. 9. Subtotal diffuse cortical necrosis with intense, astrocytic gliosis with prominent gemistocytic astrocytic and slight capillary reaction in atypical (?) case (NA 7-59 — case 26A). H.&E. ×115

Ad f). Usually proliferation of glial fibers is not seen in significant amount. Only in later stages of spongy change and severe demyelination, an increase of small fibrillary astrocytes is seen. In some spongy areas, particularly in the brain stem, moderate increase in the number of glial fibers may be present, rarely progressing to an intense fibrillary gliosis (25 A, 26 A, 31, 49) (Fig. 10B).

Ad g). There is no significant vascular response even within areas of most severe and advanced sponginess and demyelination. The relative absence of appreciable microglial and inflammatory response to the spongy lesion is a constant feature of this disease. Occasionally, fibrous thickening of vessel-walls was noted (11, 25 A).

2. Topography of the Lesions

Spongy vacuolation of tissue can extend throughout the cerebrospinal axis except for the cranial nerves, the cauda equina and the peripheral roots and nerves. While this spongy change may be more or less generalized, there are regions in which it is most marked. Among the predominantly affected areas are the subcortical white matter and adjacent deep cortical layers of the cerebrum, the cerebellar cortex, the globus pallidus, the dorsal portion of the brain stem, and the superficial white matter and gray nuclei of the spinal cord. Thus the vacuolation shows a very definite and characteristic distribution in almost all reported cases, its severity and extent varying in accordance to the duration of illness.

The sponginess is most marked at the *junction of the cortex and white matter* (2, 5, 8, 13, 25, 25 A, 31, 33, 36, 39—43, 53, 60—62, 73, 76). The convolutional white matter, including the arcuate fibers, is largely replaced by cystic spaces which extend into the deep cortical laminae (Fig. 5), whereas the rest of the cortex, the centrum ovale and the deep compact medullated structures are relatively spared. The distribution of myelin disintegration closely parallels that of the spongy degeneration. Myelin loss is most marked at the cortico-subcortical junction but, occasionally, the subcortical arcuate fibers are spared (3, 10, 13, 60, 61, 67, 72). Conversely, the general texture of myelin is often preserved in the central parts of the hemispheral white matter. The extent of demyelination accompanied by extensive sponginess, however, may vary from case to case and even in one and the same patient. Often the changes are most extreme in the occipital and parieto-occipital lobes (17, 49, 72, 73) in sharp contrast to a relative integrity of the deep frontal white matter and the centrum ovale (18, 49), whereas in other cases a more diffuse demyelination is noted (39). This local variability of the cortico-subcortical changes was conspicuous in several cases (10, 17, 49, 60—62, 73).

Within the *cerebral cortex*, large cavities are predominantly found in the deeper areas — layers IV-VI — and they are accompanied by serious loss of the intracortical myelinated fibers (Fig. 5) and by abundant proliferation of astrocytes extending into the adjacent white matter (Fig. 8B). There may be a diffuse and severe loss of cortical neurons (Fig. 9), but in most cases the architecture of the cortex is rather well preserved.

The extent to which the more compact *deep myelinated structures* are involved, also varies considerably. The centrum ovale usually is much less spongy with preservation of myelin (2, 8, 10, 17, 18, 31, 33, 40—43, 62) except in protracted cases (60, 61, 72, 73). The corpus callosum is little involved (2, 8, 9, 11, 12, 17, 18, 31, 39—43, 57, 59, 62) and severe demyelination is rare (Fig. 3B). The internal and external capsules are also very little affected (2, 8—12, 17, 21, 25A, 26A, 39—43, 60—62). They may show slight sponginess (31) but severe myelin loss is almost exceptional (18).

The *basal ganglia* show considerable variation in the extent of spongy change, demyelination and glial response. The pallidum tends to be seriously affected (2, 10, 13, 49, 57, 60—62, 73). There may be a clearly defined, bilaterally symmetrical spongy necrosis of the globus pallidus with intense loss of myelin, axons and neurons but without noticeable glial fibrosis (Figs. 3B, 7B, 10A). In other brains, however, it is less involved than the lenticular nuclei (8, 18) which usually show slight spongy alteration. Among the severely affected structures are the corpus subthalamicum (16, 25A, 57, 62), hypothalamus (70) and substantia nigra (18, 25A, 26A, 57, 60—62), but in other cases these regions are preserved (31). The thalamus shows mild to severe degrees of vacuolation and loss of neurons (Figs. 7A, 10B), sometimes with variable affection of the different nuclei.

In the *brain stem*, the spongy change is widespread along the longitudinal axis from the red nuclei to the lower medulla. In general, the tegmental parts are more severely affected than the ventral areas. Sponginess is pronounced in the tegmentum mesencephali and pontis which are poorly myelinated in contrast to the usually well preserved cerebral peduncles (10, 21, 39, 60—62). The substantia nigra and red nucleus show variable lesions, sometimes progressing to almost complete deprivation of myelin and nerve cells (25A, 26, 26A). Axonal spheroids are present in juvenile cases (60, 61, 72). Severe myelin loss accompanied by glial cell proliferation and slight fibrillary gliosis may involve the medial longitudinal fascicle, lemniscus medialis and lateralis, other sensory tracts and the middle cerebellar peduncles (13, 18, 31), while the superior cerebellar peduncles and the basis pontis are much less affected. The deep transverse fibers of the latter are pale, but the descending cerebro-spinal fiber tracts are often preserved (8, 18, 21, 25A, 41, 60—62). In the medulla the spongy change is widespread, involving the dorsal parts, the olives and the periolivary zones equally (9, 16, 31, 60—62). The pyramids are spared (49, 62) or moderately affected (9, 13, 43, 54).

The *cerebellum* usually shows striking affection, sponginess being most prominent at the junction of the molecular or Purkinje cell and internal granular layers — lamina dissecans — and to a lesser extent in the foliar white matter (Fig. 11B). The central white matter often shows only slight porosity extending to the hilus of the dentate nucleus or is spared (49). In the dentate nucleus, spongy change is often prominent (Fig. 11A). The Purkinje cell layer is dislocated and rarified, a portion of the surviving cells often being displaced into the molecular layer (5, 10, 25, 42, 43, 49). The Bergmann glia often is increased in size and number (31, 39—43, 48, 49). It may show striking hypertrophy and proliferation even in spite of lack of sponginess of the cortex

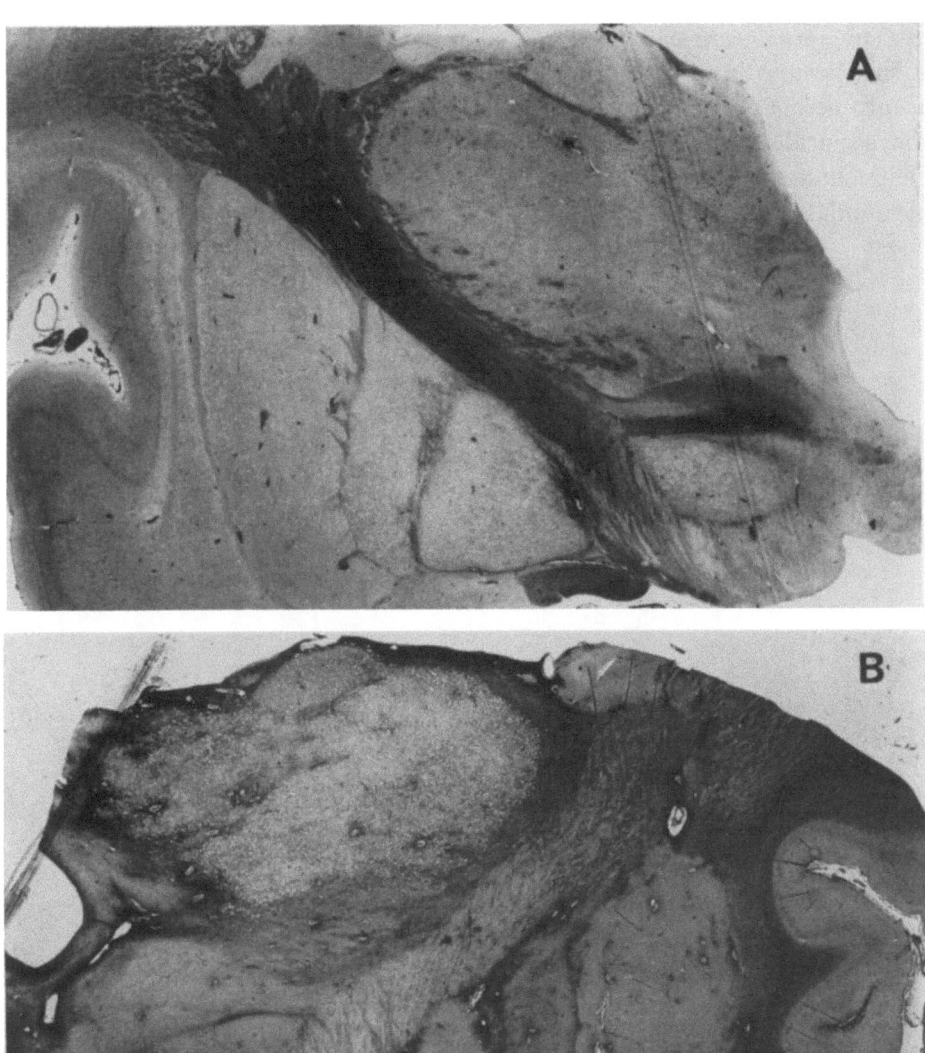

Fig. 10. A Intense spongy vacuolation of the globus pallidus and subthalamic nucleus with loss of myelin. Minor affection of other basal ganglia and claustrum (case 57). Heidenhain's myelin stain × 5. B Severe spongy vacuolation of the thalamus and diffuse fibrillary gliosis of all myelinated structures (case 25 A). Holzer's Stain × 4,5

(41). The internal granular layer is rarely normal (42). In general, it contains large cavities, particularly in the superficial parts (8, 13, 31, 39, 41, 56, 72). The spongy foliar white matter is often demyelinated (42, 43, 73), while the deep white matter shows slight spongy change (41, 73) or is spared (42). Occasionally, persistence of the external granular layer of the cerebellar cortex beyond the usual age was noted (10, 11, 24, 40, 41).

The *spinal cord* can be involved in its entirety with moderate to severe spongy lesions in all funiculi and in the gray matter, accompanied by diffuse occurrence of "naked" glia nuclei (43, 60, 61, 73). The affection may prefer the cervical and thoracic parts with preservation of the lumbar cord (31). Demyelination of the posterior and lateral columns with degeneration of the pyramidal tracts is reported (18, 31, 39, 40, 43, 60, 61), rarely unaccompanied

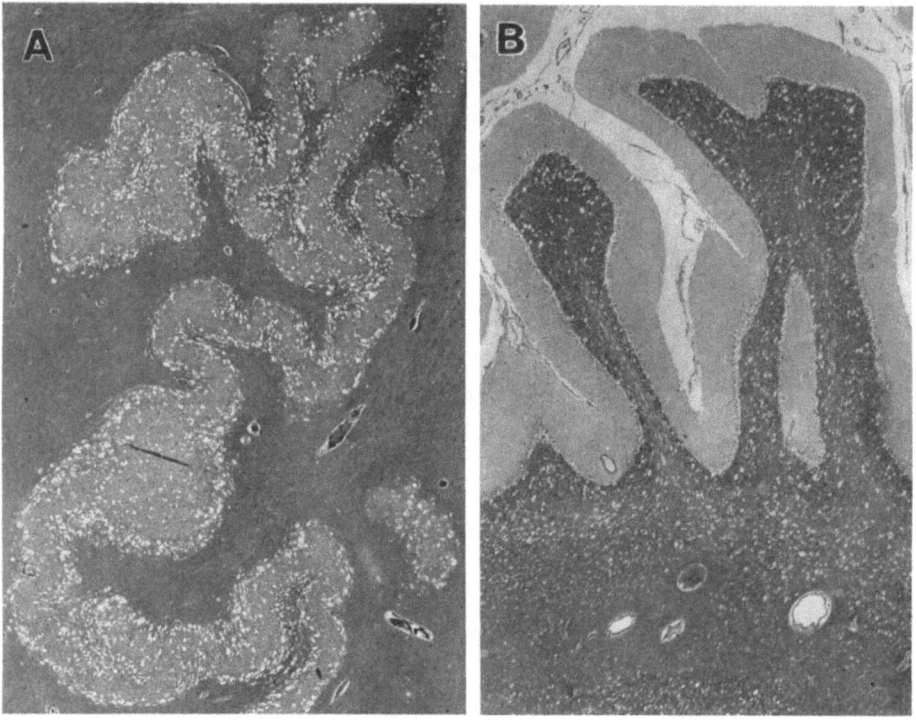

Fig. 11 A and B. Spongy vacuolation of cerebellum (case 25 A). A Clustering of vacuoles in the dentate nucleus. H. & E. × 12. B Sponginess of lamina dissecans and of the subcortical white matter. H. & E. × 12

by vacuolation (16). Often the more peripheral parts of the dorsal and lateral columns show intense sponginess. Spinal gray matter is vacuolated with preservation (25 A, 40, 60, 61) or slight loss of nerve cells (42).

The *optic system* is often involved. The optic nerves and chiasm may be intact (42, 72) or show slight vacuolation (10, 13, 60) to severe sponginess (Fig. 12 A) with partial demyelination of the central parts (39). The destroyed fibers correspond to the maculopapillary bundle (8, 21), but are not limited to this tract. Large astrocytes and "naked" nuclei are conspicuous. The optic tracts may be intact (21) or decreased in their myelin content. In cases with gross demyelination of the optic radiation severe demyelination of the optic tracts is noted (8, 10, 13). The *retina* is reported to be normal (8, 13) or to show almost total disappearance of nerve cells in the ganglion cell layer with preservation of the photoreceptor layer, changes seen in optic nerve atrophy of various origin (39). Intense vacuolation of the ganglion cell layer was reported (44).

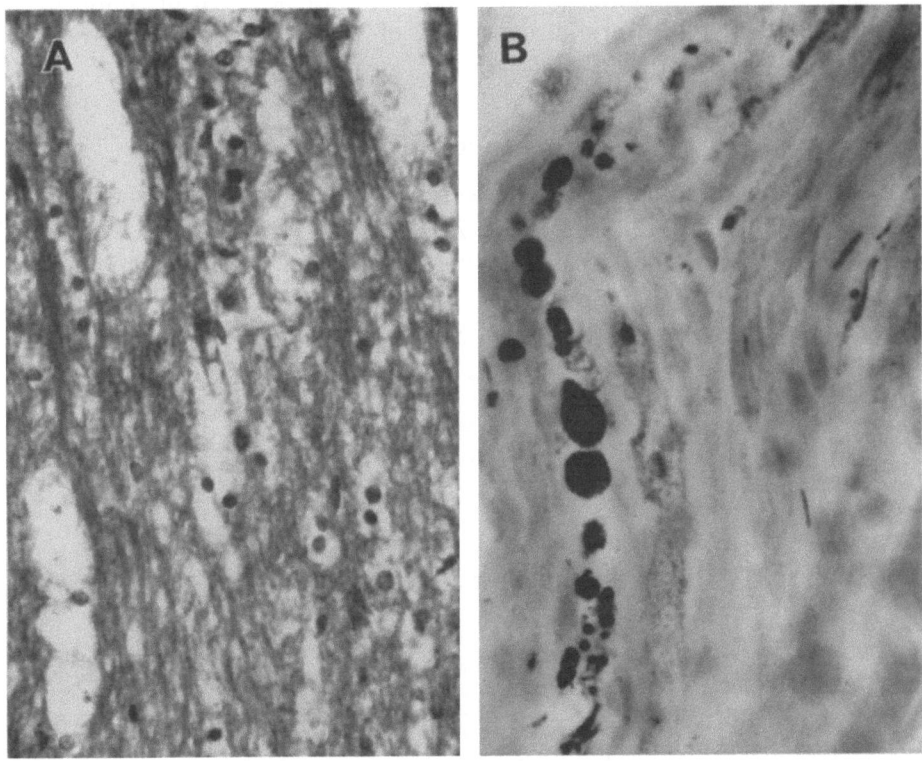

Fig. 12. A Large vacuoles in optic nerve with small islets of finely granular or amorphous PAS-positive material and adjacent oligodendrocytes (case 60). PAS × 350. B Subtotal demyelination in peripheral nerve with myelin balls and -droplets. Heidenhain × 735 (case 25 A)

3. Peripheral Nerves and Muscle

The *cranial nerves* are usually normal (8, 13, 31). No gross lesions are seen in the *spinal roots* (8, 10, 25A, 31, 43, 49, 57, 60, 61) and in the autonomic ganglia (31, 49, 73).

The *peripheral nerves* have been examined in only a few cases with no abnormalities reported (31, 44, 45, 60, 68). SUZUKI (64), however, described marked axonal changes and mild demyelination associated with abnormal cell infiltration and occurrence of vacuolated cells in the peri- and endoneurium. In one case (25 A) we saw severe demyelination with ovoids, myelin balls and breakdown products associated with proliferation of Schwann cells (Fig. 12B) but relative preservation of the axis cylinders. These changes appear to be consistent with Wallerian degeneration. The relation of these lesions to the CNS changes is not yet elucidated.

Skeletal muscle showed mild degree of neurogenic atrophy in an infantile case diagnosed by cortical biopsy (68). Electron microscopic study disclosed reduction in width of the fibrils, abundant glycogen, and abnormal mitochondria. An isolated finding was the presence within a muscle cell of round or oval profiles of undetermined origin, consisting of sheaths of parallel paired linear densities of 45 Å (GAMBETTI et al., 1969).

D. Ultrastructural Findings

Electron microscopic studies of cerebral biopsies are confined to early stages of the disease (52, 56, 68, 70, 71). NELSON and AUREBECK (1966) described vacuolation and occasional cyst formation within oligodendroglial

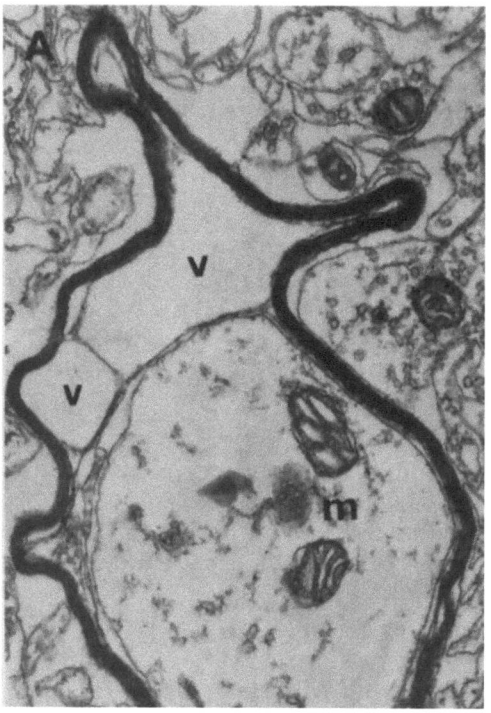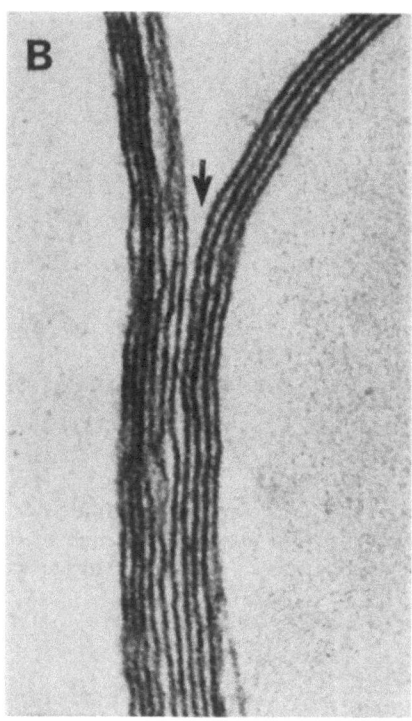

Fig. 13. A Myelinated axon with a small vacuole within the myelin sheath. Few lamellas remain contiguous to the axon; the remnant of the myelin sheath peels off forming an electron-clear space. *m* mitochondria; *v* vacuole. Electron micrograph × 29,000 (case 68). B High power electron micrograph of the myelin lamellae showing separation between the major dense lines and the obscured intraperiod lines (arrow). × 100,800 (case 49)

cytoplasm. Collapsed myelin sheaths with displacement of the axons were considered the results of progressive vacuole formation within retained glial cytoplasm. There was no evidence of myelin disintegration. Marked swelling of astrocytes, particularly of their perivascular processes, was apparent in the cortex. The cell boundaries were intact, and there was no increase in extracellular space. Some of the astrocytic processes contained large amounts of glycogen, whereas others showed abnormal mitochondria. Some cells containing large nuclei with a prominent nucleolus probably correspond to the Alzheimer cells of light microscopy. Reactive astroglia with increased numbers of intracellular fibers were infrequent.

According to ADACHI et al. (1966), the vacuoles in the subcortical white matter and deep cortex correspond to a) large spaces within myelin sheaths being present between the major dense lines of the myelin membranes and

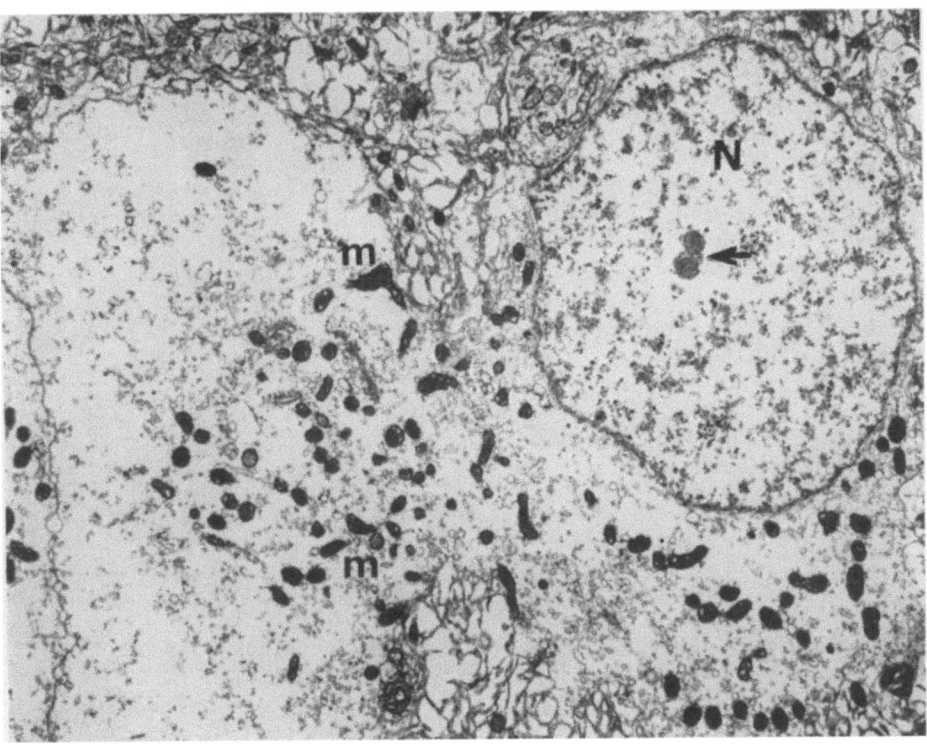

Fig. 14. Swollen astrocytic perikaryon containing abnormal mitochondria (*m*) and normal ones (arrow). × 7,000 (case 68)

resulting thus from separation of the lamellae at the intraperiod line (Fig. 13 B); b) swollen astrocytic perikarya and processes. Smaller vacuoles in the cerebral cortex resulted from enlargement of the astroglia alone. Whereas in the subcortical white matter the extracellular spaces were widened due to rupture of myelin lamellae and astrocytic cell membranes, no increased extracellular space or ruptured cell membrane were present in the cortex. The large and pale astrocytic nuclei described as Alzheimer type II by light microscopy appeared also enlarged and were seen to contain sparse nucleoplasmic granules, loss of chromatin and distinct nuclei with preserved nucleolemma. Marked changes in size and appearance of mitochondria were observed in the astrocytic processes of the cortex. The mitochondria were frequently enormously elongated and showed distention and distortion of their cristae and striation of the matrix. The latter consisted of fine electron-dense granules measuring 82 Å each which were arranged in a chain-like pattern.

These findings were confirmed by GAMBETTI et al. (1969) who observed, in addition to clefts within the myelin sheaths resulting from "split" at the intraperiod line (Fig. 13 A) and swollen astrocytic perikarya and processes, unusual mitochondria containing crystalline-like material in astrocytes

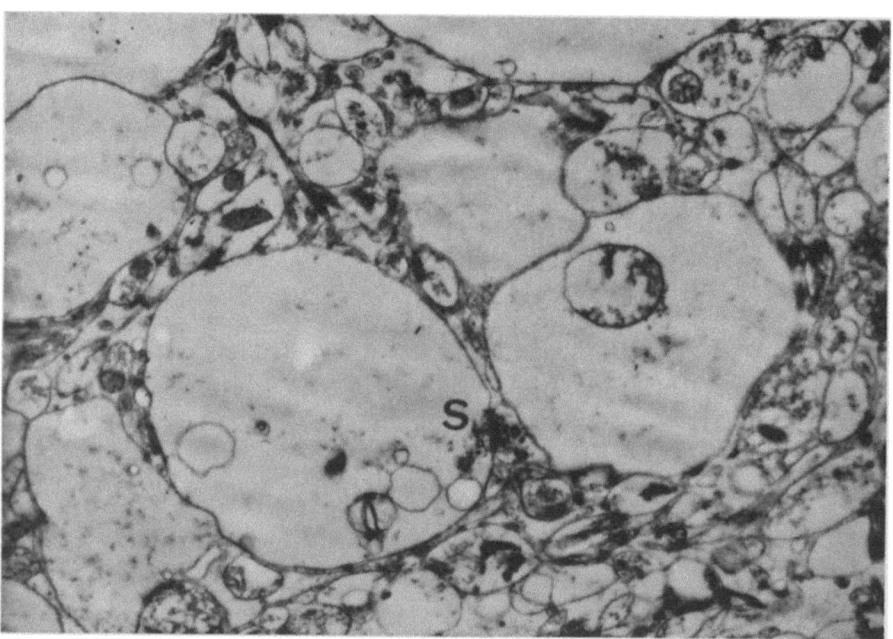

Fig. 15. Intense swelling of postsynaptic dendrites in vacuolated neuropil (N 12.751 case 70). S.-synapsis. × 12.000

(Fig. 14). The nuclei of astrocytes were normal and none of them showed a pale nucleus suggestive of Alzheimer cells. Mild focal swelling of dendrites involving frequently the postsynaptic component of axodentritic synapsis was present, the presynaptic endings being normal.

Focal swelling of the postsynaptic components of neuronal dendrites was also reported by ULE (1968) (Fig. 15). Since neurons, oligodendroglia and blood vessels were not altered (52, 68, 70), the "spongy state" was considered to be due to astroglial and dendritic swelling and to clefts within myelin sheaths. Astroglial swelling often is prominent at a distance from the capillaries, the pericapillary astroglial processes being occasionally preserved (70). Some neurons show irregular shape and dense perinuclear cytoplasm because of compression by adjacent vacuoles (68). Compressed axons, inside collapsed myelin sheaths, and empty myelin sheaths, suggesting advanced axonal degeneration, were occasionally seen in the cerebral biopsy of a rather advanced case in an 6 year-old boy (68).

VII. Biochemical Aspects

Although chemical data on brain specimens from cases of SDI are fragmentary, they have added some to our knowledge of the disease.

A. Histochemical Findings

The giant as well as the normal sized mitochondria in swollen astrocytes of the cerebral cortex show markedly decreased activities of ATPase, succinic dehydrogenase and dihydronicotinamide adenine dinucleotide diaphorase (ADACHI et al., 1966). Recently, JOHNSON (1970) detected a deficiency of the ATPase in the membranes of fibrous astrocytes in the subcortical white matter. In early stages of the disease, a decreased activity of ATPase in the basement membranes of small cerebral blood vessels has been found (ADACHI and VOLK, 1968).

B. Water Content of Brain Tissue

An *increased* water content of formalin-fixed (18) and fresh brain tissue was reported (13, 21, 52, 63, 64). The values were 92,2% for fresh white matter and 85,6 to 87% for cortical gray matter (13). In other cases, a water content of 96,8% for subcortical white matter (52) and of 86,9% for white matter (21) was found. In the cases of KAMOSHITA et al. (1968), the water content of gray matter was not elevated, but it was drastically increased in the white substance. The dry weight of the tissue was about half of the normal value in the younger patient (64) and almost one-third of the normal value in the older child (63).

C. Electrolytes

The electrolyte composition of the gray matter was essentially normal, whereas the excessive fluid accumulation in the white matter had an electrolyte composition similar to that of plasma filtrate (KAMOSHITA et al., 1968). A spectacular increase in calcium levels in the cerebral white matter and in the liver of two neonatal cases (44, 45), might be considered, however, as an artefact due to formalin fixation. Moderate increase in iron and copper levels in the liver of both latter cases were reported (SACKS et al., 1965).

D. Brain Lipids

Whereas the gray matter shows almost normal lipid composition except for a moderate decrease of cerebrosides (63, 64) or a slight depression of total lipids and phospholipids (33 — CROCKER), the chemical abnormalities are almost limited to the cerebral white matter.

Analysis of formalin-fixed (13) and of fresh material (33 — CROCKER; 34 — LEES and FOLCH-PI, 1961; 63, 64 — KAMOSHITA et al., 1968) revealed a severe loss of proteolipid protein and total lipids, particularly of galactolipids, cholesterol and total phosphatides being better preserved (KAMOSHITA et al., 1968), although CROCKER found reduced phospholipid levels. No cholesterol esters were detected, while ceramine dihexoside was greatly elevated. The total gangliosides of the gray and white matter were within normal range. There was a slight decrease of the trisialo-ganglioside G_1 and moderate increase in monosialo-gangliosides $G_{4,5,6}$[4], but both changes were considered to be non-specific (KAMOSHITA et al., 1968). According to these authors, the yields and chemical abnormalities of the isolated myelin fractions correlated well with the severity of the histological changes in the white matter: There was a significant decrease in proteolipid protein, high insoluble residue, a severe reduction of total phosphatides and glycolipids, particularly of ethanol phosphatides and cerebrosides, and a strong increase in cholesterol, while the total lipids remained relatively normal. The total gangliosides and their distribution of the isolated myelin were normal. No accumulation of small molecular weight products of myelin breakdown was found.

VIII. Differential Diagnosis

SDI is a rare neurological disorder of children often, but not exclusively, afflicting Jewish infants of Ashkenazic background. Considering the familial incidence, the racial background and the clinical features, intra vitam diagnosis can be, at least, suspected and will be confirmed by cerebral biopsy. From histological demonstration of vacuolation in the ganglion cell layer of the retina, SACKS et al. (1965) suggested that these vacuoles might be visible through the slit-lamp ophthalmoscope, thus affording a clinical method of confirming the diagnosis of SDI during life.

Among the major conditions in the differential diagnosis of the common *infantile form of SDI* are Tay-Sachs disease, several leukodystrophies, cerebral palsy, simple hydrocephalus and other cerebral space-occupying processes.

Tay-Sachs Disease: Some of the infants shown to be afflicted with SDI were originally considered as cases of TSD, although most of them appeared as "atypical" forms, since no cherry-red spot was seen in their maculae (8, 9, 10, 17, 18, 34). The need to distinguish between these two disorders was one of the impelling reasons for the earlier contribution of VAN BOGAERT and BERTRAND (1949). Their first case previously had been presented by VAN BOGAERT (1939) under the title: "Idiocy with blindness in a Polish Jew child with the outward appearance of Tay-Sachs disease". There are some areas of clinical communication between the two diseases: both are familial with a predominance of Jewish ancestry — the forebears in both disorders being derived for the most part from the same regions of north-eastern Europe — and arise in infancy, often within the first 8 months of life. Arrest in motor development and loss of acquired abilities in conjection with general hypotonia later replaced by spasticity and opisthotonus, amaurosis and idiocy predominate in each. Megalencephaly is shared by both diseases. In SDI it is frequently apparent during the initial stages, tending to recede as the disease is prolonged, while in TSD the macrocephaly is inapparent until at least the age of 20 months, following which head enlargement becomes an increasingly prominent clinical feature (ARONSON et al., 1958; KANOFF et al., 1959). Both conditions terminate fatally by the second or third year of life. Differential diagnosis is easy to make by the following features:

a) Macular degeneration with cherry-red spots is confined to TSD;

---

[4] According to the KOREY and GONATAS nomenclature.

b) serum fructose-1-phosphate aldolase levels are markedly increased in TSD, while in SDI, values of this enzyme are normal (ADACHI and VOLK, 1966);

c) demonstration of lipid storage material in rectal and brain biopsy material in TSD;

d) chromatographic demonstration of Tay-Sachs ganglioside in biopsy material, as well as in CSF (BERNHEIMER, 1968) and blood (SASTRY and STANCER, 1968).

Alexander's Disease: This leukodystrophy with diffuse formation of Rosenthal fibers is often associated with developmental retardation and early macrocephaly. It shows no predilection for Ashkenazic Jews; furthermore, blindness and optic atrophy are not common in this leukodystrophy with megalencephaly (SCHOCHET et al., 1968).

Krabbe's globoid cell leukodystrophy which is also a recessive disorder often of familial nature has a typical evolution: The onset is in the first months of life after an uneventful early development. Restlessness and irritability or apathy are said to be initial symptoms. Optic atrophy is discovered by chance. After a period of atony and of muscular weakness hypertonia of the limbs appears rapidly. Progressive spasticity is joined by pseudobulbar symptoms and tonic or clonic seizures. Myoclonus is sometimes present. The children often proceed rapidly to a cachectic state, death occurring usually between 10 and 14 months, although some cases are more prolonged in their course. CSF protein may be elevated. Peripheral nerve lesions may be recognized by clinical or bioptic investigation (LAKE, 1968; SOURANDER and OLSSON, 1968).

Metachromatic Leukodystrophy (MLD), representing a recessive familial malady of the group of generalized lipidoses, has a somewhat later onset of symptoms between 1 and 2 years. Often the disorder has been noted when the child begins to walk. More frequently, the malady appears later, between the ages of 2 and 3, or even later, with loss of motility, epileptic fits, blindness and mental deterioration, sometimes accompanied by ocular paralysis, nystagmus and deafness. An ataxo-spasmodic syndrome later gives rise to hypertonicity, the children dying with bulbar signs between 4 and 6 years of age. In MLD the rigidity is usually more marked and synchronous and there is less hyperkinesis than in SDI. Megalencephaly is never seen in MLD. Diagnosis is confirmed by demonstration of metachromatic substances in the urine and many body tissues, including nerve and rectum or dental pulp biopsies. Decreased conduction velocity in peripheral nerves is often noted. Specific early diagnosis of MLD is possible by demonstration of lack of aryl-sulfatase A in the urine (AUSTIN et al., 1965) and in leucocytes (PERCY and BRADY, 1968).

Sudanophilic leukodystrophies, including Pelizaeus-Merzbacher disease, rather often show a familial incidence but no Jewish background and usually have a later onset between the ages of 2 and 10 years, except for the congenital (SEITELBERGER) type of Pelizaeus-Merzbacher disease. Most of the cases have a longer course than is usual in SDI. Visual complaints and optic atrophy are common, as are seizures, but megalencephaly is not present (JELLINGER and SEITELBERGER, 1969b).

Hydrocephalus and Tumors: CANAVAN (1931) has already emphasized that macrocephalus can be caused by a diffuse degenerative disease which must be distinguished from hydrocephalus due to other causes and from tumor, either of which may be suggested by the clinical symptoms in some cases of SDI. Simple or communicating hydrocephalus of unknown origin was the erroneous diagnosis in some cases (21, 62); one infant (9) had surgery for a suspected tumor of third ventricle.

Myotonia congenita: The severe muscular hypotonia and flopping of the head occasionally may suggest the diagnosis of congenital myotonia or the congenital form of Werdnig-Hoffmann's disease (30, 46, 47) which also may have familial incidence. The diagnosis of SDI will be established by supplementary findings: absence of signs of neuronal affection in the EMG and presence of pathologic EEG records.

The rare *juvenile form of SDI* is characterized clinically by a progressive cerebellar syndrome and mental deterioration followed by loss of vision, optic atrophy and generalized spasticity. Megalencephaly is not observed. Since retinal pigmentation was noted, juvenile cerebro-retinal degeneration, e.g. Spielmeyer-Vogt variant of amaurotic idiocy, was considered in the differential diagnosis (60, 61).

IX. Nosological Aspects

HALLERVORDEN (1957) suggested a relationship of SDI to the group of leukodystrophies in which they would represent a special type characterized by the features of chronic brain edema. He argued that SDI was a special form of "diffuse cerebral sclerosis", whereas the majority of the more recent authors regard it as a separate entity. The characteristic and unifying feature in this disease is the histological appearance of widespread spongy cavitation of both the white and gray matter of the neuraxis. The spongy change is generalized, but is more marked in certain regions or predilection. It is associated with a marked increase in water. This excess of fluid is responsible for the megalencephaly which is one of the most characteristic features of the early stages of SDI. Another typical change is a diffuse hypertrophy of the astroglia with occurrence of Alzheimer type II cells. In later stages, there is myelin loss in the spongy areas and partial spongy necrosis of the gray matter with relative preservation of neurons and axons and without the presence of notable degradation products at any stage of the disease.

A. Atypical Cases

As invariably happens relatively soon after a new syndrome, disease or pathological entity is discovered, described or delineated, it becomes increasingly difficult to dogmatically assign a label to some cases which show new variations or fail to show supposedly essential features.

The following observations widen still further the topic of SDI because they differ in some morphological points from "typical" instances of this disorder. They are either difficult to place or may represent transitional forms to other entities.

1. Transition to Progressive Poliodystrophy

MORSE (1949) described two white siblings with histories of difficult birth. In the elder sib, a girl, the illness began 11 months before death at age 6 with head nodding attacks, jerky movements, rolling of the eyes and episodes of unconsciousness. Later tremor, ataxia, hemiparesis and convulsions developed while myoclonic jerks persisted. Her brother had a similar syndrome with onset at the age of $2^1/_2$ years with myoclonic jerks, hemiparesis, tremor, mental retardation, deafness, blindness, and death in status epilepticus. In both cases necropsy disclosed fatty infiltration of the liver. The girl's brain showed severe cortical lesions with laminar cell loss and gliosis most marked in the left hemisphere where encephalomalacia with a rudimentary glial network was present. Considerable myelin loss and giant multinucleated astrocytes were seen in the subcortical white matter. Bilateral spongy lesions were present in the cornu Ammonis, thalamus, corpus subthalamicum and substantia nigra, and were most severe in each dentate nucleus. Small spongy lesions were seen in the left caudate nucleus, putamen and pontine nuclei. There were large vacuoles with variable nerve cell loss and gliosis. Phagocytes were abundant in the gray and white matter. The medulla and spinal cord were normal. The boy's brain disclosed minimal cortical changes with neuronal swelling, cell loss in Sommer's sector and spongy rarefication of Ammon's horn. There was also spongy vacuolation of each dentate nucleus with astroglial proliferation. In spite of the severe spongy lesions, these cases were later considered by FORD et al. (1951) as "familial degeneration of the cerebral gray matter" similar to Alpers' disease.

In the brains of two siblings mentioned by SEITELBERGER (1961) striking spongy lesions were present in the cerebral cortex, in the white matter underlying cortical gyri, in symmetrical regions of the basal ganglia (ventral thalamus, subthalamic nuclei and nucleus ruber) and in the ponto-mesencephalic tegmentum. Less severe spongy changes affected the pallidum, striatum and substantia nigra, while the allocortex and medulla were almost preserved. In the elder sib (25 A) spongy degeneration of the subcortical white matter (Fig. 5) and severe vacuolation of each dentate nucleus and of the cerebellar lamina dissecans were prominent (Fig. 11). There was generalized and intense proliferation of astrocytes predominantly of the gemistocytic type with occurrence of bizarre giant cells (Fig. 8B) and "naked" clear nuclei. Gemistocytic astrocytosis was particular prominent in the younger sib (26A). In both cases striking loss of neurons was seen throughout the cortex and deep gray nuclei. In the most severely affected areas only a few neurons were left in the otherwise parenchyma-free rudimentary glial network. In the cerebral and cerebellar white matter slight generalized pallor of myelin contrasted with intense diffuse fibrillary gliosis which was also present in the brain stem and spinal cord. The lesions in both brains were almost identical in quality and distribution, but were much more severe and advanced in the younger sib (26A) who showed diffuse microcystic necrosis with prominent gemistocytic astrocytosis throughout the isocortex (Fig. 9).

Although many features of both cases were strikingly similar to those in the majority of the reported cases of SDI, the severe neuronal loss in spongy degenerated gray matter, especially in the isocortex of the younger sib with an acute illness, is not a typical feature of SDI, but rather resembles the findings in "progressive cerebral poliodystrophy". The prominent fibrillary gliosis of the cerebral white matter and brain stem, which is not recognized even in protracted cases of SDI, likewise appears more typical for the former disease group. Although the changes in the elder sib's brain were definitely consistent with those in "typical" cases of SDI, the younger child showed morphological features which could place these cases between SDI and Alpers' disease. Since the gray matter lesions were much more severe in the patient with an acute clinical course, the deviation in the histological pictures could also be due to a different intensity of the basic process. On the other hand, it should be recognized that Alpers' disease appears to include a large variety of clinico-pathological disorders of various origin.

2. Transition to Sudanophilic Leukodystrophies

BIGNAMI et al. (1966) reported two sibling cases of infantile spasms, hypsarrhythmia and mental deterioration. In one of them study of the brain revealed diffuse vacuolation and demyelination of the cerebral white matter with amounts of sudanophilic products indicating sudanophilic leukodystrophy. Although spongy changes in the subcortex and Alzheimer type II glia were not observed, a nosological relationship of this type of sudanophilic leukodystrophy to SDI was suggested (PEIFFER, 1970).

3. Spongy Degeneration and Axonal Dystrophy

NAKAI et al. (1960) published the case of a 9-year-old boy who suffered from hypoplastic anemia from the ages of 8 to 26 months, and who later developed neurologic signs of cerebellar and brain stem dysfunction (24A). Necropsy showed testicular atrophy, renal cortical fibrosis and degenerative changes in the renal tubules with deposition of chromolipid pigment in the cells of the loops of Henle. Similar pigment was found in the basal ganglia and brain stem. Since there were demyelination and gliosis of the brain stem and spinal cord associated with multiple axonal "spheroids", especially in the cerebellum, this case was considered as "spastic amaurotic axonal idiocy" or late infantile neuroaxonal dystrophy (SEITELBERGER, 1957). Reexamination of this case, however, disclosed intense spongy lesions in the basal ganglia, cerebellum and brain stem associated with multiple axonal spheroids in the vacuolated areas (Fig. 6C), suggesting an association of spongy degeneration with axonal dystrophy. The nosological position of this case and its relationship to SDI, however, are not clear.

The most conspicucos finding in juvenile cases of SDI (60, 61, 72) was the presence of axonal dystrophy, mainly in the pallido-nigral system, which BRUCHER et al. (1968) considered to be consistent with the findings in the late infantile type of Hallervorden-Spatz disease. Additional axonal spheroids were seen in the spongy white matter (60, 61) where they have been previously noted in an infantile case (62).

Axonal dystrophy is the characteristic morphologic substrate of a group of degenerative disorders of the nervous system referred to as "neuroaxonal dystrophies", but it also has been found in various neurological and non-neurological diseases and experimental conditions (cf. JELLINGER, 1968; HERMAN et al., 1969). From statistical investigations it may be regarded as a "physiological" degeneration phenomenon in the CNS which might be enhanced by various conditions (JELLINGER, 1968). Since axonal dystrophy in SDI is mainly located in its constantly affected sites (globus pallidus, substantia nigra), this association is considered not to be incidental. Neither a combination of two different diseases, i.e. late infantile neuroaxonal dystrophy and SDI, nor merely "symptomatic" dystrophic lesions of the axons in SDI can be reasonably assumed. These axonal changes are rather suggested to be due to a premature and local enhancement of axonal dystrophy in protracted forms of SDI (JELLINGER and SEITELBERGER, 1969a). The underlying pathogenic factors are not understood.

B. Relationship to Other Spongy Encephalopathies

The occurrence of vacuolation of cerebral tissue, accompanied by variable loss of myelin without considerable degradation products and by a diffuse and conspicuous increase and hyperplasia of the astroglia, in itself is *not* unique to SDI but may be found in a variety of human disease states and experimental conditions. Attention has been drawn to the morphologic similarities between SDI and the CNS changes in inborn errors of amino acid metabolism and in certain toxic encephalopathies, both in man and animals, e.g. due to hepatic failure or administration of various chemical substances to animals, such as triethylin (TET), ouabain, hydrazine monoamino oxidase inhibitors (Iproniazid), isonicotinic acid hydrazide (INH) and Cuprizone. The ultrastructural and biochemical findings in these various experimental models of "spongy dystrophies" may offer some morphologenic and etiologic clues to the basis for the spongy lesions.

1. Hepatic Encephalopathies

The combination of spongy changes in gray and/or white matter and diffuse hypertrophy of astroglia with occurrence of Alzheimer type II — and type I — cells is common in encephalopathies associated with hereditary and acquired hepato-cerebral degeneration, hemochromatosis, exogenous liver disturbances and in porto-caval encephalopathies (f. ref. STADLER, 1936; ADAMS and FOLEY, 1953; ERBSLÖH, 1958; VICTOR et al., 1965; MOSSAKOWSKI, 1966; LAHL, 1967; ADAMS, 1968).

2. Inborn Errors of Amino Acid Metabolism

Although most of these genetically determined metabolic disorders reproduce in part the histological features of SDI, a specific pattern of CNS involvement could never be established. Vacuolation is usually accentuated in the myelinated portions of the neuraxis and often associated with loss of myelin or some deficiency in myelin formation without sudanophilic substances. Various degrees of gliosis with or without pale "naked" nuclei are present.

Spongy changes of the neuraxis have been observed in phenylketonuria, Maple syrup urine disease, hyperglycinia, homocystinuria (CHOU and WAISMAN, 1965), cystin-lysinuria, Lowe's syndrome, hyperammonemia, tyrosinemia, Oasthouse urine disease and β-alaninemia (DONOHUE, 1967). Vacuolation varies from case to case but appears to be most severe in hyperglycinemia, homocystinuria and Maple syrup urine disease, where the distribution of spongy lesions may closely resemble SDI. Similar changes, however, have been observed in inborn errors of carbohydrate metabolism, e.g. galactosuria (CROME, 1962) and lipid metabolism, such as Refsum's disease (PEIFFER and SOLCHER, 1966).

a) *Phenylketonuria*: The extent of the morphological changes in brains of patients with PKU ranges from spongy lesions of the white matter accompanied by astrocytosis and diffuse or focal loss of myelin (ALVORD et al., 1950; BENDA, 1952; POSER and VAN BOGAERT, 1959; BEHAR et al., 1965; MALAMUD, 1965) to extensive demyelination resembling sudanophilic leukodystrophy (CROME, 1962). Spongy demyelination has been found to be closely related with the age of the patients, suggesting that the early effect of PKU on the CNS is to induce vacuolation in the presence o fairly intact myelin, evoking a mild gliosis, and that in adults the changes are transformed into frank demyelination with sudanophilic products and intense gliosis (MALAMUD, 1965). ZELMAN et al. (1967) noted additional spongy necrosis of the gray matter resembling Alpers' disease.

Biochemical studies usually showed an increased water content and reduced lipid content (CROME et al., 1962; MENKES, 1966). The reduction of the myelin lipids, cerebrosides and proteolipid protein, exceeded the other lipid classes (MENKES, 1968; PRENSKY et al., 1968). Lipid defects correlated well with the degree of demyelination (GERSTL et al., 1966; CUMINGS et al., 1968) and were not associated with increase of esterified cholesterol. An additional disturbance of fatty acid composition of cerebrosides and sulfatides with a reduction of the ratio of the principal unsaturated fatty acids to the principal saturated fatty acids was found (FOOTE et al., 1965; MENKES, 1966; GERSTL et al., 1966; CUMINGS et al., 1968).

b) *Maple Syrup Urine Disease*: Diffuse spongy change of the white matter with astroglial hyperplasia and myelin loss without sudanophilic degradation products have been reported in "branched chain ketoaciduria" (SILVERMAN et al., 1961; CROME et al., 1961; DIEZEL and MARTIN, 1964; SCHMIDT et al., 1965; FEIGIN et al., 1968; SANDER et al., 1968). Focal spongy lesions were also present in the dentate nuclei and throughout the brain stem (SILVERMAN et al., DIEZEL and MARTIN, MARTIN et al., 1968) and in the subcortex (SCHMIDT et al., PEIFFER and SOLCHER, 1966; DAMBSKA et al.), while DANCIS et al. (1960) reported megalencephaly. Whereas MENKES et al. (1965) could not demonstrate any abnormality in lipid composition and structure in the spongy white matter, PRENSKY and MOSER (1966) and PRENSKY et al. (1968) reported elevated water content and reduction of total lipids in the white matter with preferential loss of cerebrosides and proteolipid protein. Marked increase of the branched-chain amino acids might be consistent with storage of crystallized proteins in glial cells and tissue vacuoles (DIEZEL and MARTIN, 1964).

c) *Hyperglycinia* (familial glycinosis) is characterized by CNS lesions similar to those in MSUD (DIEZEL and MARTIN, 1964). The spongy lesions affect the white matter without subcortical predilection but severe vacuolation of cerebellar white matter, dentate nuclei and brain stem nuclei (RUSHTON, 1968; ANDERSON, 1969). In the cases of DONOHUE (1967) the lesions were more severe and devastating than in any other case of spongy degeneration associated with inborn errors of amino acid metabolism.

d) *Homocystinuria*: In this condition, CHOU and WAISMAN (1965) reported widespread spongy degeneration of the neuraxis, the pattern of which was very similar to that seen in SDI.

e) *Other Conditions*: Spongy lesions in the brain stem were seen in familial cystin-lysinuria (MARTIN et al., 1968). In *Lowe's syndrome* they may be associated with widespread demyelination resembling sudanophilic leukodystrophy (HABIB et al., 1962; PASSARGE and McADAMS, 1967). In 3 necropsy cases of a progressive cerebral disorder associated with *hyperammonemia* (RETT, 1966), we found widespread vacuolation of the cerebral and cerebellar white matter and less severe spongy changes in the cortex and brain stem, associated with moderate diffuse increase in astroglia, fibrillary gliosis and moderate cortical lesions. There was but minimal loss of myelin without sudanophilic degradation products.

3. Encephalopathy in Infantile Dystrophy

In infants who have succumbed to endogenous intoxication or acute dystrophy, a definite increase in volume and weight of the brain is often noted (ALTEGOER, 1952). Nutritional loss usually caused irreversible nerve cell damage probably due to profound hypoglycemia. A general spongy appearance, with its preference for the cortico-subcortical junction and the lamina dissecans of the cerebellum, was identical to the findings in SDI. None of the children, however, had any of the unusual glia present in the latter disease.

In two prematurely born infants without neurological abnormalities who died from apnoeic episodes at the age of 6 and 24 days, ANDERSON (1969) detected spongioform lesions only in myelinated regions of the brain and spinal cord. There was generalized poverty of myelin showing a 20 to 34 % decrease compared with other infants at the same stage of gestation. It was accompanied by an excessive accumulation of non-phagocytic lipid-filled glial cells in the parts of the brain and spinal cord in which smaller numbers of such cells are normally found in newborn babies. The etiology of the spongy degeneration in these two infants is unknown.

4. Presenile Spongiform Encephalopathy

In this progressive disorder of the presenium which is believed to be identical with Jakob-Creutzfeldt disease, spongy lesions usually involve the deep cerebral cortex, the striatum and thalamus, while the brain stem and cerebellum are rather rarely affected (f. ref. MAY, 1968; COLMANT, 1968; MENOZZI and SCARLATO, 1969). Electron microscopically, this "spongy state" is chiefly due to marked swelling of astrocytes (MARIN and VIAL, 1964; GONATAS et al., 1964; FONCIN, 1967; KIDD, 1967; SLUGA and SEITELBERGER, 1967; TORACK, 1969), probably arising from expansion of the smooth endoplasmic reticulum (FONCIN, 1967). Occasional cytoplasmic vacuolation of neurons was reported (GONATAS et al., 1964; FONCIN), but neuronal degeneration is suggested to be secondary to glial disease (KIDD, 1967; SLUGA and SEITELBERGER, 1967), while RIBADEAU et al. (1969) discuss affection of both neuron and astroglia. SLUGA (1967) mentioned swelling of oligodendroglia.

5. Border Disease of Sheep

Infantile spongy degeneration of the CNS has some pathological similarity to Border disease of sheep. This is a congenital disorder with a nervous system lesion characterized by myelin poverty and astrocytic proliferation at all levels in the brain and spinal cord, preservation of axons and nerve cells, and, in lambs less than 6 months old, accumulation of sudanophilic lipids (HUGHES et al., 1959; BARLOW and DICKINSON, 1965). Spongy change of the white matter has not been described, but vacuolation within the lamellae of myelin sheaths is seen on electron microscopy (CANCILLA and BARLOW, 1968). In animals which survive, the lesion is ultimately repaired and consequently the myelin deficit is thought to be due to retardation of myelin formation rather than demyelination. Border disease has been found to be transmissible by the inoculation into pregnant ewes of extracts of tissue from affected fetuses and newborn lambs (DICKINSON and BARLOW, 1967; SHAW et al., 1967), indicating that an infective agent is operating during intrauterine life. This raises the possibility that at least some infants with spongy degeneration of the CNS may be suffering from a transmissible disease (ANDERSON, 1969).

6. Experimental Spongy Encephalopathies

a) *Triethyltin (TET) Intoxication:* A remarkable vacuolation of the neuraxis has been observed both in man (GRUNER, 1958) and animals. Spongy change, accompanied by marked increase in water, sodium and chloride content, is predominantly a white matter phenomenon due to intramyelinic vacuoles which are produced by splits in the central myelin (ALEU et al., 1963; LEE and BAKAY, 1965; KOLKMANN and ULE, 1967). These splits are always found between the intraperiodic lines and therefore can be considered to be analogous to the embryonic extracellular space since the intraperiodic line is formed by apposition of the external surface of the plasma membrane of the myelin forming cells (PETERS, 1960). These vacuoles are, however, not continuous with the extracellular space (ALEU et al., 1963; HIRANO et al., 1968) and the study using radioactive sulfate suggests no appreciable alteration of the brain extracellular space (KATZMAN et al., 1963). In gray matter, astroglial swelling is found. The ultrastructure of the capillaries is normal. Since the permeability of the BBB for vital dyes and large molecules is not affected (MAGEE et al., 1957; KATZMAN et al., 1963; BAKAY et al., 1965), the excess fluid is considered as an ultrafiltrate of plasma (KATZMAN, 1967; CLASEN et al., 1968).

b) *INH-Induced Encephalopathy:* Administration of isonicotinic acid hydrazide to dogs and ducklings induced spongy lesions of the CNS that was most severe in the cerebellar white matter and less affected the optic lobes and spinal cord (PALMER and NOEL, 1965; CARLTON and KREUTZBERG, 1966; LAMPERT and SCHOCHET, 1968). Vacuolation was associated with demyelination and occurrence of Alzheimer type II glia. The early ultrastructural changes consisted of the formation of vacuoles in or beneath the myelin sheath due to a split of the intraperiodic lines without apparent damage to glia (LAMPERT and SCHOCHET) or occasional vacuolation of astrocytes (ULE, 1968). The vessels remained impermeable to usual tracers (LAMPERT and SCHOCHET, WEGENER et al., 1968). In advanced stages proliferation of astroglia, removal of damaged myelin sheaths by phagocytes and increased permeability of the BBB were noted. Supplemental pyridoxine which had a protective effect in INH-induced neuropathy, could not prevent the development of cerebral spongy lesions (CARLTON and KREUTZBERG, 1966).

c) *Iproniazid — Induced Encephalopathy:* Spongy lesions following similar morphologic and distribution patterns were produced in chicks and ducklings by administration of Iproniazid (Marsilid), a potent inhibitor of monoamine oxidase (CARLTON, 1967b). The sites of predilection were the deep cerebellum and optic lobes. Similar lesions with different sites of predilection were induced in dogs by several monoamine oxidase inhibitors (PALMER and NOEL, 1963). Iproniazid has been found to produce fatty metamorphosis of the liver in experimental animals (CARLTON, 1967b).

d) *Cuprizone — Induced Encephalopathy:* Oral administration of cuprizone (biscyclohexanone oxalyldihydrazone), a chelator used as a reagent for copper analysis, produced a spongy change most prominent in the cerebellar white matter and brain stem of mice associated with a prominence of large pale glial nuclei (CARLTON, 1967a). Ultrastructural study showed the spongy lesions to be due to formation of vacuoles in the myelin sheaths between the intraperiod lines and also to vacuole formation in the cytoplasm of astrocytes and oligodendroglia (SUZUKI and KIKKAWA, 1969), a feature not seen in TET- and INH-induced encephalopathies. Slight alteration of the mitochondria in swollen astrocytes and degenerating neuronal processes were not similar to those found in SDI. The mice fed with cuprizone also had giant mitochondria and proliferation of smooth endoplasmic reticulum in the hepatocytes. As the lesions in the CNS and in the liver appeared almost simultaneously, it does not appear likely that the former are secondary to the latter.

e) *Ouabain — Induced Lesions*: Intracerebral injection of ouabain, a potent inhibitor of Na^+-K^+-activated ATPase, in addition to convulsions, produces another type of spongy change with swelling of glial cells and perinuclear vacuolation of neurons in the cerebral cortex (BIGNAMI and PALLADINI, 1965, 1966), rapidly progressing to subacute necrosis (PETSCHE and SEITELBERGER, 1967). Whereas the light optical changes are considered to be similar to the spongy state in Jakob-Creutzfeldt disease (BIGNAMI et al., 1967), at the ultrastructural level, there is no close correlation between these two disorders. CORNOG et al. (1967) reported marked swelling of astroglia and of certain presynaptic processes in the rat cortex, whereas neuronal perikarya, axons, dendrites and oligodendroglia were relatively unaffected in the earlier stages of the lesion.

f) *Lesions due to Methionine Sulfoximine*: Administration of this substance, which is suggested to inhibit glutamine synthetase, a membrane-bound enzyme primarily localized in non-cholinergic nerve endings (DE ROBERTIS et al., 1967), has been shown to produce convulsions and spongy changes of the CNS due to swelling of oligodendroglia (HARRIS, 1964) and particularly of astroglia (ULE, 1968) and presynaptic endings with clustering and loss of synaptic vesicles (DE ROBERTIS et al., 1967). Occasional swelling of postsynaptic dendrites and focal cytoplasmic vacuolation of neurons in the mouse rather than in the rabbit were reported by ULE (1968).

g) *Reversible spongy lesions in respiratory acidosis*: In experimental respiratory acidosis in cats caused by arteficial CO_2 respiration of one hour, which was associated with electrocerebral silence, SCHLOTE et al. (1969) reported spongy changes of the CNS due to generalized swelling of the postsynaptic components of neuronal dendrites, whereas the presynaptic dendrites, neuronal perikarya and astroglia were unaffected. Both the neurophysiological and ultrastructural lesions were completely reversible. The etiological background of this highly selective swelling of the postsynpatic dendrites is hitherto unknown.

A critical review of the aforementioned experimental forms of spongy encephalopathy indicates that, at the ultrastructural level, there is close relation between the changes in TET-intoxication and INH-induced encephalopathy and those observed in SDI. Therefore these two conditions are generally considered as useful *experimental models of the human disorder* (ADACHI and ARONSON, 1966; KOLKMANN and VÖLZKE, 1966; LAMPERT and SCHOCHET, 1968; REIN et al., 1968). As far as we know there are no biochemical studies suggesting a similarity between SDI and cerebral edema produced by the action of TET and INH, except for recent electrolyte analysis in two cases of SDI by KAMOSHITA et al. (1968). These authors demonstrated that the excess fluid accumulation in the white matter of the pathological brains had an electrolyte composition similar to plasma, whereas the electrolyte composition of gray matter was essentially normal in both cases. The widely held assumption that the edema fluid which accumulates in the brain is an ultrafiltrate of plasma is not supported by statistical evaluation with the exception of TET poisoning. The published data in all other types of cerebral edema indicate rather that the edema fluid contains a considerable lower concentration of sodium and chloride than serum (CLASEN et al., 1968). The similarity of the electrolyte composition of white matter in SDI and TET intoxication in conjunction with the ultrastructural findings are consistent with the assumption that similar basic processes might be operative in both disorders. Recent demonstration of ATPase deficiency in astrocytes of SDI strengthens the suggestion of a parallel between SDI and TET-edema. Cuprizone-induced encephalopathy, in addition to intramyelinic vacuolation and astroglial swelling comparable with the findings in SDI, is characterized by severe vacuolation of astroglia and hepatic changes which are not seen in human SDI. The other types of experimental spongy degeneration fail to show the intramyelinic vacuolation, so typical for SDI, and thus appear to have no close morphological relationship to this entity.

X. Pathogenetic Aspects

The cause and pathogenesis of SDI are still obscure. Four hypotheses have been advanced to explain the pathogenesis of the CNS lesions in this disorder.

The first theory is that chronic edema of the white matter is the primary pathological factor (VAN BOGAERT and BERTRAND, 1949) which leads to secondary destruction of myelin (MEYER, 1950).

BLACKWOOD and CUMINGS (1954) believed that edema alone could not account for the lowering of brain lipids, the amount of which was found to be identical to that in a 6 to 7 month fetus. They concluded that the fundamental fault in this disease is a failure in myelinic maturation. Later, VAN BOGAERT (1960) also suggested a disorder of myelogenesis which he believed to originate in an antenatal pathological process. ZU RHEIN et al. (1960) postulated that the water retained in the nervous tissue interfered with the normal process of myelination or that demyelination occurred when edema progressed into previously uninvolved but already myelinated area. SDI was believed to be a disorder of myelin synthesis because of the distribution of the myelin deficiency, the paucity of surviving myelin and the modest evidence of lipid degradation.

WOLMAN (1958) proposed that this disease is another variety of "diffuse cerebral sclerosis of the degenerative type". He suggested that a rapid catabolism of possibly abnormal myelin might be the primary event. He attributed the absence of the usual myelin breakdown products to its rapid turnover resulting in the production of increased amounts of low molecular weight substances which in turn, could cause adsorption and accumulation of water.

The fourth theory was advanced by FEIGIN and BUDZILOVICH (1966) who suggested that this type of spongy change of the CNS tissue is an artefact of autolysis secondary to glycogenolysis with agonal or postmortem release of CO_2. FEIGIN et al. (1968) demonstrated excessive glycogen in all cases of a series of infantile spongy degenerations except in LEIGH's disease. They also stated that the axons had been transected by the microcysts or gas bubbles and yet there were no swellings of spheroids. They believed this was evidence that the cysts had formed after death.

All of these theories were developed on the basis of indirect data combined with rather extensive speculation. Recent morphological and biochemical data have helped to narrow down the problem by eliminating some possibilities.

First of all, the new data do *not substantiate the interpretation of the spongy state as being the result of agonal or postmortem procedures*. From the findings in biopsy material from several cases of SDI and from current data on other spongiform encephalopathies in man and animals, the intravital production of the spongy degeneration, and hence, a valid basis for delineating SDI as a nosological entity is established beyond any doubt! The other theories mentioned above merit further discussion.

A. Chronic Edema

VAN BOGAERT and BERTRAND (1949) originally suggested that the basic morphologic picture of SDI is that of a chronic edema of the white matter. This assumption was supported by MEYER (1950) who felt that the spongy change represented a chronic edema of the cerebral tissue and that it was the result of inhibition by protein-rich liquid due to an abnormal permeability of the BBB. In favor of tissue permeation by an abnormal liquid he invoked the finding that, in addition to the spaces in the brain parenchyma, there was noticeable dilatation of the adventitial spaces of Held. He proposed that the condition should be named "chronic edema disease of the brain".

The enhanced weight of the brain, when considered in connection with the vacuolation and increased water content, suggests some parallelism between this disorder and cerebral edema. Current biochemical and ultrastructural findings add weight to the assumption that the characteristic spongy lesion in SDI is associated with "edema". In the deep cortex the excess fluid accumulate in the cytoplasm of astrocytes and in neuronal dendrites, while in the subcortical white matter intramyelinic vacuoles and swelling of astroglia without distension of the extracellular spaces are prominent. Thus we are dealing with an entity entirely different from the usual cerebral edema characterized by swollen astrocytic processes in the gray matter and by distended extracellular spaces in the white substance which primarily result from abnormal permeability of the BBB, and, hence, is referred to as the "vasogenic" type (KLATZO, 1967) or — more accurately — the "vasoglial" type of brain edema (JELLINGER, 1969). The ultrastructural changes in SDI are more akin to the findings in various experimental forms of "cytotoxic" edema in which *no primary hyperpermeabiltiy of the BBB* for vital dyes or macromolecules is recognized. The earlier implication of MEYER (1950) that in SDI edema was the result of an abnormal vascular permeability, therefore, has not been substantiated.

1. Myelin Swelling

The precise mechanism by which intramyelinic vacuoles develop in SDI and in any of the comparable experimental conditions is unknown.

Splitting of myelin sheaths at the intraperiodic lines has been observed in several unrelated conditions associated with fluid accumulation in the CNS. In addition to the edema produced by TET, INH, and cuprizone, these lesions have also been observed to a lesser degree in edema associated with glioma (ALEU et al., 1966; LONG et al., 1966), following silver nitrate implantation (HIRANO et al., 1965), cryptococcus polysaccharide implantation (GONATAS et al., 1964), asphyxia (VAN HARREVELD and KHATTAB, 1967), extradural balloon compression (RAIMONDI et al., 1962; LONG et al., 1966), trauma (SCHRÖDER and WECHSLER, 1965), and other forms of white matter edema (SLUGA, 1967). Therefore, vacuolation of myelin might be interpreted, at least in some instances, to be secondary to different types of edema.

In cerebral edema produced by epidural compression, TANI et al. (1969), in addition to a significant increase of sodium precipitates on the plasma membrane of the endothelial cell and on the internal surface of the astrocytic plasma membrane opposing the capillary, noted fine dense sodium precipitates in the myelin lamellae. They differed in appearance from dense precipitates on the plasma membranes of cellular compartments and in the intramyelinic clear space in TET poisoning.

It has been known for some years that TET acts as a powerful uncoupler of oxidative phosphorylation *in vitro* (ALDRIDGE, 1958) and that it causes inhibition of ATP *in vivo* (MOORE and BRADY, 1961). TORACK (1965) has demonstrated that TET inhibits a glutaraldehyde resistent Mg^{++}-activated, specific, Na^+-dependent ATPase which is normally present on most surface membranes, while no alteration in Na^+-Mg^{++}-dependent ATPase was noted in TET edema by KATZMAN et al. (1963). Electrolyte analysis in this condition showed marked increase of Na^+, Cl' and water content in the white matter (ALEU et al., 1963; SCHEINBERG et al., 1966). In TET poisoning, TANI et al. (1969) reported the occurrence of large amounts of Na^+-precipitates in the intramyelinic clear space and at its border, namely on the intraperiodic dense line. No significant increase of sodium precipitates was evident in other cellular compartments as compared with normal brain tissue. Since many of these precipitates may indicate the localization of the sodium necessary for the activation of Na^+-K^+-activated ATPase (KAYE et al., 1965; TANI et al., 1969), this was thought to indicate an alteration in this enzyme system. Since the myelin sheath is enzymatically relatively inactive (ADAMS, 1965) and shows no ATPase activity (TORACK, 1965; SLUGA and TOMONAGA, 1969), the sodium precipitates in the myelin sheath are believed not to be associated with any enzymatic structures. Recent data, however, indicate that whereas glial or Schwann intercellular clefts may not be critical barriers in solute exchange they may form a type of traffic bottleneck, at least for some ions. One has thus the impression that the spaces between cells of the ensheathment for nerve fibers are thoroughfares for solute movement (BUNGE, 1968). The demonstration of Na^+-K^+-activated ATPase at the membrane of the Schmidt-Lantermann clefts in the peripheral nerve (SLUGA and TOMONAGA, 1969) adds weight to the suggestion that this enzymatic ion-transport system may be present also at the periodic interruptions of central myelin at the nodes of Ranvier. Hence, an alteration in this enzyme system can be responsible for intramyelinic deposition of sodium and water.

The capacity of cerebral lipids to bind inorganic cations is of considerable significance in the maintenance of ion balance in normal brain tissue. When the lipids are extracted by organic solvents, they may remove up to 50 micro-Eq. of inorganic salts per gram of brain (MCILWAIN, 1966). It is conceivable that the separation of the intraperiodic line would either free previously bound cations or permit additional cations to be fixed by the newly exposed lipid. Under these circumstances the influx of water, rendering the salt solution isotonic, could result in vacuole formation within the myelin sheath (LAMPERT and SCHOCHET, 1968). Biochemical and ultrastructural data in TET-edema confirmed that there was no evidence of a connection between the intramyelinic vacuoles and the extracellular space, and the increase of sodium in the white matter was ascribed to a decrease of efflux of Na^+ (KATZMAN et al., 1963). WOLMAN et al. (1965) indicated that an excess of Na^+ in the medium was associated with lengthening of the *in vitro* myelin. In TET-intoxication and INH-encephalopathy, the split myelin was not interrupted through the full length and no change was seen in the periodicity of the myelin lamellae, indicating a marked increase in the length of myelin lamellae. It could be assumed, therefore, that in TET poisoning the sodium in the myelin sheath might be released and at the same time water might be formed from the hydrophilic group in myelin lamellae.

We are unaware of biochemical studies suggesting a similarity between the action of INH and that of TET. The group of hydrazines and hydroxylamines to which INH belongs, is known for its potent reactivity with carbonyl groups, for interference with the synthesis of nucleic acids, proteins and a lipid component in the membranes (cf. LAMPERT and SCHOCHET, 1968), and for inhibition of amine oxidases. In a recent discussion of amine oxidases, NARA and YASUNOR (1966) have cited references establishing that these enzymes are inhibited by both isoniazid and iproniazid, thus invalidating the older classification based on the apparent fact that monoamine oxidases are inhibited by isoniazid, but not by iproniazid. From the light optical identity of the lesions in INH-encephalopathy and those found after administration of various monoamine oxidase inhibitors, CARLTON (1967b) argued that the pathogenetic mechanism in the development of the neural changes may be the same in the two intoxications and may reside in the common biochemical activity of amine oxidase inhibition. Accumulation of substrates of amine oxidases (histamine, serotonine) appear to be especially toxic to the astroglia.

From currently available data it therefore remains speculative, whether the inhibition of ATPase or of another enzyme-dependent system by TET, INH or any other substance can produce focal intramyelinic accumulation of sodium ions and water associated with myelin split.

2. Astroglial Reactions

Besides the splitting of myelin sheaths, severe and widespread swelling of the astroglia and peculiar changes of astrocytic mitochondria characterize the ultrastructural picture of SDI. The diffuse hyperplasia of protoplasmic astroglia and the occurrence of Alzheimer type II cells present in almost all the reported cases suggest that an important component of the disease is a metabolic disorder of astroglia. Since the astrocytes are considered to play a key role in the fluid balance of the CNS (f. ref. FARQUHAR and HARTMANN, 1957; MUGNAINI and WALBERG, 1964; DE ROBERTIS, 1965; FRIEDE, 1966), GAMBETTI et al. (1969) argued that the astrocytes may be primarily responsible for the fluid accumulation in spongy degeneration, and the myelin swelling may be a secondary lesion.

The peculiar changes of astrocytic mitochondria with distension and distorsion of their cristae, striation of the matrix and chain-like arrangement of electron-dense granules with enzymatic abnormalities (decreased activity of ATPase and oxidative enzymes) seen in SDI probably indicate a biologic dysfunction of these organelles. Mitochondrial changes similar to those observed in SDI have been occasionally reported in different cells and unrelated conditions (cf. SUZUKI and MOSTAFI, 1967; CHOU, 1969; GAMBETTI et al., 1969), but, to the best of our knowledge, they have never been seen in normal or pathological conditions of the CNS other than the spongy degeneration.

Whatever the cause of the morphological alterations in the mitochondria, they must be related to disorders in the metabolism of the astroglia, since mitochondria are known to contain the organized enzyme systems of the Krebs citric cycle, electron transport, and oxidative phosphorylation, and many of these enzyme systems are located in the mitochondrial membranous system (LENINGER, 1964). In cerebral cortex it has been shown that 30 to 40%

of the energy produced by mitochondrial respiration is coupled to the so-called ionic pump, i.e. Na^+-K^+-dependent ATPase (WHITTAM and BLOND, 1964), which regulates the permeability of the plasma membrane to ions and water (SKOU, 1965; VAN HARREVELD, 1966). It can be speculated that, if the astrocytic mitochondria fail in their role of energy supply, a disturbance in the ionic pump mechanism could occur with resulting accumulation of fluid. Conversely, a long-standing impairment of the ionic pump could produce changes in mitochondria. The role and significance of the observed abnormalities of astroglial mitochondria, however, are uncertain at present.

It is proposed that astroglia are high-sodium cells (KATZMAN, 1961; HARTMANN, 1966), since it is known that, in general, the amount of membrane-bound ATPase is inversely proportional to the sodium content of the cell (SKOU, 1964). As pointed out by DAVSON (1963), however, high sodium cells would still presumably require the active removal of sodium to meet the requirements of Donnan equilibrium, and might even be expected to be unusually sensitive to inhibition of the sodium pump because any influx of sodium in such cells would not be even partly balanced by the efflux of potassium, as is the case with the high-potassium cell. Since a *deficiency of the ATPase activity in astrocytes* was noted in comparatively early stages of SDI (ADACHI et al., 1966; JOHNSON, 1970), it is possible that this *enzyme defect in the astroglia may be an important factor in the pathogenesis* of this rare disorder. No conclusions can yet be drawn as to whether this presumed astrocytic enzyme failure represents a primary lesion of SDI.

The significance of Alzheimer type II cells in SDI also remains uncertain. JERVIS (1942) expressed the opinion, based on the work of ROBACK and SCHERER (1935), that the peculiar morphology of these large astrocytic nuclei indicates an immaturity of the astroglia. According to KOLKMANN (1968), however, in SDI brains, the development of glia is not disturbed. In the younger patients the so-called myelination glia predominantes, whereas in the older cases mature glia is abundant. In three infants with spongy CNS lesions, one with hyperglycinemia, ANDERSON (1969) saw an excessive accumulation of non-phagocytic lipid-laden glial cells in the myelinated areas of the brain and spinal cord. In each of the three infants with spongy disease the quantity of lipid present was much greater than normal, yet it was found only within the normal distribution, and the morphology of the fat-containing cells was normal and was not that of phagocytic microglia. Other authors suggested that these nuclei represented the end products of a specific type of degeneration of astrocytes, and have mentioned the resemblance of these cells to Alzheimer type II glia seen in hepatic encephalopathies. Although several of the post mortem cases of SDI have shown some degree of fatty degeneration of the liver, none has had the degree of hepatic disease which would justify considering these glial cells as being secondary to liver disease. On the other hand, one may speculate that the pathologic process that affects the astroglia also involves the liver, but that the latter is less sensitive to the defect, whatever it may be, and reacts to a lesser degree in clinical cases of SDI.

It is of interest that unusual giant cells were noted in protracted cases of SDI in addition to Alzheimer type II cells. Since morphologic and enzymatic abnormalities were reported in the astroglia during the early stages of the disease, it might be conjectured that these giant cells are derived from Alzheimer type II astrocytes having abnormal intracellular metabolism (ADACHI and VOLK, 1968).

B. Pathogenesis of Myelin Destruction

In advanced stages of the disorder, a progressive increase in number and size of the vacuoles in the cerebral gray and white matter is associated with increasing megalencephaly and with myelin disintegration progressing to severe or almost complete myelin loss. Progressive degeneration and loss of the white matter in late stages of the disease are thought to be responsible for the decline of brain weight in more protracted cases. BANKER et al. (1964) attempted to establish a relationship between the intensity of the demyelination and the duration of the disease, but this appears possible only in few cases with a prolonged course (ADACHI and VOLK, 1968; BRUCHER et al., 1968; JELLINGER and SEITELBERGER, 1969a).

Since ultrastructural findings in progressive phases of the disorder are not available, the course and pathogenesis of myelin loss and other changes of the nervous parenchyma are not clear at present. From the demonstration of many ruptured myelin lamellae and astrocytic cell membranes and from the markedly increased extracellular spaces, even in earlier stages of the disease, ADACHI et al. (1966) argued that, in the protracted phase, the progressively increasing intracellular fluid subsequently overflows into the extracellular spaces. The increased extracellular fluid then spreads along the bundles of myelinated fibers into the deep white matter, in turn, causing degeneration of myelin and promoting destruction of the axonal fibers, thus contributing to the pathogenesis of the severe degeneration of the white matter in the terminal stage. Accordingly, GAMBETTI et al. (1969), saw occasionally empty myelin sheaths, suggesting advanced axonal degeneration.

Similar changes have been observed in severe and progressive stages of various types of cerebral edema in man and animals (ALEU et al., 1966; SCHRÖDER and WECHSLER, 1965; LONG et al., 1966; HIRANO et al., 1967). Light optical analysis of the course of lesions in the white matter and currently available ultrastructural findings in SDI, therefore, are in agreement with the hypothesis that *destruction of myelin is secondary to edema*.

This assumption has recently received strong support from biochemical findings. KAMOSHITA et al. (1968) investigated the chemical composition of the white matter and of isolated central myelin from two biopsy cases of SDI. There was a drastic loss of total lipid and proteolipid protein which is the chemical manifestation of severe myelin loss in these brains. No accumulation of small molecular weight products of myelin breakdown was found. These results did not substantiate WOLMAN's (1958) theory proposing that rapid catabolism of abnormal myelin might be the primary event. Furthermore, the yields and chemical abnormalities of the isolated myelin correlated well with the severity of the pathological changes in the white matter. These abnormalities consisting of reduction of proteolipid protein and of phosphatides and glycolipids, particularly of ethanolamine phosphatide and cerebroside were of the same nature as those found in the myelin of subacute sclerosing panencephalitis (SSPE), which was described as "typical of severe demyelination" (NORTON et al., 1966), and in certain types of cerebral lipidoses with severe white matter change (f. rev. SUZUKI et al., 1969); hence, they were considered to represent the transitional state of myelin undergoing non-specific secondary degeneration. Similar decrease in total phospholipids, ethanolamine phosphatides and cerebrosides was found in edematous white matter of human brains in connection with tumors or infarctions (YANAGIHARA and CUMINGS, 1968, 1969).

Conversely, the chemical composition found in the myelin of SDI was not that of normal immature myelin (SUZUKI et al., 1967, 1968) and these findings did not substantiate the theory of BLACKWOOD and CUMINGS (1954) suggesting a disorder of myelogenesis as the fundamental fault in this disease.

No information is available at present on the fatty acid composition of cerebrosides and sulphatides in brains of patients with SDI. In edematous areas of white matter, YANAGIHARA and CUMINGS (1969) found a decrease in C 24 non-hydroxy fatty acids of cerebrosides which they considered to be a reflection of early stages in secondary demyelination. A decrease in long chain fatty acids, including C 24, reported in cerebrosides and sulphatides in various types of leukodystrophies (O'BRIEN, 1964; GERSTL et al., 1965; MENKES, 1966), in SSPE (STÄLLBERG-STENHAGEN and SVENNERHOLM, 1965), etc. is thought to be non-specific and to be a consequence of demyelination (YANAGIHARA and CUMINGS, 1969).

The total ganglioside level in SDI was within normal range (KAMOSHITA et al., 1968). There was a slight increase in monosialo-gangliosides $G_{4, 5, 6}$ (according to the Korey system of nomenclature). Since similar changes have been found in brains of metachromatic leukodystrophy, so-called juvenile and adult lipidoses, Hurler's and Niemann-Pick's disease (SUZUKI et al., 1967; SUZUKI and CHEN, 1967), in SSPE (LEDEEN et al., 1968), and in Jakob-Creutzfeldt disease (SUZUKI and CHEN, 1966), these changes are considered to be non-specific.

The chemical abnormalities found in the myelin fractions of SDI are considered to be characteristic of myelin in the process of undergoing destruction due to nonspecific cause. It is suggested then that *myelin loss in SDI is secondary to water accumulation*. Neither the data presented by KAMOSHITA et al. (1968) in SDI nor those reported by YANAGIHARA and CUMINGS (1968, 1969) in human brain edema, however, can establish the possible causal relationship between the edema and myelin loss. The latter authors admit that they cannot conclude whether demyelination was caused by the same noxious stimulus which produced the cerebral edema, or whether demyelination occurred as the result of the cerebral edema.

C. Myelin Deficit in Other Spongy Encephalopathies

Current biochemical data in SDI do not substantiate the theory of BLACKWOOD and CUMINGS (1954) that the basic defect in this disorder might be the arrest of myelination at an early age, but, instead, give support to the assumption that myelin destruction in this disorder is non-specific and secondary to edema. Similar problems arise with regard to the pathogenesis of myelin loss associated with spongy degeneration in various inborn errors of amino acid metabolism. Two hypotheses have been suggested about this question:

The first theory proposed by ALVORD et al. (1950), SCHOLZ (1957), POSER and VAN BOGAERT (1959), FOOTE et al. (1965), DONOHUE (1967) a. o. suggests that the pathologic process is essentially one of retardation or arrest in development of myelin formation. This assumption is supported by the observation that sudanophilic myelin breakdown products are not prominent in these spongy dystrophies characterized by variable myelin loss. The degree of spongy change is supposed to be related to the degree of failure of myelination (RUSHTON, 1968). An excess accumulation of non-phagocytic lipid-filled glial cells associated with myelin poverty in spongioform areas of newborn infants also suggests that in infantile spongy disease of various etiology there is a diminished rate of incorporation of lipid into the myelinating brain (ANDERSON, 1969).

According to the second theory, proposed by MALAMUD (1966), the demyelinating lesions become more pronounced with advancing age and are due to myelin breakdown. Presuming that myelin destruction in SDI is nonspecific and secondary to edema, KAMOSHITA et al. (1968) would expect to find similar abnormalities in the myelin in genetic amidoacidurias. In samples of spongy areas from younger patients with PKU, GERSTL et al. (1967) found more moderate lipid defects with preferential deficits of cerebroside and cerebron acid, than they found in samples with severe demyelination from an older patient. This would support the view of CROME et al. (1962) of gradual demyelination and MALAMUD's theory of myelin breakdown. It should be stressed, however, that an absence of esterified cholesterol (CUMINGS et al., 1968) makes the latter seem unreasonable.

The first view has received support from biochemical findings by PRENSKY and MOSER (1966) and PRENSKY et al. (1968): In patients with MSUD and PKU, the myelin lipids, cerebroside and proteolipid protein, were reduced more profoundly than total lipids. In patients over one month of age, the greatest reduction was found in the proteolipid protein. From these data, it was suggested that an abnormality of amino acid metabolism diminishes the synthesis of proteolipid proteins which form part of the neurokeratin network of myelin, at a time when they are normally formed most rapidly, and that the resulting deficiency of proteolipids limits the formation of myelin. MENKES (1968) also postulated a reduction of the proteolipid fractions to result from the disorder in amino acid environment in PKU.

Recent studies suggest a mechanism by which high plasma levels of one or more amino acids could interfere with the synthesis of myelin. *In vitro*, high levels of phenylalanine or leucine in the surrounding media restrict the uptake of other essential amino acids in brain slices (NEAME, 1961); *in vitro* (APPEL, 1965) and *in vivo* (LINNEWEH and SOLCHER, 1965) the synthesis of protein is also reduced under these circumstances.

DAVISON and DOBBING (1966) have indicated that the vulnerable period in human myelination extends from the 7th month of intrauterine life into the first few months of postnatal life and that even small restrictions imposed during this period may cause permanent damage to the developing CNS. It would appear that inborn errors of amino acid metabolism may play an important role of disturbed myelination during this period (DAVISON, 1968).

These data support the belief that the cerebral white matter pathology in spongy degeneration associated with inborn errors of amino acid metabolism is, for the most part, restricted to the myelin membrane. It is concluded that there is a deficiency of myelin in the brain of untreated patients with MSUD and PKU which has been referred to as a delay in myelin formation. The data of PRENSKY et al. (1968), however, suggest that myelination is not merely delayed but interrupted. They further appear to indicate that, if the normal schedule of myelination is interrupted at a critical period and for a sufficient time, irreversible changes ensue.

Furthermore, the data reported by FOOTE et al. (1965), GERSTL et al. (1967), and CUMINGS et al. (1968) in PKU brain tissue suggest that there may be a disturbance in the build-up of long chain fatty acids from the shorter chain fatty acids. It is well known that the length of the fatty acid chains of cerebrosides and sulfatides increase during brain maturation (f. ref. O'BRIEN and SAMPSON, 1965; MENKES et al., 1966; PILZ, 1968). A disturbance of the intracerebral elongation process of both monounsaturated and saturated fatty acids from C-16 or C-18 to C-22 or C-24, however, was also seen in other demyelinating conditions (f. ref. GERSTL et al., 1967).

It is suggested that a disturbance of the elongation process of both monounsaturated and saturated fatty acids may prevail in PKU and in other inborn errors of amino acid metabolism. It is at least possible that the accumulation of abnormal levels of various metabolites in the early stages of these disorders affects enzymatic processes involved in the laying down of normal myelin in infancy, and thus is associated with the loss of cerebrosides and cholesterol found biochemically in these conditions. In contradiction to the view of KAMOSHITA et al. (1968) one may speculate that in congenital cases of SDI a similar interference of the hitherto unknown noxious agent with myelin formation takes place.

Reviewing the current date on the pathogenesis of myelin deficit in SDI and spongy encephalopathies associated with inborn errors of amino acid metabolism, it becomes obvious that further investigations of the CNS along both biochemical and ultrastructural lines are required before the nature of the earliest changes in myelin and their further evolution can be definitely established in these and related disorders.

D. Localization Problems

The cause of the typical localization and the spread of the spongy lesion in SDI and comparable spongy degenerations of the CNS is unknown. Its preferential site at the arcuate fibers is in accordance with the preferential site of cerebral edema of various origin. Since there is no longer any evidence to implicate serous inbibition due to a primary disorder of vascular permeability, the topographic pattern of spongy lesions cannot be determined by peculiarities of local angio-architectonic arrangement. Two problems arise in this respect. The first suggests some relationship with regard to location of the excess fluid to the ultraarchitectonic arrangement and density of the white and gray matter of the CNS (cf. HAGER, 1968) and its different biochemical peculiarities, especially the enzymatic composition of the nervous tissue (FRIEDE, 1966). The second — which is in some ways related to it — is concerned with determination of the fundamental mechanism which is responsible for this remarkable change.

The close relationship between biochemical architectonics of the CNS tissue and the action of a noxious agent to produce the topographic pattern of the resulting tissue lesion has been demonstrated in many examples of human and experimental neuropathology, particularly in anoxic and toxic conditions leading to strictly confined alterations (f. ref. FRIEDE, 1966; HIRANO et al., 1967; HAGER, 1968). However, it cannot be determined at present whether the tissue alterations result from a direct or an indirect action of the noxious agent on the neural tissue. The focal occurrence of spongy lesions resulting from myelin splitting after direct implantation of TET into the brain indicates that this agent produces its unique effect by *direct action* on neural tissue and not by any other indirect mechanism (HIRANO et al., 1968). In other comparable experimental disorders, it appears likely that both liver and CNS damage is produced simultaneously and directly by the noxious agents (SUZUKI and KIKKAWA, 1969), whereas encephalopathies associated with liver disease are considered to be secondary to the hepatic disorder. Since the morphological lesions in SDI are usually confined to the CNS, it seems reasonable to assume a *direct* action of the hitherto unknown etiologic agent on the neural tissue.

XI. Etiological Problems

While histologic features presently hold the key to clinical understanding of this disease, and biochemistry and electron microscopy have added important information toward understanding the pathogenesis of some of its characteristic lesions, the etiology of SDI remains enshrouded in mystery. Various researchers have pointed out the resemblance of pathologic features of SDI to those in inborn errors of amino acid metabolism. Yet studies of urine and serum for abnormalities of amino acid metabolism have been unrewarded. Other observers have considered the possibility of an inborn error of trace metal metabolism as the basis of this rare disorder (ZU RHEIN et al., 1960; SACKS et al., 1965) but exceptional elevations in the trace metal levels in urine or brain tissue have not been confirmed by other authors. Two currently available experimental models seem to reproduce the lesions found in SDI, that of TET poisoning and INH-induced encephalopathy. Whereas the pathogenesis of the latter condition is still uncertain, recent demonstration of ATPase deficiency in astrocytes of SDI strengthens the suggestion of a parallelism between this human disorder and TET-induced spongy lesions of the CNS which are considered to result from disturbance in the ionic pump mechanism. Yet, abnormal levels of tin have not been found in human cases. The significance of decreased enzyme activity, notably that of ATPase, in the mitochondrial matrix and in the membranes of astrocytes in two biopsy cases of SDI (ADACHI et al., 1966; JOHNSON, 1970) is not understood at present, nor can we say if they are primary or secondary changes, although the possibility of a biological dysfunction of the organelles must be considered. Isolation of the abnormal astrocytic mitochondria noted in SDI, study in their biochemical properties, and investigations on the Na-K-dependent ATPase in biopsy material from cases of SDI may provide further information on this problem. The familial nature and racial background of this disorder highly suggest a genetically determined metabolic abnormality which presumably affects mechanism involved in the energetic supply of those functional compartments of the CNS which are concerned with transcellular fluid and ion transport. At present while we may offer the hypothesis that some enzyme system (or systems) is congenitally deficient in SDI and that the same enzyme systems are inhibited or inactivated by TET and presumably by INH, we can offer no evidence whatsoever to substantiate this hypothesis. Until some biochemical alterations can be constantly demonstrated in this rare genetic disorder, the etiology of SDI must be left in abeyance.

Acknowledgements

We wish to express our gratitude to Dr. I. KLATZO, chief of the Laboratory of Neuropathology and Neuroanatomical Sciences, NINDB, Bethesda, Md., for the cases 25A and 26A, to Prof. G. PETERS, director of the Max-Planck-Institute of Psychiatry, Munich, for slides of case 48, to Dr. B. H. LANDING, Div. of Pathology, Children's Hospital, Cincinnaty, Ohio, for slides of case 24A, to Dr. M. ADACHI, Isaac Albert Research Institute of the Jewish Chronic Disease Hospital, Brooklyn, N.Y., for providing Fig. 13B, and to Dr. N. K. GONATAS, Dept. of Neuropathology, Univ. of Pennsylvania School of Med., Philadelphia, Pa, for providing Fig. 13A and for allowing us to reproduce Fig. 14, previously published by GAMBETTI et al. (Acta neuropath. 12, 103—115, 1969). We are further indebted to Prof. G. ULE, director of the Institute of Neuropathology, Heidelberg, for providing Fig. 15. We also thank Prof. H. ASPERGER, director of the Pediatric Clinic, Univ. Med. School of Vienna, and Doz. A. RETT, head of the Dept of Retarded Children, Lainz-Hospital, Vienna, for the clinical data of cases 57—60. Our thanks are due to Dr. WALTER C. BECK, visiting pathologist to the Neurol. Inst., for revising the English manuscript.

References

ABDEL-LATIF, A. A., BRODY, J., RAMAHI, H.: Studies on sodium-potassium adenosine triphosphatase of the nerve endings and appearance of electric activity in developing rat brain. J. Neurochem. 14, 1133—1141 (1967).

ADACHI, M., ARONSON, S. M.: Studies on spongy degeneration of the central nervous system (Van Bogaert-Bertrand type). In: Inborn disorders of sphingolipid metabolism (S. M. ARONSON and B. W. VOLK, eds.), p. 129—147. Oxford and New York 1966.

— VOLK, B. W.: Protracted form of spongy degeneration of the central nervous system (Van Bogaert and Bertrand type). Neurology (Minneap.) 18, 1084—1092 (1968).

ADACHI, M., WALLACE, B. J., SCHNECK, L., VOLK, B. W.: Fine structure of spongy degeneration of the central nervous system (Van Bogaert and Bertrand type). J. Neuropath. exp. Neurol. 25, 598—610 (1966).
ADAMS, C. W. M.: Neurohistochemistry. Amsterdam: Elsevier 1965.
ADAMS, R. D.: Hereditary hepatocerebral degeneration of Wilson-Westphal-Strümpell with reference to acquired hepato-cerebral degeneration. In: Zukunft der Neurologie, H. BAMMER (Hrsg.), p. 45—69. Stuttgart: G. Thieme 1967.
— Acquired hepatocerebral degeneration. In: Handbook of clinical neurology (P. J. VINKEN and G. W. BRUYN, eds.), vol. 6. Amsterdam: North Holland Publ. Comp. 1968.
— FOLEY, J. M.: The neurological disorders associated with liver disease. Ass. Res. nerv. Dis. Proc. 32, 198—237 (1953).
ALBERS, R. W., RODRIGUEZ DE LORES ARNAIZ, G., DE ROBERTIS, E.: Sodium-potassium activated ATPase and potassium-activated p-nitrophenyl-phosphatase. A comparison of their subcellular localization in rat brain. Proc. nat. Acad. Sci. (Wash.) 53, 557—564 (1965).
ALDRIDGE, W. N.: The biochemistry of organotin compounds; trialkyltins and oxidative phosphorylation. Biochem. J. 69, 367—376 (1958).
ALEU, F. P., KATZMAN, R., TERRY, R. T.: Fine structure and electrolyte analysis of cerebral edema induced by alkyl tin intoxication. J. Neuropath. exp. Neurol. 22, 403—413 (1963).
ALEU, F., SAMUELS, S., RANSOHOFF, J.: The pathology of cerebral edema associated with gliomas in man. Amer. J. Path. 48, 1043—1061 (1966).
ALPERS, B. J.: Diffuse progressive degeneration of the gray matter of the cerebrum. Arch. Neurol. Psychiat. (Chic.) 25, 469—505 (1931).
ALTEGOER, E.: Zur Morphologie und Genese des akuten Hirnödems bei ernährungsgestörten Säuglingen. Beitr. path. Anat. 112, 205—215 (1952).
ALVORD, E. C., JR., STEVENSON, L. D., VOGEL, ST., EGLE, L. R.: Neuropathological findings in phenyl-pyruvic oligophrenia (phenylketonuria). J. Neuropath. exp. Neurol. 9, 298—310 (1950).
ANDERSON, J. M.: Spongy degeneration in the white matter of the central nervous system in the newborn: pathological findings in three infants, one with hyperglycinaemia. J. Neurol. Neurosurg. Psychiat. 32, 328—337 (1969).
APPEL, S. H.: In vitro inhibition of brain protein synthesis: An approach to the molecular pathology of maple syrup urine disease and phenylketonuria. J. clin. Invest. 44, 1026—1035 (1965).
ARONSON, S. M., ARONSON, B. E., (eds.): Clinical neuropathological conference. Dis. nerv. Syst. 28, 828—835 (1967).
— LEWITAN, A., RABINER, A. M., EPSTEIN, N., VOLK, B. W.: The megalencephalic phase of infantile amaurotic familial idiocy. Arch. Neurol. Psychiat. (Chic.) 79, 151—163 (1958).
— VOLK, B. W.: Genetic and demographic considerations concerning Tay-Sachs disease. In: Cerebral sphingo-lipidoses (S. M. ARONSON and B. W. VOLK, eds.), p. 375—394. New York: Academic Press 1962.
AUSTIN, J., MCAFEE, D., SHEARER, L.: Metachromatic form of diffuse cerebral sclerosis. IV. Low sulfatase activity in the urine of nine living patients with metachromatic leukodystrophy (MLD): Arch. Neurol. (Chic.) 12, 447—456 (1965).
BAKAY, L., LEE, J. C.: Cerebral edema. Springfield, Ill.: C. C. Thomas 1965.
— — The effect of acute hypoxia and hypercapnia on the ultrastructure of the central nervous system. Brain 91, 697—706 (1968).
BANKER, B. Q., ROBERTSON, J. T., VICTOR, M.: Spongy degeneration of the central nervous system in infancy. Neurology (Minneap.) 14, 981—1001 (1964).

BARLOW, R. M., DICKINSON, A. G.: On the pathology and histochemistry of the central nervous system in Border disease of sheep. Res. Vet. Sci. **6**, 230—237 (1965).
BECHAR, M., BORNSTEIN, B., ELIAN, M., SANDBANK, U.: Phenylketonuria presenting an intermittent progressive course. J. Neurol. Neurosurg. Psychiat. **28**, 165—170 (1965).
BENDA, C. E.: Developmental disorders of mentation and cerebral palsies, p. 451 ff. New York: Grune & Stratton 1952.
BERNHEIMER, H.: Ganglioside im Liquor cerebrospinalis und Tay-Sachssche Erkrankung. Klin. Wschr. **46**, 258—261 (1968).
BIELSCHOWSKY, M.: Über Markfleckenbildung und spongiösen Schichtenschwund in der Hirnrinde der Paralytiker. J. Psychol. Neurol. (Lpz.) **25**, 72—100 (1919).
BIGNAMI, A., MARINACCI, F., ZAPPELLA, M., TINGEY, A. H.: Familial infantile spasms and hypsarrhythmia associated with leukodystrophy. J. Neurol. Neurosurg. Psychiat. **29**, 129—134 (1966).
— PALLADINI, G.: Subacute spongiform encephalopathy. An experimental study. Proc. Vth. Int. Congr. Neuropath. Excerpta med. I.C.S. **100**, 572—575, Amsterdam 1966 (a).
— — Experimentally produced cerebral status spongiosus and continuous pseudorhythmic electroencephalographic discharges with a membrane-ATPase inhibitor in the rat. Nature (Lond.) **209**, 413—414 (1966b).
— — APPICCIUTOLI, L., MACCAGNANI, F.: Etude expérimentale de la spongiose cérébrale. Acta neuropath. (Berl.), Suppl. III, 119—126 (1967).
BLACKWOOD, W., BUXTON, P. H., CUMINGS, J. N., ROBERTSON, J., TUCKER, S. M.: Diffuse cerebral degeneration in infancy (Alpers' disease). Arch. Dis. Childh. **38**, 193—204 (1963).
— CUMINGS, J. N.: A histological and chemical study of 3 cases of diffuse cerebral sclerosis. J. Neurol. Neurosurg. Psychiat. **17**, 33—49 (1963).
BOGAERT, L. VAN: Idiotie avec amaurose chez un enfant d'Israélites polonais en dehors de la maladie de Tay Sachs. J. belge Neurol. Psychiat. **39**, 470—471 (1939).
— Les dégénérescences spongieuses du système nerveux infantile. Deux aspects anatomo-cliniques particuliers. Wld Neurol. **1**, 396—408 (1960).
— Familial spongy degeneration of the brain. Complementary study of family R. Acta psychiat. scand. **39**, 107—113 (1963).
— BERTRAND, I.: Sur une idiotie familiale avec dégénérescence spongieuse du névraxe. Note préliminaire. Acta neurol. belg. **49**, 572—585 (1949).
— — Spongy degeneration of the brain in infancy. Amsterdam: North Holland Publ. Comp. 1967.
BONTING, S. L.: Na-K activated ATPase and active cation transport. In: Water and electrolyte metabolism, p. 35—68. Amsterdam: Elsevier 1964.
BRAUNMÜHL, A. VON: Alterserkrankungen des Zentralnervensystems. In: Handbuch der speziellen pathologischen Anatomie, Bd. XIII/1 A, S. 337—539. Berlin-Göttingen-Heidelberg: Springer 1957.
BRUCHER, J. M., DOM, R., ROBIN, A.: Dégénérescence spongieuse juvénile du système nerveux central. Ses rapports avec la maladie d'Hallervorden — Spatz et les dystrophies neuro-axonales. Rev. neurol. **119**, 425—444 (1968).
BUBIS, J. J., LUSE, S. A.: An electron microscopic study of experimental allergic encephalomyelitis in the rat. Amer. J. Path. **44**, 299—317 (1964).
BUCHANAN, D. S., DAVIS, R. L.: Spongy degeneration of the nervous system. A report of four cases with a review of the literature. Neurology (Minneap.) **15**, 207—222 (1965).
BUNGE, R. P.: Glial cells and the central myelin sheath. Physiol. Rev. **48**, 197—251 (1968).

CANAVAN, M.: Schilder's encephalitis periaxialis diffusa. Report of a child aged sixteen and one-half month. Arch. Neurol. Psychiat. (Chic.) 25, 229—308 (1931).
CANCILLA, P. A., BARLOW, R. M.: An electron microscopic study of the spinal cord in Border disease in lambs. Res. Vet. Sci. 9, 88—90 (1968).
CARLTON, W. W.: Studies on the introduction of hydrocephalus and spongy degeneration by cuprizone feeding and attempts to antidote the toxicity. Life Sci. 6, 11—19 (1967a).
— Iproniazid-induced encephalopathy in ducklings and chicks. Exp. molec. Path. 7, 133—144 (1967b).
— KREUTZBERG, G.: Isonicotinic acid hydrazide-induced spongy degeneration of the white matter in the brains of Pekin ducks. Amer. J. Path. 48, 91—105 (1966).
CHOU, S. M.: "Megaconial" mitochondria observed in a case of chronic polymyositis. Acta neuropath. (Berl.) 12, 68—89 (1969).
— WAISMAN, H. A.: Spongy degeneration of the central nervous system. Case of homocystinuria. Arch. Path. 79, 357—363 (1965).
CHRISTENSEN, E., HOJGAARD, K.: Poliodystrophia cerebri progressiva infantilis. Acta neurol. scand. 40, 21—40 (1964).
— KRABBE, K. H.: Poliodystrophia cerebri progressiva (infantilis). Arch. Neurol. Psychiat. (Chic.) 61, 28—43 (1949).
CLASEN, R. A., PANDOLFI, S., RUSSELL, J., STUART, D., HASS, G. M.: Hypothermia and hypotension in experimental brain edema. Arch. Neurol. (Chic.) 19, 472—486 (1968).
COLMANT, J. H.: Spongiöse Dystrophien. Verh. dtsch. Ges. Path. 52, 126—142 (1968).
CORNOG, J. L., JR., GONATAS, N. K., FEIERMAN, J. R.: Effects of intracerebral injection of ouabain on the fine structure of rat cerebral cortex. Amer. J. Path. 51, 573—590 (1967).
CROME, L.: The association of phenylketonuria with leucodystrophy. J. Neurol. Neurosurg. Psychiat. 25, 149—153 (1962).
— DUTTON, G., ROSS, C. F.: Maple syrup urine disease. J. Path. Bact. 81, 379—384 (1961).
— PARE, C. M. B.: Phenylketonuria. A review and report of the pathological findings in four cases. J. ment. Sci. 106, 862—883 (1960).
— TYMMS, V., WOOLF, L. I.: A chemical investigation of the defects of myelination in phenylketonuria. J. Neurol. Neurosurg. Psychiat. 25, 143—148 (1962).
CROMPTON, M. R.: Spongiform subacute necrotizing encephalomyelopathy. Acta neuropath. (Berl.) 13, 294—298 (1969).
CUMINGS, J. N.: Some lipid diseases of the brain. Proc. roy. Soc. Med. 58, 21—28 (1965).
— GRUNDT, I. K., YANAGIHARA, T.: Lipid changes in the brain in phenylketonuria. J. Neurol. Neurosurg. Psychiat. 31, 334—337 (1968).
DAMBSKA, M., SZELOZYNSKA, K., KAMRAJ-MAZURKIEWICZ, K.: Kliniczno-morfologiczne opracowanie przypadku choroby syropu klonowego. Neurol. Neurochir. Pol. 19, 323—326 (1969).
DANCIS, J., LEVITZ, M., WESTALL, R. G.: Maple syrup urine disease. Branched chain ketoaciduria. Pediatrics 25, 72—79 (1967).
DAVISON, A. N.: Myelination. In: F. LINNEWEH (hrsg.) Fortschritte der Pädologie, S. 65—87. Berlin-Heidelberg-New York: Springer 1968.
— DOBBING, J.: Myelination as a vulnerable period in brain development. Brit. med. Bull. 22, 40—44 (1966).
DAVSON, H.: The cerebrospinal fluid. Ergebn. Physiol. 52, 20—73 (1963).
DE ROBERTIS, E.: Some new electron microscopical contributions to the biology of neuroglia. Progr. Brain Res. 15, 1—11 (1965).
— ALBERICI, M., DE LORES ARNAIZ, G. R.: Astroglia swelling and phosphohydrolases in cerebral cortex of metrazol convulsant rats. Brain Res. 12, 461—466 (1969).

DE ROBERTIS, E., SELLINGER, O. Z., DE LORES ARNAIZ, G. R., ALBERICI, M., ZIEHRER, L. M.: Nerve endings in methionine sulphoximine convulsant rats, a neurochemical and ultrastructural study. J. Neurochem. 14, 81—89 (1967).

DE VRIES, E., BOGAERT, L. VAN, EDGAR, G. W. F.: Nouvelles observations d'idiotie familiale avec dégénérescence spongieuse des centres nerveux. (Maladie oedémateuse progressive cérébrale de la première enfance). Rev. neurol. 98, 271—295 (1958).

DICKINSON, A. G., BARLOW, R. M.: The demonstration of the transmissibility of border disease of sheep. Vet. Rec. 81, 114 (1967).

DIEZEL, P. B., MARTIN, K.: Die Ahornsirupkrankheit mit familiärem Befall. Virchows Arch. path. Anat. 337, 425—445 (1964).

— — Hyperglycinämie (Glycinose) mit familiärer idiopathischer Hyperglycinurie. Dtsch. med. Wschr. 91, 2249—2254 (1966).

DONOHUE, W. L.: Lesions in the CNS associated with inborn errors of amino acid metabolism. Acta paediat. (Uppsala) 56, 116—117 (1967).

DREIFUSS, F. E., NETSKY, M. G.: Progressive poliodystrophy. The degeneration of cerebral gray matter. Amer. J. Dis. Child. 107, 649—656 (1964).

EISELSBERG, F.: Über frühkindliche familiäre diffuse Hirnsklerose. Z. Kinderheilk. 58, 702—725 (1937).

ERBSLÖH, F.: Das Zentralnervensystem bei Leberkrankheiten. In: Handbuch der speziellen pathologischen Anatomie und Pathologie, Bd. XIII/2B, S. 1645—1698. Berlin-Göttingen-Heidelberg: Springer 1958.

FAHN, S., COTE, L. J.: Regional distribution of sodium-potassium activated adenosine triphosphatase in the brain of the Rhesus monkey. J. Neurochem. 15, 433—436 (1968).

FARQUHAR, M. D., HARTMANN, J. F.: Neuroglial structure and relationships as revealed by electron microscopy. J. Neuropath. exp. Neurol. 16, 18—39 (1957).

FEIGIN, I., BUDZILOVICH, G.: The spongy state: a form due to the agonal or postportem evolution of gaseous carbon dioxide from glycogen. Acta neuropath. (Berl.) 7, 136—148 (1966).

— PENA, C. E., BUDZILOVICH, G.: The infantile spongy degenerations. Neurology (Minneap.) 18, 153—167 (1968).

FISCHER, O.: Der spongiöse Rindenschwund, ein besonderer Destruktionsprozeß der Hirnrinde. Z. ges. Neurol. Psychiat. 7, 1—33 (1911).

FONCIN, J. F.: Electron microscopic observations in Creutzfeldt-Jakob disease. In: Brain edema (I. KLATZO and F. SEITELBERGER, eds.), p. 171—177. Vienna and New York: Springer 1967.

— GACHES, J., LE BEAU, J.: Encéphalopathie spongiforme (Biopsie, étudiée au microscope électronique; confirmation autopsique). Rev. neurol. 111, 507—515 (1964).

FOOTE, J. L., ALLEN, R. J., AGRANOFF, B. W.: Fatty acids in esters and cerebrosides of human brain in phenylketonuria. J. Lipid Res. 6, 518—524 (1965).

FORD, F. R., LIVINGSTON, S., PRYLES, C. V.: Familial degeneration of the cerebral gray matter in childhood, with convulsions, myoclonus, spasticity, cerebellar ataxia, choreoathetosis, dementia, and death in status epilepticus. Differentiation on infantile and juvenile types. J. Pediat. 39, 33—43 (1951).

FRIEDE, R. L.: Topographic brain chemistry. New York: Academic Press 1966.

— JONG, R. DE: Neuronal enzyme failure in Creutzfeldt-Jakob disease. Arch. Neurol. (Chic.) 10, 181—195 (1964).

GABURRO, D., MARTIN, J. J., SCARPA, P., VOLPONE, S.: Forme congénitale de la dégénérescence spongieuse familiale. Rev. neurol. 112, 15—29 (1965).

GAMBETTI, P., MELLMANN, W. J., GONATAS, N. K.: Familial spongy degeneration of the central nervous system (van Bogaert-Bertrand disease). An ultrastructural study. Acta neuropath. (Berl.) 12, 103—115 (1969).

GERSTL, B., MALAMUD, N., ENG, L. F., HAYMAN, R. B.: Lipid alterations in human brains in phenylketonuria. Neurology (Minneap.) 17, 51—58 (1967).
— — HAYMAN, R. B., BOND, P. R.: Morphological and neurochemical study of Pelizaeus-Merzbacher disease. J. Neurol. Neurosurg. Psychiat. 28, 540—547 (1965).
GLOBUS, J. H., STRAUSS, I.: Progressive degenerative subcortical encephalopathy (Schilder's disease). Arch. Neurol. Psychiat. (Chic.) 20, 1190—1228 (1928).
GONATAS, N. K., TERRY, R. D., WEISS, M.: Electron microscopic study in two cases of Jakob-Creutzfeldt disease. J. Neuropath. exp. Neurol. 24, 575—598 (1964).
— ZIMMERMAN, H. M., LEVINE, S.: Ultrastructure of inflammation with edema in the rat brain. Amer. J. Path. 42, 455—469 (1963).
GREENHOUSE, A. H., NEUBUERGER, K. T.: The syndrome of progressive cerebral poliodystrophy. Arch. Neurol. (Chic.) 10, 46—57 (1964).
GRUNER, J. E.: Lésions du névraxe secondaires à l'ingestion d'éthyl-étain (Stalinon). Rev. neurol. 98, 109—116 (1958).
HABIB, R., BARGETON, E., BRISSAUD, H. E., RAYNAUD, J., LE BALL, J. C.: Constatations anatomiques chez un enfant atteint d'un syndrome de Lowe. Arch. franç. Pédiat. 19, 945—960 (1962).
HAGER, H.: Allgemeine morphologische Pathologie des Nervengewebes. In: Handbuch der allgemeinen Pathologie, Bd. III/3. Berlin-Heidelberg-New York: Springer 1968.
— Morphological compartments in the central nervous system. In: Brain edema (I. KLATZO and F. SEITELBERGER, eds.), p. 285—302. Vienna and New York: Springer 1967.
HALLERVORDEN, J.: Die degenerative diffuse Sklerose. 2. Diffuse Sklerose mit Beziehung zum Hirnödem. In: Handbuch der speziellen pathologischen Anatomie und Histologie, Bd. XIII/1A, S. 770—773. Berlin-Göttingen-Heidelberg: Springer 1957.
HARREVELD, A. VAN: Brain tissue electrolytes. Washington: Butterworths 1968.
— KHATTAB, F. I.: Electron microscopy of asphyxiated spinal cords of cats. J. Neuropath. exp. Neurol. 26, 521—536 (1967).
HARRIS, B.: Cortical alterations due to methionine sulfoximine. Arch. Neurol. (Chic.) 11, 388—407 (1964).
HARTMANN, J. F.: High sodium content of cortical astrocytes. Arch. Neurol. (Chic.) 15, 633—642 (1966).
HENN, R., GERKEN, H., WIEDEMANN, H.-R.: Über die cerebrale Ödemkrankheit des frühen Kindesalters. Z. Kinderheilk. 93, 277—292 (1965).
HERMAN, M. M., HUTTENLOCHER, P. R., BENSCH, K. G.: Electron microscopic observations in Infantile Neuroaxonal Dystrophy. Arch. Neurol. (Chic.) 20, 19—34 (1969).
HIRANO, A., LEVINE, S., ZIMMERMAN, H. M.: Experimental cyanide encephalopathy. Electron microscopic observations of early lesions in white matter. J. Neuropath. exp. Neurol. 26, 200—213 (1967).
— ZIMMERMAN, H. M., LEVINE, S.: The fine structure of cerebral fluid accumulation. IX. Edema following silver nitrate implantation. Amer. J. Path. 47, 537—548 (1965).
— — — Myelin in the CNS as observed in experimentally induced edema in the rat. J. Cell. Bioll 31, 397—411 (1966).
— — — Fine structure of cerebral fluid accumulation. X. A review of experimental edema in white matter. In: Brain edema (I. KLATZO and F. SEITELBERGER, eds.), p. 569—589. Vienna and New York: Springer 1967.
— — — Intramyelinic and extracellular spaces in triethyl tin intoxication. J. Neuropath. exp. Neurol. 27, 571—580 (1968).

HIRNER, A.: Elektronenmikroskopische Untersuchungen zur formalen Genese der Balkenläsionen nach experimenteller Cyanvergiftung. Acta neuropath. (Berl.) 13, 350—368 (1969).

HOGAN, G. R., RICHARDSON, E. P., JR.: Spongy degeneration of the nervous system (Canavan's disease). Report of a case in an Irish-American family. Pediatrics 35, 284—294 (1965).

HOOFT, C., VALCKE, R., HERPOL, J., BOGAERT, L. VAN, GUAZZI, G. C.: Neurologie et neuropathologie du syndrome de Lowe: J. neurol. Sci. 3, 353—373 (1966).

HUGHES, L. E., KERSHAW, G. F., SHAW, I. G.: "B" or border disease. Vet. Rec. 71, 313—317 (1959).

HYDEN, H.: The neuron and its glia- a biochemical and functional unit. Endeavour 1962, 144—155.

ISHINO, H., GUAZZI, G. C., BOGAERT, L. VAN: Histoire naturelle de l'état spongieux. Sa significance en cytopathologie optique. Arch. Psychiat. Nervenkr. 211, 289—307 (1968).

JELLINGER, K.: Neuroaxonale Dystrophien. Verh. dtsch. Ges. Path. 52, 92—126 (1968).

— Morphologische und pathogenetische Aspekte beim Hirnödem. Referat Symposium Österr. A. G. Angiologie, 1. 3. 1969.

— Glio-neuronal dystrophy in infancy and childhood. Joint Meet. British. Austrian and Swiss Neuropathologists, Gstaad, Jan. 29.—31. 1970.

— SEITELBERGER, F.: Different types of infantile encephalopathy. Proc. Ist. Congr. Int. Assoc. Sci. Stud. Ment. Deficiency, Montpellier 1967, p. 950—951. Surrey: Jackson Publ. Comp. 1968.

— — Juvenile form of spongy degeneration of the CNS. Acta neuropath. (Berl.) 13, 276—281 (1969a).

— — Pelizaeus-Merzbacher disease. Acta neuropath. (Berl.) 14, 108—117 (1969b).

— — Subacute necrotizing encephalomyelopathy (Leigh). Erg. inn. Med. Kinderheilk., N. F. 29, 155—219 (1970).

JERVIS, G. A.: Early infantile diffuse sclerosis of the brain (Krabbe's type). Report of two cases with a view of the literature. Amer. J. Dis. Child. 64, 1055—1072 (1942).

— Pers. Commun. to B. Q. BANKER (1964).

JOHNSON, A. B.: Deficiency of ATPase-positive astrocytic processes in spongy degeneration of the nervous system (Canavan's disease). Abstr. 45th. Ann. Meet. Amer. Ass. Neuropath. June 20—22, 1969, p. 22—23.

KAMOSHITA, S., REED, G. B., JR., AGUILAR, M. J.: Axonal dystrophy in a case of Canavan's spongy degeneration. Neurology (Minneap.) 17, 895—898 (1967).

— RAPIN, I., SUZUKI, K., SUZUKI, K.: Spongy degeneration of the brain: A chemical study of two cases including isolation and characterization of myelin. Neurology (Minneap.) 18, 975—985 (1968).

KANOFF, A., ARONSON, S. M., VOLK, B. W.: Clinical progression of amaurotic familial idiocy. Anthropometric studies. Amer. J. Dis. Child. 97, 656—662 (1959).

KATZMAN, R.: Electrolyte distribution in mammalian central nervous system. Are glia high sodium cells? Neurology (Minneap.) 11, 27—36 (1961).

— Effect of electrolyte distribution on the central nervous system. Rev. Med. 17, 197—212 (1966).

— Biochemical correlates of cerebral edema. In: Brain edema (I. KLATZO and F. SEITELBERGER, eds.), p. 461—467. Vienna and New York: Springer 1967.

— ALEU, F., WILSON, C.: Further observations on triethyltin edema. Arch. Neurol. (Chic.) 9, 178—187 (1963).

KAYE, G. I., COLE, J. D., DON, A.: Electron microscopy: Sodium localization in normal and ouabain-treated cells. Science 150, 1167—1168 (1965).

KIDD, M.: Some electron microscopical observations on status spongiosus. Acta neuropath. (Berl.), Suppl. III, 137—144 (1967).
KLATZO, I.: Neuropathological aspects of brain edema. J. Neuropath. exp. Neurol. 26, 1—14 (1967).
— SEITELBERGER, F. (eds.): Brain edema. Vienna and New York: Springer 1967.
KLEIN, H., DICHGANS, J.: Familiäre juvenile glio-neurale Dystrophie. Akut beginnende progressive Encephalopathie mit rechtsseitigen occipito-parietalen Herdsymptomen und Status epilepticus. Arch. Psychiat. Nervenkr. 121, 400—422 (1969).
KNUDSON, A. G., JR., KAPLAN, W. D.: Genetics of the spingolipidoses. In: Cerebral sphingolipidoses (S. M. ARONSON and B. W. BOLK, eds.), p. 395—411. New York: Academic Press 1962.
KOLKMANN, W.: Gliabefunde bei den diffusen und fokal-disseminierten Formen der spongiösen Neurodystrophien des frühen Kindesalters. Acta neuropath. (Berl.), Suppl. IV, 105—108 (1968).
— u. R. A. OKPARA: Über die Ultrastruktur der Striatumveränderungen bei der Natriumazid-Vergiftung der Ratte. Virchows Arch. Abt. A 349, 179—194 (1970).
— ULE, G.: Tin poisoning edema. In: Brain edema (I. KLATZO and F. SEITELBERGER, eds.), p. 530—535. Vienna and New York: Springer 1967.
— VÖLZKE, E.: Über die spongiösen Dystrophien des Nervensystems im frühen Kindesalter. I. Die diffuse Form: Typ Canavan. Z. Kinderheilk. 97, 222—239 (1966).
KOREY, S. R., GONATAS, J.: Separation of human brain gangliosides. Life Sci. 2, 296 (1963).
LAHL, R.: Zur Häufigkeit astrozytärer Gliaveränderungen ("Leberglia") bei hepatogenen Erkrankungen, insbesondere Leberzirrhosen, und ihre Abhängigkeit vom Funktionszustand des Organs. Zbl. allg. Path., path. Anat. 110, 518—545 (1967).
LAKE, B. D.: Segmental demyelination of peripheral nerves in Krabbe's disease. Nature (Lond.) 217, 171—172 (1968).
LAMPERT, P. W., EARLE, K. M., GIBBS, C. J., JR., GAJDUSEK, D. C.: Experimental Kuru encephalopathy in chimpanzees and spider monkeys: electron microscopic studies. J. Neuropath. exp. Neurol. 28, 353—370 (1969).
— FOX, J., EARLE, K.: Cerebral edema after Laser radiation. J. Neuropath. exp. Neurol. 25, 531—541 (1966).
— SCHOCHET, S. S., JR.: Electron microscopic study on experimental spongy degeneration of the cerebellar white matter. J. Neuropath. exp. Neurol. 27, 210—220 (1968).
LAURENCE, K. M., CAVANAGH, J. B.: Progressive degeneration of the cerebral cortex in infancy. Brain 91, 261—280 (1968).
LEDEEN, R., SALSMAN, K., CABRERA, M.: Gangliosides in subacute sclerosing leukoencephalitis: isolation and fatty acid composition of nine fractions. J. Lipid Res. 9, 129—136 (1968).
LEE, J. C., BAKAY, L.: Ultrastructural changes in the edematous central nervous system. I. Triethyltin edema. Arch. Neurol. (Chic.) 13, 48—57 (1965).
LEES, M. B., FOLCH-PI, J.: A study of some human brains with pathological changes. In: Chemical pathology of the nervous system (J. FOLCH-PI, ed.), p. 75—82. New York: Pergamon Press 1961.
LEIGH, D.: Subacute necrotizing encephalomyelopathy in an infant. J. Neurol. Neurosurg. Psychiat. 14, 216—221 (1951).
LENINGER, A. L.: The mitochondrion. New York: W. A. Benjamin Inc. 1964.
LING, C. V. M., ABDEL-LATIF, A. A.: Studies on sodium transport in rat brain nerve-ending particles. J. Neurochem. 15, 721—729 (1968).
LINNEWEH, F., SOLCHER, H.: Über den Einfluß diätetischer Prophylaxe auf die Myelogenese bei der Leucinose (maple syrup disease). Klin. Wschr. 43, 926—930 (1965).
LONG, D. M., HARTMANN, J. F., FRENCH, L. E.: The ultrastructure of human cerebral edema. J. Neuropath. exp. Neurol. 25, 373—395 (1966).

Lüers, Th., Spatz, H.: Picksche Krankheit. In: Handbuch der speziellen pathologischen Anatomie und Histologie, Bd. XIII/1 A, S. 614—715. Berlin-Göttingen-Heidelberg: Springer 1957.

Magee, P. N., Stoner, H. B., Barnes, J. M.: Experimental production of oedema in the central nervous system of the rat by triethyltin compounds. J. Path. Bact. **73**, 107—124 (1957).

Malamud, N.: Neuropathology of phenylketonuria. J. Neuropath. exp. Neurol. **25**, 254—268 (1966).

Marin, O., Vial, J. D.: Neuropathological and ultrastructural findings in two cases of subacute spongiform encephalopathy. Acta neuropath. (Berl.) **4**, 218—229 (1964).

Martin, J. J., Bogaert, L. van, Guazzi, G. C.: Déterminations cérébrales des amino-aciduries. Confin. neurol. **30**, 97—111 (1968).

Maxwell, D. E., Kruger, L.: The reactive oligodendrocyte. An electron microscopic study of cerebral cortex following alpha particle irradiation. Amer. J. Anat. **118**, 437—459 (1966).

May, W. W.: Creutzfeldt-Jakob disease. Survey of the literature and clinical diagnosis. Acta neurol. scand. **44**, 1—32 (1968).

McIlwain, H.: In: Biochemistry and the central nervous system. Boston: Little, Brown & Co., 3rd edit. 1966.

Menkes, J. H.: Cerebral lipids in phenylketonuria. Pediatrics **37**, 967—978 (1966).
— The pathogenesis of mental retardation in phenylketonuria and other inborn errors of amino-acid metabolism. Pediatrics **39**, 297—308 (1967).
— Cerebral proteolipids in phenylketonuria. Neurology (Minneap.) **18**, 1003—1008 (1968).
— Phillippart, H., Fiol, R. E.: Cerebral lipids in maple syrup disease. J. Pediat. **66**, 584—594 (1965).

Menozzi, C., Scarlato, G.: La malattia di Jakob-Creutzfeldt. Arch. Suisse Neurol. **103**, 47—91 (1969).

Meyer, J. E.: Über eine „Ödemkrankheit" des Zentralnervensystems im frühen Kindesalter. Arch. Psychiat. Nervenkr. **185**, 35—51 (1950).

Morcaldi, L., Salvati, G., Giordano, G. G., Guazzi, G. C.: Idiotie spongieuse familiale (van Bogaert-Bertrand) du type congénital dans une souche non-Juive. Acta Genet. med. (Roma) **18**, 142—157 (1969).

Morse, W. I.: Hereditary myoclonus epilepsy. Two cases with pathological findings. Bull. Johns Hopk. Hosp. **84**, 116—133 (1949).

Mossakowski, M. J.: Some aspects of the morphology and histochemistry of the cerebral changes in hepatic coma. Proc. Vth. Int. Congr. Neuropath., p. 981—986. Exc. Med. I.C.S. 100, Amsterdam-New York-London 1966.

Mugnaini, E., Walberg, F.: Ultrastructure of neuroglia. Ergebn. Anat. Entwickl.-Gesch. **37**, 194—236 (1964).

Nakai, H., Landing, B. H., Schubert, W. K.: Seitelberger's spastic amaurotic axonal idioty. Report of a case in a 9-year-old boy with comment on visceral manifestations. Pediatrics **25**, 441—449 (1960).

Nara, S., Yasunor, K. T.: Some recent advances in the field of amine oxidases. In: Biochemistry of copper (J. Persach, P. Aisen, and W. E. Blumberg, eds.), p. 423—441. New York: Academic Press 1966.

Neame, K. D.: Phenylalanine as inhibitor of transport of amino acids in brain. Nature (Lond.) **192**, 173 (1961).

Nelson, E., Aurebeck, G.: Electron microscopic observations on the leukodystrophies. Proc. Vth Int. Congr. Neuropath., p. 838—841. Exc. Med. ICS Nr. 100, Amsterdam-New York-London 1966.

Norton, W. R., Poduslo, S. E., Suzuki, K.: Subacute sclerosing leukoencephalitis. II. Chemical studies including abnormal myelin and abnormal ganglioside pattern. J. Neuropath. exp. Neurol. **25**, 582—597 (1966).

O'Brien, J. S.: A molecular defect of myelination. Biochem. biophys. Res. Commun. 15, 484—490 (1964).
— Sampson, E. L.: Fatty acid and fatty aldehyde composition of the major brain lipids in normal human gray matter and myelin. J. Lipid Res. 6, 545—551 (1965).
O'Leary, J. L., Harris, A. B., Fox, R. R., Smith, J. M., Tidwell, M.: Ultrastructural lesions in rabbit hereditary ataxia. Arch. Neurol. (Chic.) 13, 238—262 (1965).
Palmer, A. C., Noel, P. R.: Neuropathological effects of prolonged administration of some hydrazine monoamine oxidase inhibitors in dogs. J. Path. Bact. 86, 463—476 (1963).
— — Neuropathological effects of dosing dogs with isonicotinic hydrazid and with its methanosulphonate. Nature (Lond.) 205, 506—507 (1965).
Pant, S. S., Ashbury, A. K., Richardson, E. P., Jr.: The myelopathy of pernicious anemia. A neuropathological reappraisal. Acta neurol. scand., 44, Suppl. 35 (1968).
Passarge, E., McAdams, A. J.: Cerebro-hepato-renal syndrome. A newly recognized hereditary disorder of multiple congenital defects, including sudanophilic leukodystrophy, cirrhosis of the liver, and polycystic kidneys. J. Pediat. 71, 691—702 (1967).
Peiffer, J.: Orthochromatic leukodystrophies. In: Handbook of clinical neurology. (P. J. Vinken and G. W. Bruyn, eds.), vol. 10. Amsterdam: North Holland Publ. Comp. (1970).
— Solcher, H.: Zur Morphologie der Ahornsirupkrankheit. Proc. Vth. Int. Congr. Neuropath., Exc. Med., ICS Nr. 100, p. 164—167. Amsterdam-New York-London 1966.
Percy, A. K., Brady, R. O.: Metachromatic leukodystrophy: Diagnosis with samples of venous blood. Science 161, 594 (1968).
Peters, A.: The structure of myelin sheaths in the central nervous system of Xenopus laevis (Daudin): J. biophys. biochem. Cytol. 7, 121—126 (1960).
Petsche, H., Seitelberger, F.: Hirnelektrische Tätigkeit und Rindenstruktur. Wien. klin. Wschr. 79, 492—496 (1967).
Pilz, H.: Dünnschichtchromatographische Lipoidstudien von normalem Hirngewebe und Myelin des Menschen. Dtsch. Z. Nervenheilk. 194, 150—166 (1968).
Poser, C. M., Bogaert, L. van: Neuropathological observations in phenylketonuria. Brain 82, 1—9 (1959).
Prensky, A. L., Carr, S., Moser, H. W.: Development of myelin in inherited disorders of amino acid metabolism. A biochemical investigation. Arch. Neurol. (Chic.) 19, 552—558 (1968).
— Moser, H. W.: Brain lipids, proteolipids, and free amino acids in maple syrup urine disease. J. Neurochem. 13, 863—874 (1966).
Raimondi, A. J., Evans, J. P., Mullan, S.: Studies of cerebral edema. III. Alteration in white matter: electron microscopic study using ferritin as labelin compound. Acta neuropath. (Berl.) 2, 177—197 (1962).
Rapin, I., Suzuki, K., Suzuki, K.: Chemical pathology of spongy degeneration of the white matter. Neurology (Minneap.) 17, 302 (1967).
Rein, H., Kolkmann, F.-W., Sil, R., Ule, G.: Zur Feinstruktur der INH-Encephalopathie der Ente. Klin. Wschr. 46, 1060—1062 (1968).
Rett, A.: Über ein zerebral-atrophisches Syndrom bei Hyperammonämie. Wien: Hollinek 1966.
Reulen, H. J., Baethmann, A.: Das Dinitrophenol-Ödem. Ein Modell zur Pathophysiologie des Hirnödems. Klin. Wschr. 45, 149—154 (1967).
Ribadeau-Dumas, J. L., Escourolle, R., Castaigne, P.: Syndrome de Creutzfeldt-Jakob: Etude ultrastructurale de trois observations. Rev. neurol. 121, 405—422 (1969).

ROBACK, H. N., SCHERER, H. J.: Über die feinere Morphologie des frühkindlichen Gehirns. Virchows Arch. path. Anat. **294**, 365—413 (1935).

ROBERTSON, D. M., WASAN, S. M., SKINNER, D. B.: Ultrastructural features of early brain stem lesions of thiamine-deficient rats. Amer. J. Path. **52**, 1081—1097 (1968).

ROBINSON, N.: Creutzfeld-Jacob's disease: A histochemical study. Brain **92**, 581—588 (1969).

RODRIGUEZ DE LORES ARNAIZ, G., ALBERICI, M., DE ROBERTIS, E.: Ultrastructural end enzymatic studies of cholinergic and noncholinergic synaptic membranes isolated from brain cortex. J. Neurochem. **14**, 215—225 (1967).

RUSHTON, D. I.: Spongy degeneration of the white matter of the central nervous system associated with hyperglyinuria. J. clin. Path. **21**, 456—462 (1968).

SACKS, O., BROWN, W. J., AGUILAR, M. J.: Spongy degeneration of white matter. Canavan's disease. Neurology (Minneap.) **15**, 165—171 (1965).

SAMAHA, F. J.: Studies on Na^+-K^+-stimulated ATPase of human brain. J. Neurochem. **14**, 333—341 (1967).

SAMSON, F. E., JR., QUINN, D. J.: Na^+-K^+-activated ATPase in rat brain development. J. Neurochem. **14**, 421—427 (1967).

SANDER, C., CLOTTEN, R., NOETZEL, H., WEHINGER, H.: Zur Klinik und pathologischen Anatomie der Ahornsirupkrankheit ("branched chain ketoaciduria"). Bericht über zwei Fälle in einer Familie. Dtsch. med. Wschr. **93**, 895—903 (1968).

SASTRY, P. S., STANCER, H. C.: Blood gangliosides in infantile amaurotic idiocy. Clin. chim. Acta **20**, 487—489 (1968).

SCHEINBERG, L. C., HERZOG, I., TAYLOR, J. M., KATZMAN, R.: Cerebral edema in brain tumors: ultrastructural and biochemical studies. Ann. N.Y. Acad. Sci. **159**, II, 509—532 (1969).

— TAYLOR, J. M., HERZOG, I., MANDELL, S.: Optic and peripheral nerve response to triethyltin intoxication in the rabbit. Biochemical and ultrastructural studies. J. Neuropatdh. exp. Neurol. **25**, 202—213 (1966).

SCHLOTE, W., BETZ, E., KNEBEL, U., NGUYEN-DUONG, H.: EEG-Veränderungen und Dendritenschwellung bei schwerer respiratorischer Acidose. Herbsttagg Dtsch. Path. Wiesbaden, 10.—12. Okt. 1969.

SCHMIDT, G. W., BENECKE, G., PEIFFER, J.: Über einen diätetisch langfristig behandelten Säugling mit Valin-Leucin-Urie und Debilität (Ahornsirup-Krankheit). Helv. paediat. Acta **20**, 147—168 (1965).

SCHOCHET, S. S., JR., LAMPERT, P. W., EARLE, K. M.: Alexander's disease: A case report with electron microscopic observations. Neurology (Minneap.) **18**, 543—549 (1968).

SCHOLZ, W.: Contribution à l'anatomie pathologique du système nerveux central dans l'oligophrénie phénylpyruvique. Encéphale **46**, 668—680 (1957).

SCHRÖDER, J. M., WECHSLER, W.: Ödem und Nekrose in der grauen und weißen Substanz beim experimentellen Hirntrauma. Licht- und elektronenmikroskopische Untersuchungen. Acta neuropath. (Berl.) **5**, 82—111 (1965).

SEITELBERGER, F.: Discussion. J. Neuropath. exp. Neurol. **20**, 317—318 (1961).

— Zur allgemeinen Histopathologie degenerativer Prozesse des Nervensystems. Acta med. Acad. Sci. hung. **21**, 450—459 (1965).

— Die Hallervorden-Spatzsche Krankheit. Nervenarzt **37**, 482—493 (1966).

— The problem of status spongiosus. In: Brain edema (I. KLATZO and F. SEITELBERGER, eds.), p. 152—169. Wien and New York: 1967.

— General neuropathology of degenerative processes of the nervous system. In: Neurosciences research, vol. 2, p. 253—299. New York: Academic Press 1969.

— JELLINGER, K.: Spongiöser Typ der Leukodystrophien. In: GERLACH, J., H. P. JENSEN, W. KOOS, and H. KRAUS, Pädiatrische Neurochirurgie, S. 845—846. Stuttgart: G. Thieme 1967.

SEITELBERGER, F., WEINGARTEN, K.: Zur Beteiligung des Nervus opticus bei einigen degenerativen Hirnprozessen. J. Génét. hum. 15, 284—301 (1966).
SHAW, I. G., WINKLER, C. E., TERLECKI, S.: Experimental reproduction of hypomyelinogenesis congenita of lambs. Vet. Rec. 81, 115—116 (1967).
SILVERMAN, J., DANCIS, J., FEIGIN, I.: Neuropathological observations in maple syrup urine disease, branched chan ketonuria. Arch. Neurol. (Chic.) 5, 351—363 (1961).
SKOU, J. C.: Enzymatic aspects of active linked transport of Na^+ and K^+ through the cell membrane. Progr. Biophys. 14, 133—146 (1964).
— Enzymatic basis for active transport of Na^+ and K^+ across the cell membrane. Physiol. Rev. 45, 595—617 (1965).
SLUGA, E.: Observations on the white matter in human brain edema. In: Brain edema (I. KLATZO and F. SEITELBERGER, eds.), p. 223—239. Vienna and New York: Springer 1967.
— SEITELBERGER, F.: Beitrag zur spongiösen Encephalopathie. Acta neuropath. (Berl.), Suppl. 3, 60—72 (1967).
— TOMONAGA, M.: Elektronenoptische Befunde zur Darstellung und Lokalisation der Mg-ATPase. (Abstr.). Wien. klin. Wschr. 81, 440 (1969).
SOURANDER, P., OLSSON, Y.: Peripheral neuropathy in globoid cell leucodystrophy (Morbus Krabbe). Acta neuropath. (Berl.) 11, 69—86 (1968).
SPIELMEYER, W.: Histopathologie des Nervensystems, S. 335 ff. Berlin: Springer 1922.
STADLER, H.: Histopathologische Untersuchungen zur Frage der Beziehung zwischen Leber und Gehirnveränderungen. Z. ges. Neurol. Psychiat. 154, 626—658 (1936).
STÄLLBERG-STENHAGEN, S., SVENNERHOLM, L.: Fatty acid composition of human brain sphingomyelins: Normal variation with age and changes during myelin disorders. J. Lipid Res. 6, 146—155 (1965).
STRÄUSSLER, E., KOSKINAS, G.: Über den spongiösen Rindenschwund, den Status spongiosus und die laminären Hirnrindenprozesse. Z. ges. Neurol. Psychiat. 105, 55—71 (1926).
SUZUKI, K.: Peripheral nerve lesions in spongy degeneration of the central nervous system. Acta neuropath. (Berl.) 10, 95—98 (1968).
— CHEN, G. C.: Chemical studies on Jakob-Creutzfeldt disease. J. Neuropath. exp. Neurol. 25, 396—408 (1966).
— — Brain ceramide hexosides in Tay-Sachs disease and generalized gangliosidosis (G_{M1}-gangliosidosis). J. Lipid Res. 8, 105—113 (1967).
— KIKKAWA, Y.: Status spongiosus of CNS and hepatic changes induced by Cuprizine (biscyclohexanone oxalyl-dihydrazone). Amer. J. Path. 54, 307—325 (1969).
— PODUSLO, J. F., PODUSLO, S. E.: Further evidence for a specific ganglioside fraction closely associated with myelin. Biochim. biophys. Acta (Amst.) 152, 576—586 (1968).
— PODUSLO, S. E., NORTON, W. T.: Gangliosides in the myelin fraction of developing rats. Biochim. biophys. Acta (Amst.) 144, 375—385 (1967).
— SUZUKI, K., KAMOSHITA, S.: Chemical pathology of G_{M1}-gangliosidosis (generalized gangliosidosis). J. Neuropath. exp. Neurol. 28, 25—73 (1969).
SUZUKI, T., MOSTAFI, F. K.: Intramitochondrial filamentous bodies in the thick limb of Henle of the rat kidney. J. Cell Biol. 33, 605—623 (1967).
TANI, E., AMETANI, T., HANDA, H.: Sodium localization in the adult brain. I. Normal. brain tissue. II. Triethyltin intoxication and cerebral edema produced by epidural compression. Acta neuropath. (Berl.) 14, 137—160 (1969).
TARISKA, S.: Recent case of familial idiocy with spongy degeneration of the neuraxis. Proc. IVth. Int. Congr. Neuropath., vol. III, p. 75—80. Stuttgart: G. Thieme 1962.

Torack, R. M.: Adenosine triphosphatase activity in rat brain following differential fixation with formaldehyde, glutaraldehyde, and hydroxyladipaldehyde. J. Histochem. Cytochem. **13**, 191—205 (1965).
— Ultrastructural and histochemical studies of cortical biopsies in subacute dementia. Acta neuropath. (Berl.) **13**, 43—55 (1969).
— Barrnett, R. J.: Nucleoside phosphatase activity in membranous fine structures of neurons and glia. J. Histochem. Cytochem. **11**, 763—772 (1963).
— — The fine structural localization of nucleoside phosphatase activity in the blood-brain garrier. J. Neuropath. exp. Neurol. **23**, 46—59 (1964).
— Dufty, M. L., Gordon, J. S.: Specifity of electron microscopic localization of phosphatase activity to cerebral fine structures. In: Brain edema (I. Klatzo and F. Seitelberger, eds.), p. 491—506. Wien and New York: Springer 1967.
Ule, G.: Ultrastrukturelle Befunde bei verschiedenen Formen des Hirnödems. In: Hydrodynamik, Elektrolyt- und Säure-Basen-Haushalt im Liquor und Nervensystem (G. Kienle, Hrsg.), S. 223—227. Stuttgart: G. Thieme 1967.
— Zur Ultrastruktur der Astroglia und des Status spongiosus. Acta neuropath. (Berl.), Suppl. **4**, 98—104 (1968a).
— Feinstruktur der spongiösen Dystrophie der grauen Substanz. Verh. dtsch. Ges. Path. **52**, 142—152 (1968b).
— Kolkmann, F. W.: Zur Ultrastruktur des perifokalen und histotoxischen Hirnödems bei der Ratte. Acta neuropath. (Berl.) **1**, 519—526 (1962).
— — Experimentelle Untersuchungen zur Wernickeschen Encephalopathie. Acta neuropath. (Berl.) **11**, 361—367 (1968).
Verhaart, W. J. C.: Sponzige ontaarding von de hersenen bij kleinen kinderen. Ned. T. Geneesk. **106**, 2250—2251 (1962).
Vernandakis, A., Woodbury, D. M.: Electrolyte and amino acid changes in rat brain during maturation. Amer. J. Physiol. **203**, 748—752 (1963).
Victor, M., Adams, R. D., Cole, M.: The acquired (non-Wilsonian) type of chronic hepato-cerebral degeneration. Medicine (Baltimore) **44**, 345—396 (1965).
Wegener, K., Kolkmann, F. W., Rein, H.: Autohistoradiographische Untersuchungen zur Frage der Bluthirnschrankenfunktion bei experimentell ausgelösten spongiösen Encephalopathien. Virchows Arch. Abt. A. Path. Anat. **345**, 352—364 (1968).
Whittam, R., Blond, D.: Respiratory control by an adenosine triphosphatase involved in active transport in brain cortex. Biochem. J. **92**, 147—158 (1964).
Wolman, M.: The spongy type of diffuse sclerosis. Brain **81**, 243—247 (1959).
— Wiener, H.: Structure of myelin sheath as function of concentration of ions. Biochim. biophys. Acta (Amst.) **102**, 269—279 (1965).
Yanagihara, T., Cumings, J. N.: Lipid metabolism in cerebral edema associated with human brain tumor. Arch. Neurol. (Chic.) **19**, 241—247 (1968).
— — Fatty acid composition of cerebrosides and cerebroside sulphatides in cerebral edema. Acta neuropath. (Berl.) **12**, 62—67 (1969a).
— — Alterations of phospholipids, particularly plasmalogens, in the demyelination of multiple sclerosis as compared with that of cerebral oedema. Brain **92**, 59—70 (1969b).
Zadunaisky, J. A., Wald, F., De Robertis, E. D. P.: Osmotic behaviour and glial changes in isolated dog brains. Progr. Brain Res. **15**, 196—218 (1965).
Zelman, I. B., Czochanska-Kruk, J., Borowicz, K.: Neuropathologia fenyloketonurii. Neuropat. pol. **5**, 509—518 (1967).
Zu Rhein, G. M., Eickman, P. L., Puletti, F.: Familial idiocy with spongy degeneration of the central nervous system of van Bogaert-Bertrand type. Neurology (Minneap.) **10**, 998—1006 (1960).

The Myothelia (Myoepithelial Cells)*

Normal State; Regressive Changes; Hyperplasia; Tumors

H. HAMPERL**

With 29 Figures

Table of Contents

I. Shape and Function of Normal Myothelia (Mt) 162
   1. Shape and Occurrence 162
   2. Development and Histology 164
   3. Function and Biochemistry 165
   Conclusions 167

II. Regressive Changes 167
   1. Uptake of Water 167
   2. Glycogen Storage 168
   3. Pigment Deposition 170
   4. Fat Deposition 173
   5. Myothelia in Cases of Atrophy 174
   Conclusions 175

III. Hyperplasia 176
   1. Circumscribed Proliferation 176
   2. Rosette-Shaped Hyperplasia 176
   3. Diffuse Hyperplasia 178
   4. Epimyothelial Islands 181
   5. Fibrosing Adenosis of the Mamma 182
   6. Intracanicular Hyperplasia 183

IV. Benign Tumors Containing Myothelia 184
   1. Benign Tumors Containing Mt Occurring only in the breast 185
   2. Benign Tumors Containing Mt Occurring only in the Skin 188
   3. Benign Tumors Containing Mt Occurring only in the Salivary Glands . 189
   4. Tumors Containing Mt Occurring in Several Organs 189
      a) Mixed Tumor of the Salivary Gland Type 190
      b) Cylindroma (Adenoid Cystic Carcinoma) 192
      c) Adeno-Myothelioma 194

V. Malignant Tumors Containing Myothelia 199
   1. Malignant Mixed Tumors of the Salivary Gland Type 199
   2. Sarcomas of the Mammary Gland 200

---

* With the generous support of the Nordrhein-Westfalen Office for Research. I dedicate this paper in gratitude to my technical assistants, Countess M. MATUSCHKA and M. HALAND, and also to all fellow-workers in Vienna, Berlin, Prague, Salzburg, Marburg, Bonn and Bogotá who prepared the necessary sections.

** Patholog. Institute, Bonn University, 5300 Bonn 1, (Germ. Fed. Rep.) Postfach.

3. Malignant Adeno-Myotheliomas 203
4. Myothelia in Typical Carcinomas 205
5. Carcino-Sarcomas 208
VI. Final Considerations 209
VII. Summary 211
References 213

The myoepithelial cells are indeed a fascinating type of cell, in that they appear to belong to two widely divergent types of tissues, namely the epithelium and the mesenchyma. This two-sided nature is expressed not only by their position (on the one hand they are connected in typical manner with the secreting epithelium, whereas on the other hand they interact with the stroma and the basal membrane in the same way as smooth muscle fibres), but also by their possession of potentialities of both kinds of tissue, although these potentialities become apparent only under pathological conditions of growth. This concept is the key-note of the following paper, whose purpose is to report a comparative study of the myoepithelia of various organs. Many phenomena that were detectable and detected in only one organ, will be used to elucidate certain otherwise obscure changes in other organs. First we shall examine the normal myoepithelia of various tissues (I), then consider regressive changes (II) and hyperplasia (III), in order to apply the information thus obtained to the problem of tumors (IV, V). To some extent, therefore, this paper constitutes a continuation of my paper from 1939 "On the myothelia of the mammary gland". Additional material has been collected since then; unfortunately, however, some of the relevant documents were lost during the war and in the post-war period.

Even in the first publication (1939) the name "myoepithelial cells" was recognized to be too long, because it could give rise to tongue-twisters such as "epi-myo-epithelial proliferation". It was therefore proposed that the special nature of these cells should be indicated by the term "myothelia" (and by the adjective "myothelial"); accordingly, that term (abbreviated to: "Mt") will be used in the following discussion.

I. Shape and Function of the Normal Myothelia

1. Shape and Occurrence

Mt have been described in the secretory structures and excretory ducts of numerous glands in man and animals.

In the *secretory parts* of the sweat glands, the Mt appear long and spindly thus closely resembling smooth muscle cells (Fig. 1a); they envelop the mammary and salivary glands with star-shaped intertwining tentacles (Fig. 1b), hence these cells are often called "basket-cells". The glands of the buccal mucous membrane, trachea, oesophagus, lacrimal gland and the

Bartholin's glands also contain Mt like the larger salivary glands (parotid, submaxillary, and sublingual). Recently, Mt were described in the prostate (ROWLATT and FRANKS, 1964); they are not found, however, in the pancreas (ZIMMERMANN, 1927).

Some spindle-shaped and even more cuboid Mt have been described in the *excretory ducts* of the above mentioned glands. As to the cuboid Mt, however,

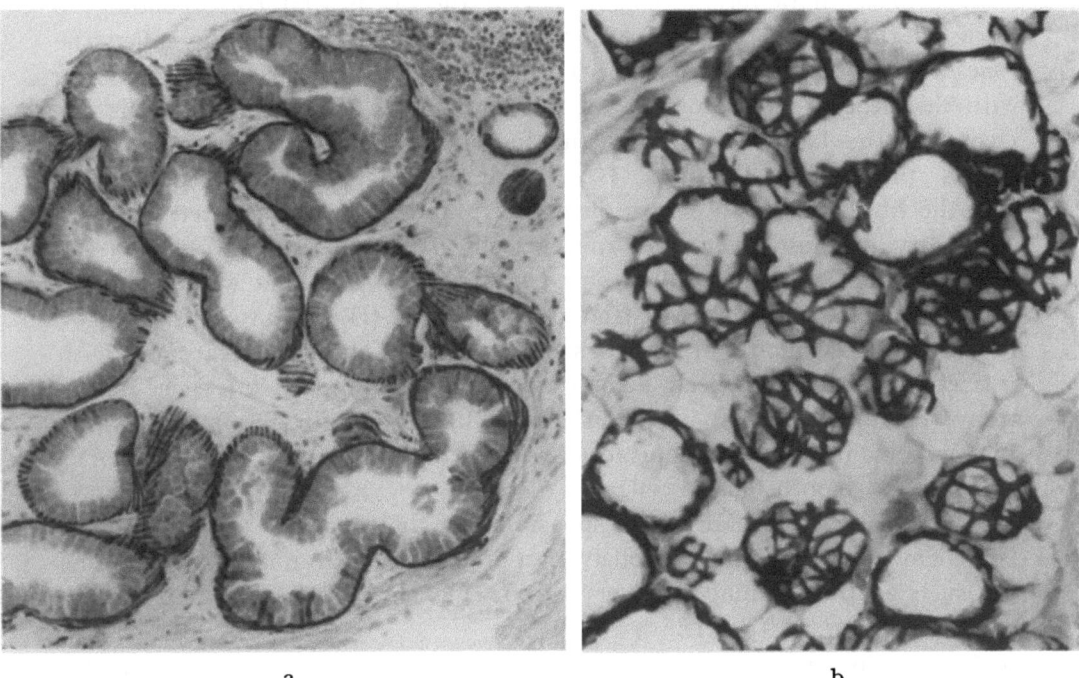

a b

Fig. 1a and b. Various types of normal Mt. a Spindle-shaped Mt in sweat gland. (Modified iron-hematoxylin method of Heidenhain.) Section Prof. BESEZNY †, Prag. 80×. b Basket-cells in the mammary gland of the rat. Alkaline phosphatase (Gomori's method). Section Prof. BÄSSLER, Mainz. 190×

some doubts might arise whether these really are myothelial cells or merely basal cells, which — to a certain extent — would represent only homologues (LENNOX et al., 1952) of Mt. Their behaviour in hyperplastic growth, and the results of more recent studies (see below), however, strongly suggest that these cuboid forms really are myothelial cells.

Mt have been described not only in man, but also in the mammary and salivary glands of rodents, such as the rat and the mouse, in the mammary glands of the sheep (RICHARDSON, 1949), and in the parotid of the cow (SILVER, 1954); surprisingly, SCOTT and PEASE (1959) found Mt only in the submaxillary and sublingual glands of the rat, but not in their parotid.

Perhaps, one should include among the Mt the epithelial muscle cells of the dilator pupillae as well as certain elements of crocodile derma (MASSON and PEYRON, 1914).

2. Development and Histology

Mt become apparent in human sweat glands at the 22. week of embryonic life (HASHIMOTO et al., 1966). From then onwards, the basal cells of the epithelial cords arising from the epidermis differentiate into the basal Mt and the secreting cells that form the lumen. From the histogenetic point of view, the Mt are undoubtedly of ectodermal origin and of epithelial nature.

The most characteristic constituent of the Mt is that corresponding to fibrils of the smooth muscle cells, and which could therefore be called the *"mesenchymal"* one. LANGER and HUHN (1958) first succeeded in detecting with the electron-microscope a fine felt of fibrils in the parts of the Mt adjacent to the basal membrane; the individual fibrils measured 50—80 Å (ELLIS, 1965, 50 Å; TANDLER, 1965, 40 Å); ELLIS (1965) has demonstrated that the fibrils possess a certain degree of uniformity, as compared with the variability of those in smooth muscle cells (see WEISS, 1968: 30—200 Å). The fibrils have irregularly distributed transverse stripes that were compared with I- and Z-stripes of cross-striated muscle cells (HAGUENAU, 1959; ELLIS, 1965); they terminate at the basal membrane. Through treatment with antiactomyosin, it has been demonstrated with immuno-fluorescence-microscopy (ARCHER and KAO, 1968), that the fibrils contain actomyosin which is so important in muscle contraction. Thus that part of the Mt corresponds exactly to a smooth muscle cell.

The fibrils of the Mt are responsible for their special color reactions. These can be used for the demonstration of both smooth muscle cells and the Mt, such as the staining with erythrosin, fuchsin, PTAH (DEMPSEY et al., 1947), crystal-violet (BERTKAU, 1907).

Various silver impregnation methods have also been applied and have revealed that at least a fair proportion of the Mt are argyrophilic (RICHARDSON, 1949; LINZELL, 1952; FEYRTER, 1961).

The presence of parallel filaments is also responsible for the birefringence of Mt, which has been reported by BUNTING et al. (1948) and GOLDSTEIN (1961).

The *"epithelial"* part of the Mt situated towards the lumen is remarkably poor in cell-organelles, and therefore looks very pale under the electron microscope and even under the light microscope. The Mt cells are linked to the secreting epithelial cells by desmosomes, and to the basement membrane by hemidesmosomes, in the same manner as smooth muscle fibres are.

Other peculiarities detectable through the electron microscope include the regular presence of glycogen granules and pinocytotic vesicles on the cell-surface adjacent to the basement membrane, which similarly occur in smooth muscle cells (WEISS, 1968). The nucleus is relatively rich in chromatin, and is characterised by deep indentations (HOLLMANN, 1959; HAGUENAU and ARNOULT, 1959).

The description given above applies to the Mt of the secretory glands. The situation is rather different, however, when we consider the *Mt of the ducts*. In the mammary gland, for example, cuboid cells are often closely packed to form an unbroken basal layer on the basement membrane. These cells fail to stain with any of the techniques that are characteristic of the fibrils of smooth muscle cells, owing to the scarcity or absence of fibrils. The mesenchymal components of the Mt are to some extend replaced by epithelial ones: the Mt occupy the place of basal cells in the stratified epithelium. Indeed, transitions between basal cells and Mt have been described (see below).

3. Function and Biochemistry

One function of the Mt now appears to be established beyond any doubt, namely its *ability to contract like muscle fibres*. Apart from the detection by electron-microscopy and fluorescence-microscopy of myofibrils, the contraction and even the effect of such a contraction of the Mt has actually been observed both macroscopically and microscopically.

RICHARDSON (1949) and also LINZELL (1955) were able to determine the decrease in the volume of the lobules of the mammary gland when they applied drops of various compounds. Oxytocin was particularly active in this respect; by means of the electron-microscope BÄSSLER et al. (1967) and BÄSSLER and BRETHFELD (1968) observed changes in the shape of the Mt after contraction, and showed that on contraction they squeeze the glands. The Mt move apart from one another, and thus allow a contact between the secretory epithelia and the basement membrane, so that the epithelia protrude in a characteristic manner (DEMPSEY et al., 1947; GOLDSTEIN, 1961; ELLIS, 1965; BÄSSLER et al., 1967). An action similar to that of oxytocin is exerted by all stimuli that normally induce a contraction of smooth muscle cells (HURLEY and SHELLEY, 1954; LINZELL, 1955).

The Mt arranged longitudinally or spirally in the excretory ducts will, on contraction, give rise to a dilatation of the ducts, and thus exert a kind of *pumping-effect* in unison with the acinar Mt.

In the mammary gland the contraction results from a *humoral stimulus* and is held responsible for the so-called "let-down" of the milk. This explains the fact that, even after denervation, this contraction can be induced by oxytocin (LINZELL, 1952). The functional importance of the Mt in lactation is further corroborated by the increase in their processes during pregnancy (BÄSSLER et al., 1967), although their numbers are said to show no increase (WAUGH and V. D. HOEVEN, 1962).

In salivary and sweat glands a *neural stimulus* rather than a humoral stimulus, is mainly involved. Nerve-endings in the region of the Mt have indeed been observed by SCOTT and PEASE (1959) in the sublingual gland, and by TAMARIN (1964) in the submaxillary gland of the rat. According to HURLEY and SHELLEY (1954), the Mt in human sweat glands are equipped with adrenergic nerve-fibres; they observed such fibres in the region of the tips of the Mt.

Thus we encounter a difference between the "basket-cell" Mt of the mammary gland and the Mt of the salivary and sweat glands, although they are in other respects morphologically similar; no experimental data are available about the function of the Mt in the salivary glands.

Because the Mt lie sandwiched between the secretory epithelial cells and the stroma containing the nutrient vessels, one can reasonably conclude that they may fulfil some kind of *transport-function* and/ or control of the metabolism (ELLIS, 1965), which is also manifested in the presence of pinocytotic vesicles on the side nearest to the basement membrane.

No evidence has yet been obtained of the production of any secretion of hormones, not even in the sense of a paracriny (HOLLMANN, 1959).

A participation of the Mt in the *formation of the basement membrane*, similar to that for the smooth muscle cells, has been suggested (ELLIS, 1965; GOLDSTEIN, 1961).

When the Mt contain few fibrils or even none, they are not only difficult to distinguish from the so-called *basal cells*, but they may actually function as basal cells, in that through division they provide a substitute for the secretory cells situated near the lumen (BÄSSLER and SCHÄFER, 1969). One should, therefore, expect to find transitions between Mt and the other cells in the glands and their ducts. This question is, however, an open one.

For example, GOLDSTEIN (1961) and also ELLIS (1965) do not mention any transitions between the Mt and the secretory cells, such as HIBBS (1958) observed in human sweat glands. MURAD and VAN HAAM (1968) observe transitions between light Mt and dark myothelial cells, which may correspond to the B and A cells of CASPERSSON and SANTESSON. Furthermore, MURAD and VON HAAM (1967) emphasize that, during pregnancy, Mt are transformed into secretory epithelia, and thus to some extent function as replacement-cells. TANNENBAUM et al. (1969) are unable to find with the electronmicroscope any "essential differences" between epithelium and Mt in the human mammary ductule. Finally TANDLER (1965) describes transitions between Mt and special light cells. Thus it is by no means clear what changes into what, or what is capable of changing.

The *alkaline phosphatase* activity in the Mt can also be connected with a metabolic function; the presence or absence of that activity however should not be regarded as a decisive criterion for the identification of Mt; first, because that activity is present also in the cytoplasm of the secretory cells of the human mammary gland (NEWMAN et al., 1950) and the submaxillary gland (NOBACK and MONTAGNA, 1947), and second, because that activity can be absent in normal Mt (O'HARA et al., 1966). The studies of BÄSSLER and BRETHFELD (1968) and also our own Fig. 1b show, however, that the alkaline phosphatase activity at times is very impressive. Generally, the azo-methods are preferred, but good results can also be obtained with cobalt-silver methods (see Fig. 1b).

In man, alkaline phosphatase has been studied mainly in the sweat glands. SHELLEY and MESCON (1952) and also KOPF (1957) found alkaline phosphatase in the Mt of exocrine and apocrine sweat glands, but not in the excretory ducts. BUNTING et al. (1948), BUNTING (1948) and also PIRILÄ and ERÄNKÖ (1950) described a positive reaction in the cytoplasm of the secretory cells and in Mt and basal membranes. Moreover, ELLIS (1965), and also DEMPSEY et al. (1947) have detected a close local relationship of the alkaline phosphatase activity to the pinocytotic vesicles at the base of the Mt, and have related that activity to a transporting function of these cells. The activity does not appear to be connected with the fibrils.

In animals, positive alkaline phosphatase activity has been detected in the Mt of the mammary gland of the rat (DEMPSEY et al., 1947; BÄSSLER and BRETHFELD, 1968), in the Mt of the salivary glands of the rat (DEWEY, 1958; SHEAR, 1964; BOGART, 1968; MÜLLER, 1969), in the extraorbital glands and Harders's glands of the rat (LEESON, 1960), and in the mammary glands of the rat, rabbit and sheep (SILVER, 1954), as well as in the parotid gland of the sheep. BOGART (1968) found the alkaline phosphatase activity in the submandibular gland of the rat connected with the pinocytotic vacuoles and on the tip of the cellular processes of the Mt; the side of the Mt towards the lumen exhibits greater activity than the side towards the basement membrane. It is remarkable that alkaline phosphatase activity disappears in the salivary glands of the rat after hypophysectomy (DEWEY, 1958).

Conclusions

Reviewing all that has been said so far about the Mt, we must admit that even normally they show very different pictures, which vary according to the qualities predominating in each instance. If however, we admit that these cells exhibit a wide range of forms and possible reactions, then we may justifiably wonder how a cell belonging to this group can definitely be recognized. This is, of course, accomplished best by the detection of the myofibrils and by the positive results of all methods and tests which depend on their presence. But can we say that all cells, in which detection of myofibrils and other tests fail, are definitely not Mt? Most certainly not! First, because very few myofibrils may go undetected, either because they are just not found, or because their quantity is insufficient to produce a suitable color or enzyme reaction. Second, because Mt may even exist that are completely devoid of fibrils; their epithelial aspect is then so predominant that they appear to be pure basal cells or even transition-cells to secretory epithelia. Their inclusion in the Mt group is then based more on their shape and their position between the basement membrane and the secretory epithelium, and especially on their ability to form basement-membrane-like substances.

II. Regressive Changes

The intermediary role of the Mt in the metabolism of glands and ducts imposes at the same time the possibility that the cells take up and store different substances in their cytoplasm. Usually that process is confined to the Mt and does not involve the covering epithelia. A certain similarity or even identity in the reaction of the Mt of different organs is unmistakable.

1. Uptake of Water

The Mt of the glands (Fig. 2b) and ducts of the salivary glands (FEYRTER, 1961) and of the mammary gland (Fig. 2a) may swell to a balloon-like shape through *incorporation of watery fluid*. The nucleus appears to float in an empty bubble; the covering epithelial cells with their darker stained cytoplasm are then very easy to differentiate from the Mt.

2. Glycogen Storage

The Mt under normal conditions contain already some *glycogen*, as has been shown by electron-microscopy. The content of glycogen however can be greatly increased (Fig. 3c) under very different conditions, so that the Mt stand out as clear elements. That is especially evident in atrophy of the glands (s. below).

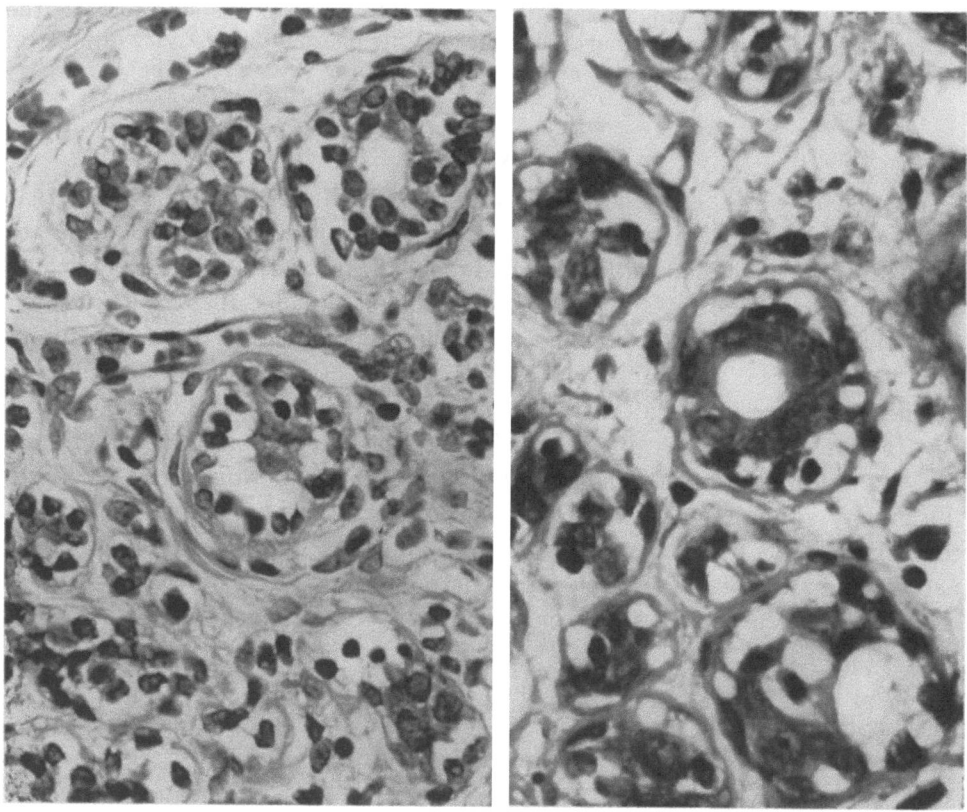

Fig. 2a and b. Hydropic swelling of Mt in a Human mammary gland (Oldenburg, No. 5638/69). HE 480 ×. b In salivary gland after irradiation (Bonn, A 3786/58). HE 600 ×

The cells described by SKORPIL in salivary glands (1940) and the mammary gland (1953) as *"lamprocytes"* probably can be explained by such a glycogen storage in Mt. In the mammary gland one may find whole lobules composed of clear cells, full of glycogen (Fig. 3b). SKORPIL mentioned that the epithelial cells in lobules composed of his lamprocytes were arranged only in a single layer. The question is thus: have the epithelia stored glycogen and the Mt disappeared or have the Mt stored glycogen and the epithelia disappeared? I would like to assume the latter possibility, considering the special metabolic role of Mt. Besides, pictures exist supporting that assumption, as Fig. 3a shows, where the basal myothelial layer of a small duct seems to continue without interruption into the glycogen containing layer of cells.

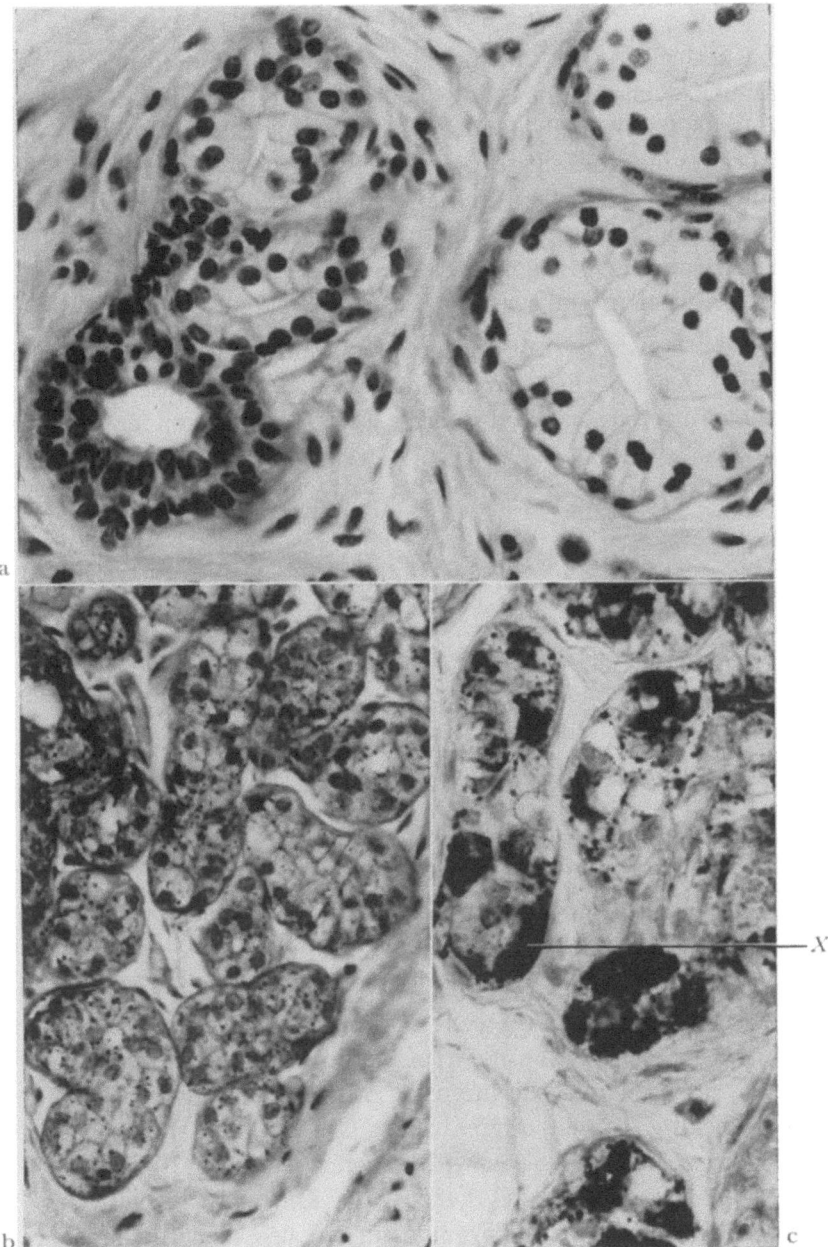

Fig. 3 a—c. Glycogen-containing cells. a "Lamprocytes" in the mammary gland. Transition of the basal myothelial layer of a duct into lamprocytes (left below). Section Prof. SKORPIL †, Prag. 300 ×. b "Lamprocytes" containing granular glycogen (Gyn. Köln, 1142/68). PAS 300 ×. c Glycogen-storage in sweat gland in a case of athyreosis. Many of the cells (X) by their shape and position correspond to Mt (Marburg, S 506/51). Best-Carmin. 480 ×

3. Pigment Deposition

The basket cells of the salivary glands especially in old age may contain a finely granular, yellow-fluorescing pigment that reacts like *lipofuscin* (HAMPERL, 1931, 1934). The cells appear swollen owing to their content of pigment-granules occupying the entire cytoplasm (Fig. 4). The Mt resemble in this respect smooth muscle cells which also under certain conditions, e.g. old age, may contain abundant lipofuscin granules that crowd out the contractile fibrils. Such deposits of pigment are never demonstrable in the Mt of the mammary gland or in the sweat glands.

One meets, however, rather frequently another pigment in the mammary gland, that is reacting like *ceroid* (HAMPERL, 1969). These pigment granules are round, of different size and fluoresce bright yellow under ultraviolet light

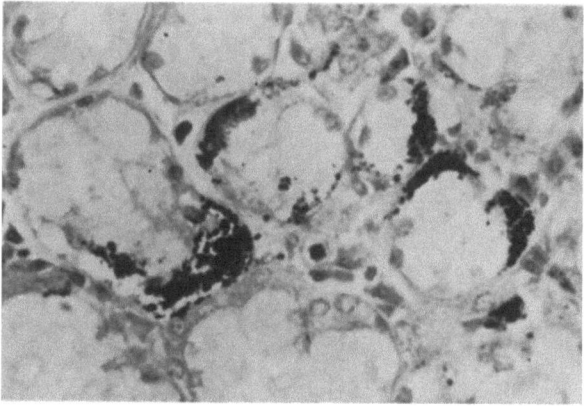

Fig. 4. Lipofuscin granules in Mt (basket cells) of submandibular gland (Wien, S 328/30). Silver stain Masson-Hamperl. Ca. 400 ×

(Fig. 5). I, therefore, called the cells containing such a ceroid pigment fluorocytes (HAMPERL, 1950). The color of the pigment granules varies between pale yellow and brown — the intensity of the yellow fluorescence decreasing with the deepening of their original color. The granules stain most intensively with PAS, even after digestion with diastase (Fig. 6b, d) and are acid- and alcohol-resistant, as shown by the positive ZIEHL-NIELSON stain. The iron-reaction varies: sometimes the granules in one cell react strongly positive; in another cell they are only weakly positive, or not stained at all. The argent-affine reaction, using the method of MASSON-HAMPERL, yields only a deep-brown color at best; with the Bodian silver-stain they appear pale brown. Their argentaffinity and argyrophylia is thus weak and irregular. Fat stains give positive results also after treatment of the tissue with alcohol and xylene — the quality characteristic for ceroid.

GEDIGK and FISCHER (1959) explained the ceroid as the result of oxidation and polymerisation of highly unsaturated fatty acids. The occurrence of that pigment in the vicinity of older extravasates of blood and the almost always positive iron-reaction — although sometimes only very weak — induced me in 1950 to explain this kind of pigment as an "expression of a peculiar transformation of the substances liberated during the desintegration of erythrocytes". HARTROFT and PORTA (1965) pointed to the high oxygen level in tissues with local hemorrhage. These high levels could favor the oxidation of unsaturated fatty acids. HARTROFT (1951) accordingly succeeded in producing ceroid in rats by the crushing of fat tissue accompanied by hemorrhage. MAEDA (1968) stressed the importance of glycoproteins (phospholipids and cerebrosides) which he thinks are responsible for the positive PAS-reaction. He traces these substances to the membranes of erythrocytes; they are thought to combine with the unsaturated fats.

Cells containing ceroid pigment (fluorocytes) are found in the mammary gland in three places: as rounded elements in the lumen of distended ducts

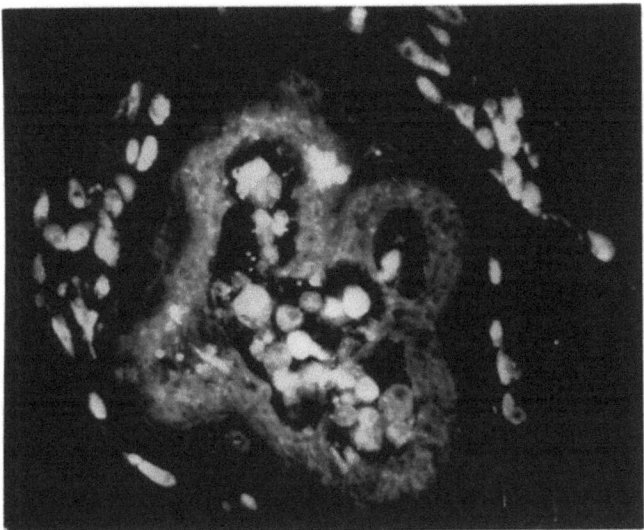

Fig. 5. Autofluorescence of ceroid-containing cells (Fluorocytes) in the lumen and in the stroma around a mammary duct. 190 ×

(Fig. 5), in the epithelium lining these ducts (Fig. 6a) and, finally, in the surrounding stroma (Fig. 6b, d). They usually appear after some bleeding into the ducts has occurred, either from intraductal papillomas or from other sources. Since the rounded fluorocytes in the lumen obviously come from the wall of the ducts one should look for their origin first there. In fact there are cells to be found here lying immediately above the basement membrane and containing ceroid (Fig. 6a). Usually they are covered by a continous layer of epithelial cells, sometimes thinned out and pushed towards the lumen (Fig. 6b) by the pressure exerted by the bulging pigmented cells lying beneath them. Occasionally one may find that the thin epithelial layer has ruptured, allowing the pigment cells to escape through the defect into the lumen.

The basal location of the pigment cell within the epithelial layer correspond exactly to that of the Mt. One may assume therefore, that they represent transformed Mt. According to what we know about the origin of ceroid in other

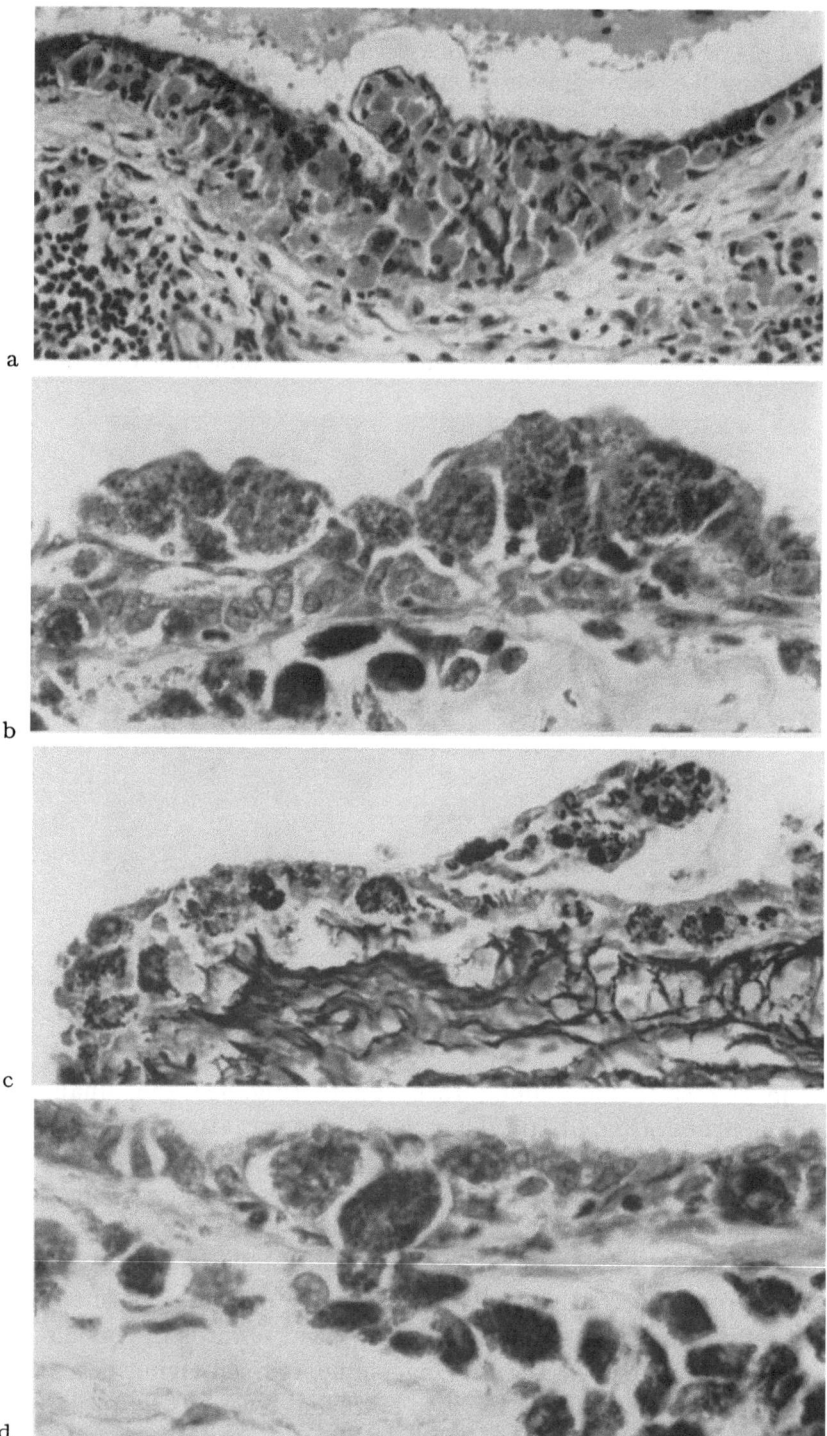

Fig. 6a—d. Ceroid containing cells (Fluorocytes) in a human mammary gland. a Forming a basal layer (Gyn. Köln, 1790/67) HE. ca 300 ×. b Within the epithelial layer immediately before their breakthrough; thinned and stretched epithelium (Gyn. Köln, 1790/67). PAS 380 ×. c Disrupted basement membrane beneath the ceroid-containing cells (Gyn.

sites we may further surmise, that hemoglobin diffused from the lumen into the epithelial lining and was taken up and metabolized by the Mt.

The cells in the surrounding stroma that contain ceroid are more difficult to explain. In Fig. 6d a ceroid-containing cell is visible above the basement membrane but protrudes through a gap in the basement membrane into the stroma. With silver-stains these gaps are easy to demonstrate: the basement membrane appears fragmented, being interrupted in several places (Fig. 6c). Therefore it seems as if the ceroid-containing cells could emigrate into the stroma. Actually just in these places one finds ceroid-containing cells distributed as single elements in the stroma; some are round, some are spindly especially those lodged between collageous fibers.

Considering all these histological pictures it seems reasonable to assume, that hemoglobin coming from the lumen is taken up by the Mt, digested and converted into ceroid. Finally some of these cells are desquamated into the lumen; others emigrate into the stroma. Such changes would roughly correspond to the situation in the lung where dust particles are phagocytized by cells lining the alveoli; later these cells may be desquamated and expectorated or may enter the stroma of the alveolar wall.

The interpretation of the origin and distribution of the ceroid-containing cells given here seems to be reasonable and corresponds most probably to the facts. Another interpretation is possible however, and should at least be taken into consideration: hemoglobin may penetrate from the lumen of ducts through the epithelial lining *and* basement membrane and pass into the stroma where histiocytes may take it up and digest it into ceroid. These cells may then emigrate through the basement membrane and epithelial layer into the lumen of the ducts. It is impossible to refute such an explanation, but it seems far less probable than the one adopted above.

The pigmented ceroid-containing cells within the epithelial lining have received little notice in the literature; the corresponding cells in the stroma were firsted seen by von Saar (1941) who interpreted them as mesenchymal phagocytes; Dyx (1941) described their argentaffinity. A. Schultz (1933) undoubtedly had seen these cells too; he described their pale original color, their content of insoluble fats and their occasional positive reaction for iron. His presentation is, however, not very clear, since he confuses these cells with the foam-cells occurring at almost the same places (see below).

4. Fat Deposition

In paraffin sections Mt enlarged by their *content of lipids* differ from hydropic swollen Mt by the foamy appearance of their cytoplasm (Fig. 7). The double refractile lipids give a positive reaction for cholesterol (Schultz,

---

Köln, 1790/67). Foot silver stain. 300×. d Ceroid containing cells within the epithelial layer and in the stroma. One cell protruding through the basement membrane (emigrating) into the stroma (Gyn. Köln, 1790/67). PAS 480×

1933). They push the overlying epithelium towards the lumen, which becomes stretched and gradually thinned until it breaks. Through the resulting gaps the foamy cells escape into the lumen. Smaller ducts may be completely filled by them.

Evidently the basal myothelial layer regenerates as do the covering epithelial cells independent of each other. The newly formed Mt may take up lipids anew, hence the epithelial lining may contain foam cells at different levels and may at some places be reduced to a kind of network, whose gaps are filled by the lipid-containing cells.

One can thus assume that the lipids found in these cells penetrated the epithelial lining from the lumen and were taken up by phagocytic cells and as is the case with hemoglobin taken up and transformed in the ceroid containing cells.

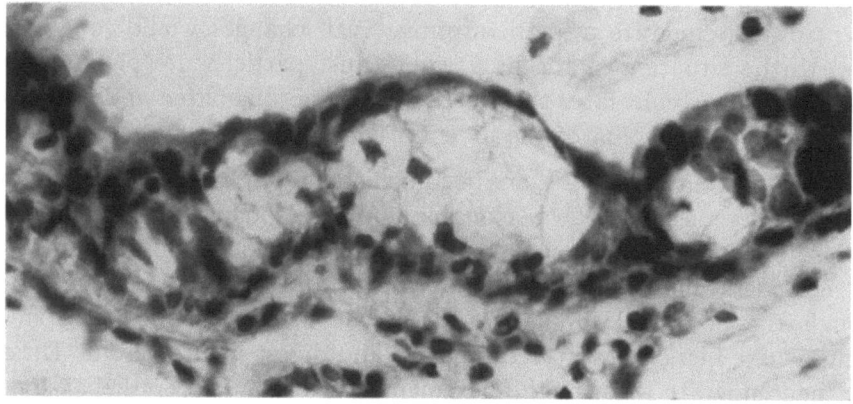

Fig. 7. Foam-cells within the epithelium of a mammary duct (Berlin Charité, S. 168/36). HE 480 ×

Foamy cells were already observed by von Saar (1907) in cases of chronic mastopathy; in his opinion they represented cells that migrated from the stroma towards the lumen and ingested on their way all kind of pigments and cellular debris. Schultz (1933) on the other hand, thinks that foamy epithelial cells — our Mt — penetrate into the stroma when the basement membrane is destroyed — a statement I was unable to verify, but applies very well to the ceroid containing cells as pointed out earlier.

Archer and Omar (1969) observed in cases of mastopathy the same *oncocytic transformation in Mt* as in the covering pink epithelia. Their myofibrils are enhanced in number and prominence.

5. Myothelia in Cases of Atrophy

The role played by the Mt in *atrophy* is best observed in the mammary gland, be it physiological involution or atrophy caused by irradiation or otherwise. In involution the epithelial cells become smaller faster than the

Mt (BÄSSLER and BRETHFELD, 1968). The latter may even enlarge by taking up watery fluid and therefore appear very clear.

The Mt remain intact longer than the epithelial cells in the process of atrophy, possibly owing to their close attachment to the basement membrane. When the epithelial cells of the mammary gland have disappeared some lobules may consist almost entirely of the residual Mt (Fig. 8). The same changes can be observed in sclerosing adenosis or in fibroadenomas undergoing fibrous obliteration.

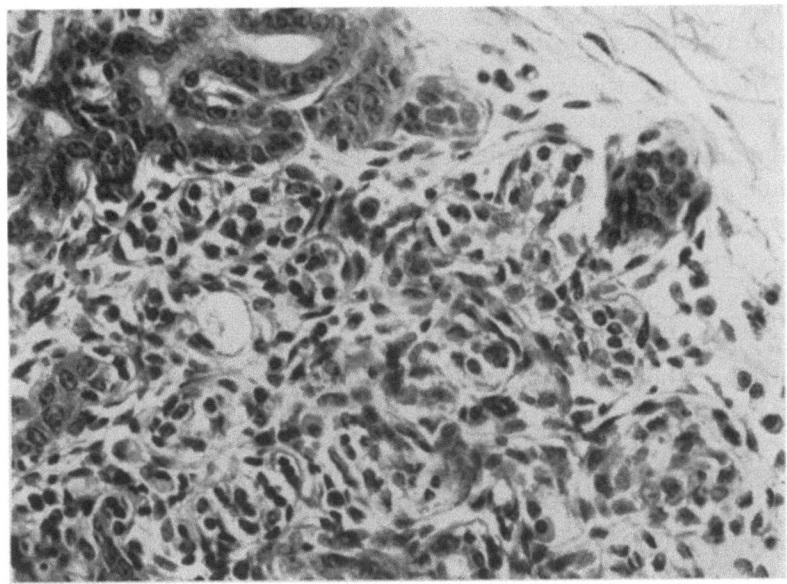

Fig. 8. Atrophy of a lobule of human mammary gland; only the hydropic Mt are left (Gyn. Erlangen, 1515/66). HE 300×

Even in the atrophic mammary tissue of men the Mt prove more resistant than the cylindrical epithelial cells (WEBER, 1949/50) to such an extent, that eventually the ducts are lined exclusively by Mt (KARNAUCHOW, 1954). The Mt thus behave according to the mesenchymal side of their nature, since mesenchymal cells generally are more resistant than epithelial cells.

Conclusions

In summarizing the changes described in this section one is rather surprised by the role Mt may play in the life of some glands, especially in the mammary gland. Disturbances in the metabolism of the Mt are reflected in their uptake of watery fluid, carbohydrates, lipids and substances from the ductal lumen, like hemoglobin with its conversion into ceroid pigment. The Mt correspond in this respect to the "active" smooth muscle-cells (WEISS, 1968), also capable of phagocytosis and of transforming themselves into foam cells. We must keep in mind all these qualities belonging to the mesenchymal side of the Mt when dealing with some peculiarities of their neoplastic growth.

III. Hyperplasia

Isolated hyperplasia of Mt, i.e., a hyperplasia of Mt not accompanied by epithelial proliferation, takes several forms:

1. Circumscribed Proliferation

Circumscribed hyperplasias of Mt in the lining of a duct may either protrude outwards, i.e., towards the stroma, or-covered by epithelium-inwards toward the lumen. KARNAUCHOW (1954) speaks in this context of centrifugal and centripetal myothelial outgrowth.

Centrifugal myothelial outgrowths are rather infrequent; they occur mostly in the mammary gland. FEYRTER (1961) saw them in salivary glands and in the mammary gland (FEYRTER and HARTMANN, 1963), where they may show some argyrophilia.

Centripetal myothelial outgrowths are frequently found in the female mammary gland. They protrude hillock-like towards the lumen (Fig. 9a) and eventually may lead to its complete occlusion.

Both forms of hyperplasia occur in gynecomastia (KARNAUCHOW, 1954), where on the whole Mt are more prominent than in the female mammary gland (BÄSSLER and SCHÄFER, 1969).

2. Rosette-Shaped Hyperplasia

One of my pupils, R. GÜNTHER (1937) was the first to describe a peculiar proliferation of the Mt around medium-sized and small excretory ducts in proliferating mastopathy. The longitudinally arranged Mt proliferate irregularly around the unchanged epithelial cells lining the lumen. They form cords, each of which consists of several Mt cells that protrude into the stroma (see Fig. 9b). These Mt resemble normal Mt in their staining and chemical properties (Fig. 12d). The basement membrane follows and surrounds the protrusions, so that a silver staining produces the typical picture of a rosette (see Fig. 12c). This type of hyperplasia of the Mt might, therefore, be called a *cord-* or *rosette-shaped hyperplasia*.

The rosette structures may become somewhat obscured when the myothelial cords are larger and lie so close to one another that the myothelial masses seem to be surrounded by a smooth basal membrane. In that case the rosette shape is recognizable only by the septa projecting into the myothelial mass (Fig. 11 c).

Fig. 9a—d. Hyperplasia of Mt. a Localized hyperplasia in the mammary gland x (Marburg, J. 700/53). HE 190×. b Rosette shaped hyperplasia in a mammary duct: at the right hand in transversal section, at the left hand in tangential section (Gyn. Köln, 225/68). HE 190×. c Diffuse hyperplasia in mammary gland (Bogotá, 2995/63). HE; d same area as c, Foot silver stain. Ca. 190×

The Myothelia (Myoepithelial Cells) 177

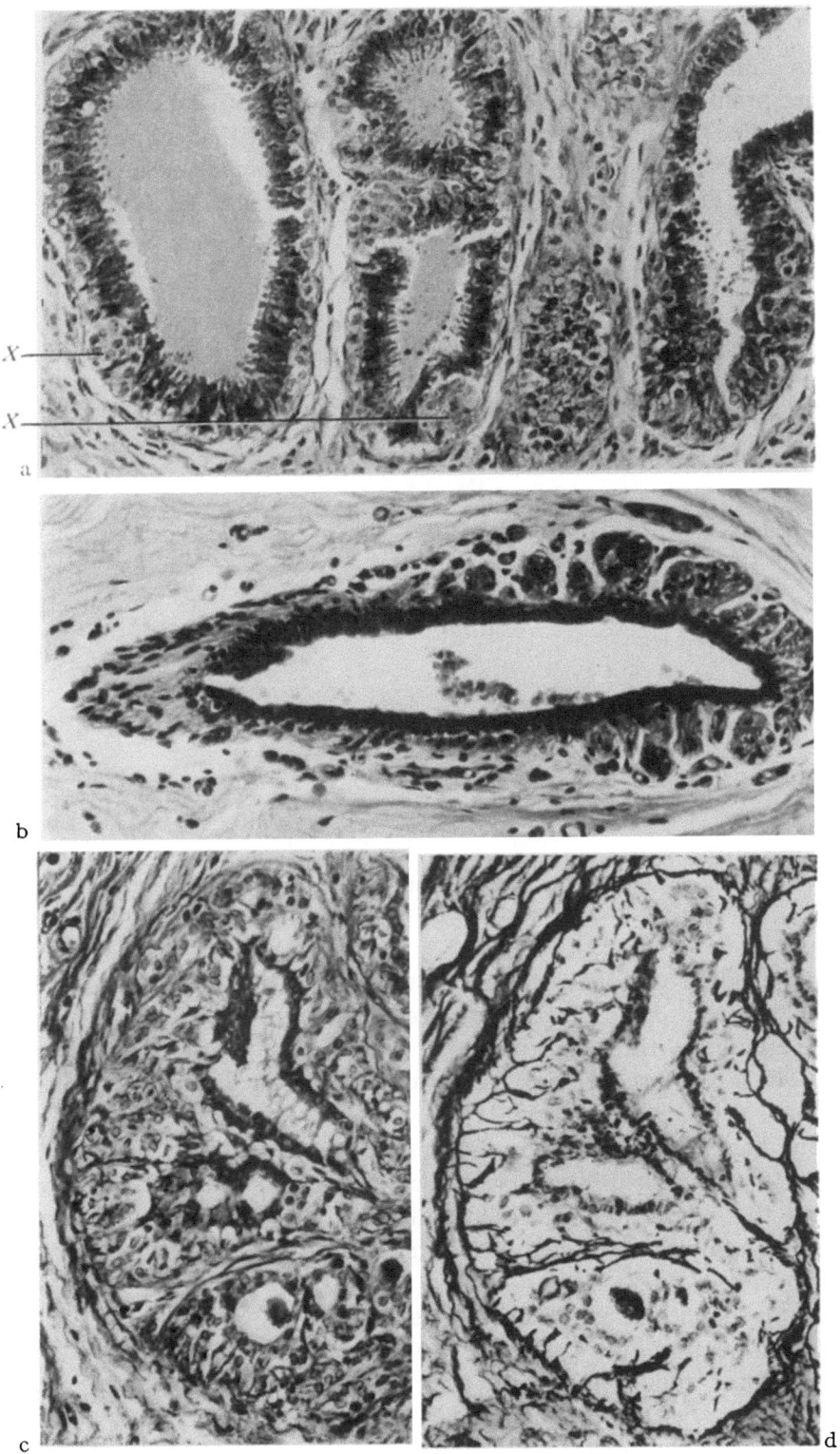

3. Diffuse Hyperplasia

In chronic mastopathy a more *diffuse hyperplasia* of the Mt can be seen around proliferated small excretory ducts (Fig. 9c, d). Several layers of cuboidal cells are lodged between cylindrical epithelial cells that surround the lumen and the smooth basement membrane. These cuboidal cells possess a clear cytoplasm (Fig. 9c). At first glance they might be regarded as a duplication or

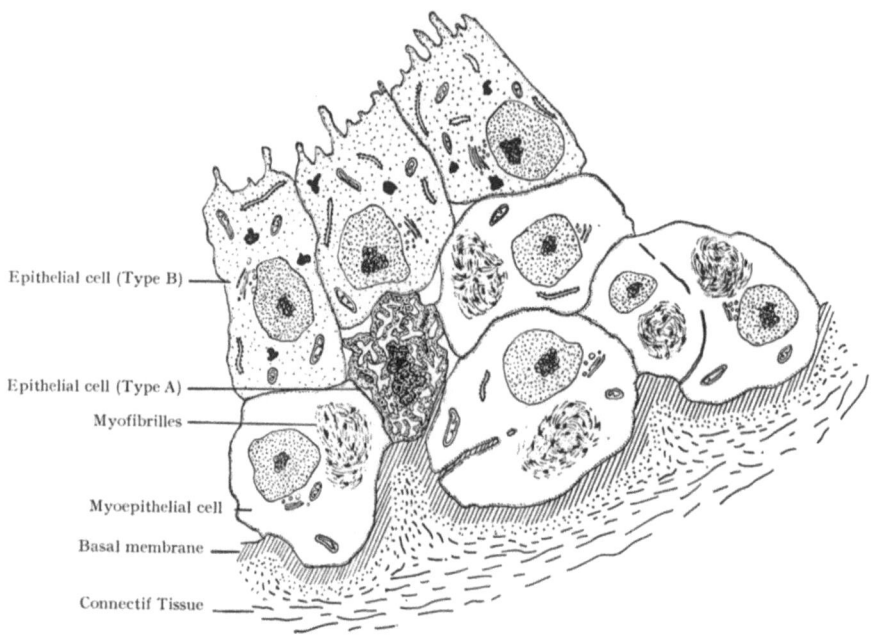

Fig. 10. Schematic drawing of the electron-microscopic findings in diffuse hyperplasia of Mt in the mammary gland. (After HAGUENAU and ARNOULT, 1959)

a multiplication of the basal layer. HAGUENAU and ARNOULT (1959) and BERGER (1960) however demonstrated by electromicroscopy that typical myofibrils may be found in these cells inspite of their clear cytoplasm (Fig. 10).

A similar diffuse hyperplasia of the Mt occasionally may be seen around the ducts of *sweat glands* (Fig. 11).

The basement membrane is of particular interest in this kind of hyperplasia. It sharply delineates the canaliculi from the stroma; processes originate from it that extend between the proliferated Mt (Fig. 9d), reminiscent of the spike-like projections of the basement membrane in rosette-shaped hyperplasia (see above).

Tangential sections indicate that some of these processes are incomplete septa arising from the basement membrane; other processes are in reality narrow cords and even filiform structures that terminate with a round or ovoid swelling within the myothelial layer (Fig. 12a), as silver stains clearly reveal. Once attention has been drawn to these round or ovoid inclusions, they are easily recognized even with the usual collagen stains. The ovoid bodies may represent the end result of disintegration of a septum, which is reduced so much that only a filiform link remains between the part nearest the lumen and the basement membrane. The ovoid bodies look then like a cherry hanging from a stem. Should this thin filament also disappear, then the ovoid terminal part would lie free within the myothelial layer. On the other hand, one is not always able to differentiate between another possibility: masses similar to the basement membrane might be deposited primarily between the myothelial cells, i.e., be independent of the basement membrane and thus assume a variety of shapes, e.g., that of a septum, a filament, or a round or ovoid body.

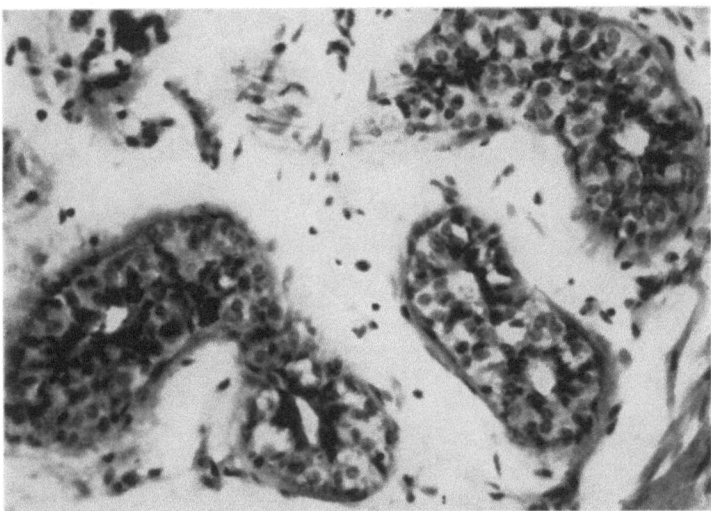

Fig. 11. Diffuse hyperplasia of Mt in the sweat gland (Prag E 285/44). HE 190 ×

The ovoid bodies may enlarge and swell; at the same time their affinity for collagen stains decreases, whereas their affinity for mucus stains is enhanced. Silver stains (see Fig. 12b) may then demonstrate filiform or radially arranged structures owing to a radial coagulation of the mucus. This picture matches exactly that of inclusions in a cylindroma (see page 92) and might even be regarded as a model of the development of rounded and otherwise shaped structures in cylindromas. FEYRTER's schematic drawing of the development of such inclusions in cylindromas (Fig. 20) also applies to these changes in the mammary gland.

The diffuse proliferation of the Mt and their "cylindromatous transformation" may occasionally be observed in the whole of the circumference of a duct. At other times the proliferation may be purely focal, analogous to the focal hyperplasia described above. Sometimes, a small excretory duct can even become completely obliterated, so that it gives the impression of a minute cylindroma (see below). It may also happen that the epithelium is compressed by the expanding inclusions to such an extent that it becomes necrotic and only the ovoid inclusions finally remain.

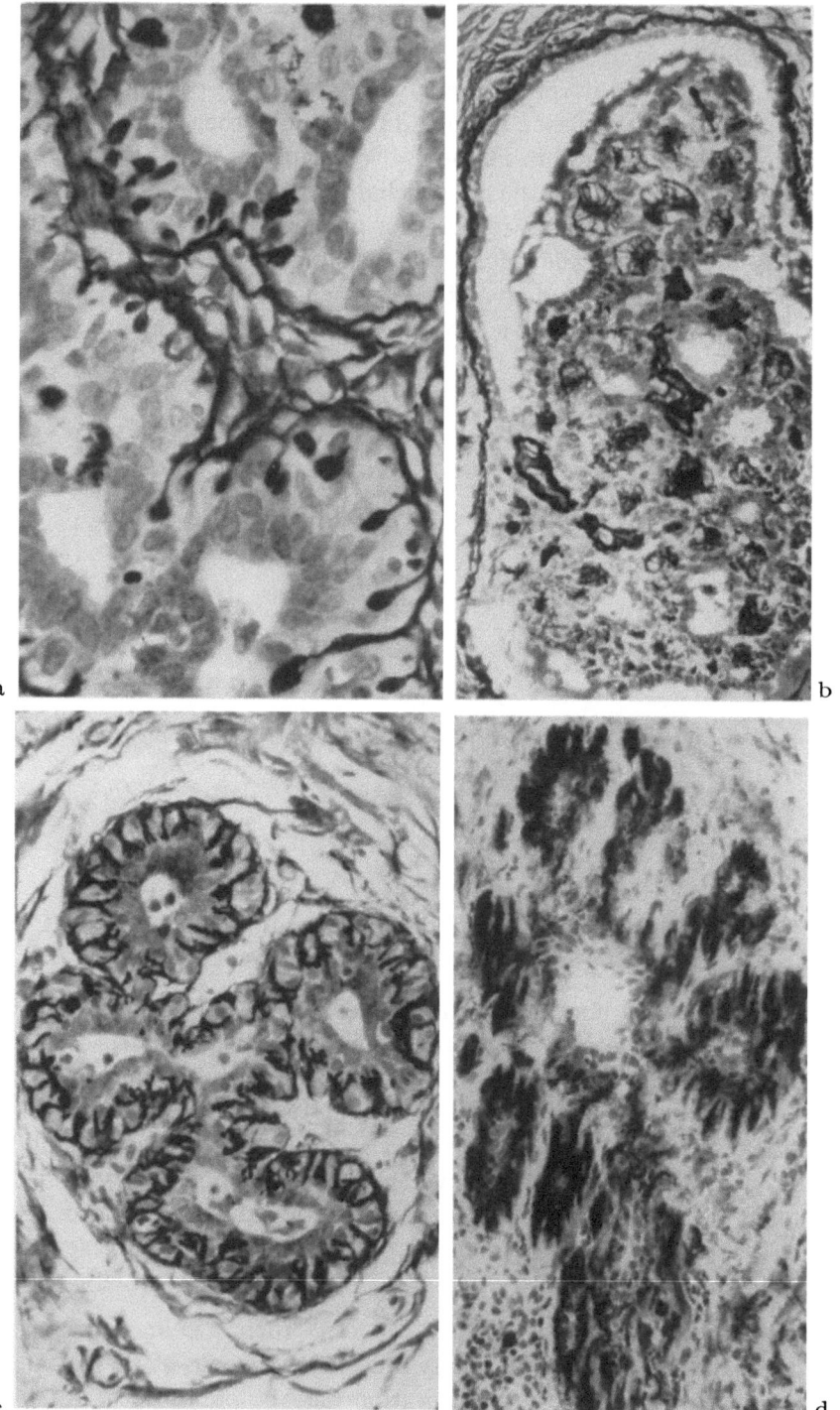

Fig. 12. a Diffuse hyperplasia of Mt in the mammary gland with formation of ovoid inclusions (Gyn. Köln, 662/67). Foot silverstain. 190×. b Cylindroma-like transformation of inclusions in intracanalicular hyperplasia of Mt (Gyn. Köln, 662/67). Foot silverstain. 190×. c Rosette-shaped hyperplasia of Mt (Gyn. Köln, 40/69). Foot silverstain. 300×. d Rosette-shaped hyperplasia of Mt. Alcaline phosphatase reaction (Azo-method). 190×

Taking into account the present state of our knowledge it seems futile to argue whether these septa, intercellular filaments, and corpuscles ought to be considered as excretion products of the Mt (similar to the preformation of collagenous fibriles as filaments in fibroblasts and their subsequent extrusion), or whether the cells by excretion of enzymes only stimulate the production of these structures in the fluid surrounding them. The ways and means may be different in either case, but the end-product is similar. The statement that Mt "produce" reticular and basement membrane-type structures must thus be taken in this wider sense. In any case, the Mt share this ability or activity with the smooth muscle cells, which are thought to take part in the production of the fibrous structures that surround them (WEISS, 1968).

4. Epimyothelial Islands

The hyperplasias described so far concerned only the Mt — the epithelial cells took no part in them. In some types of hyperplasia, however, both cells participate though in varying degree. Localized hyperplasia of Mt *and* epithelium produces the epimyothelial island.

Such islands occur in the *mammary gland* in cases of proliferating mastopathy. They represent cell clusters that are sharply delineated from the stroma (Fig. 13a) and consist of closely intermingled, spindle-shaped cells and cuboidal epithelial cells surrounding lumina. When the basement membrane or the reticular structures are properly stained, the two components can easily be distinguished: an irregular network of reticular fibres is found to have developed between the spindle-shaped myothelial cells, whereas the epithelial cords and ducts are surrounded by a smooth basement-membrane; silver-stained masses may occasionally enlarge and form ovoid or even cylindroma-like structures.

This description may be applied almost literally to the epimyothelial islands in the *salivary glands* (Fig. 13b), except that they may contain lymphocytes. These islands lie, in fact, in stroma infiltrated by lymphocytes; the stroma contains as well disintegrated glandular structures.

LÖWENSTEIN (1910) was the first to describe such islands in the salivary glands. He observed intercellular inclusions of collagen and of structures of the basement membrane type, which were found to enlarge and produce cylindroma-like formations. SKORPIL (1942) confirmed these findings. MORGAN and CASTLEMAN (1953), SEIFERT and GEILER (1957), and CRUICKSHANK (1965) studied the occurrence of these islands in rheumatic disorders, ERICSON (1968) in Sjögren's syndrome and Mikulicz's disease. GODWIN (1952) introduced the term "benign lymphoepithelial lesion" in the Anglo-American literature. MORGAN and CASTLEMAN (1953) speak of "epi-myo-epithelial" proliferations or islands, a term which might with advantage be abbreviated to "epi-myothelial" proliferations or islands.

SEIFERT and GEILER (1957) investigated the genesis of these islands. They thought that cushions of Mt first appear that eventually cause an obliteration of the ducts with subsequent glandular atrophy. Ligation of a duct according to DIETZ (1955) may lead to similar changes. In the view of SEIFERT and GEILER (1957) a periductal lymphocytic infiltration can be

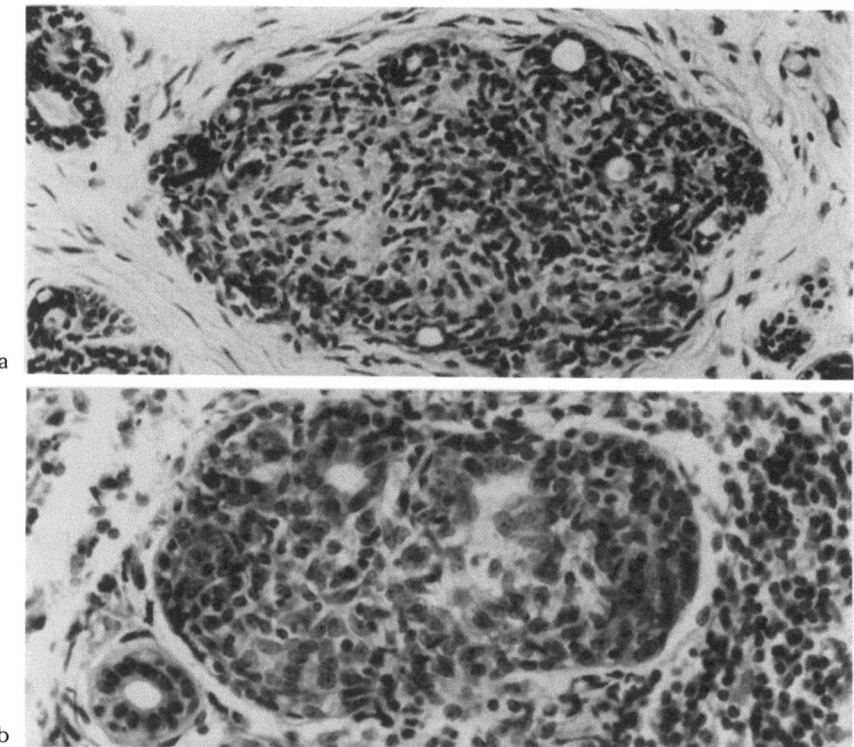

Fig. 13a and b. Epi-myothelial islands. a In proliferating mastopathy (Gyn. Köln, 40/69). HE 300×. b In parotid gland (Bonn, A 672/55). HE 480×

functionally analogous to ligation of the duct and may trigger an epimyothelial proliferation as an adaptive hyperplasia. The authors, therefore, propose the term "lymphoid-myo-epithelial sialadenitis", as the islands are no more than a partial symptom in the picture of an chronic inflammation of the salivary glands.

CRUICKSHANK (1965) claimed to have seen similar islands in inflammations of the *prostate*.

5. Fibrosing Adenosis of the Mamma

The most extensive combined proliferation of Mt and epithelium is found in the mammary gland in *fibrosing adenosis*. This condition is so well known and has been described so frequently with regard to the Mt (HAMPERL, 1939; KUZMA, 1943; STEWART, 1950) that I can limit myself to a brief discussion of their role. As a rule, myothelial proliferation begins as "hyperplasie myoide" (MASSON, 1956) in the center of such a focus, around a medium-sized excretory duct. In the periphery smaller ducts radiating from the central duct may predominate whereas the centre contains a tightly packed mixture of Mt and epithelial structures. The intermingling becomes quite evident when reticulin stains are used. Reticulin fibres smoothly surround the glandular tubuli in the periphery; instead in the center a network of reticulin fibres enclose the proliferated Mt and epithelial ducts. MASSON (1956) pointed out that the Mt, in spite of their epithelial nature, assume the form of mesenchymal cells and behave like connective tissue cells as soon as they lose contact with the epithelium. They are, nevertheless, recognizable as Mt by electronmicroscopy (MURAD and VON HAAM, 1968a), because of their content of fibrils.

The peripheral tubuli in a focus of fibrosing adenosis may, though rarely, exhibit a distinct myothelial layer or even a preponderance of Mt (Fig. 14), so that they seem to consist mainly of spindle-shaped cells.

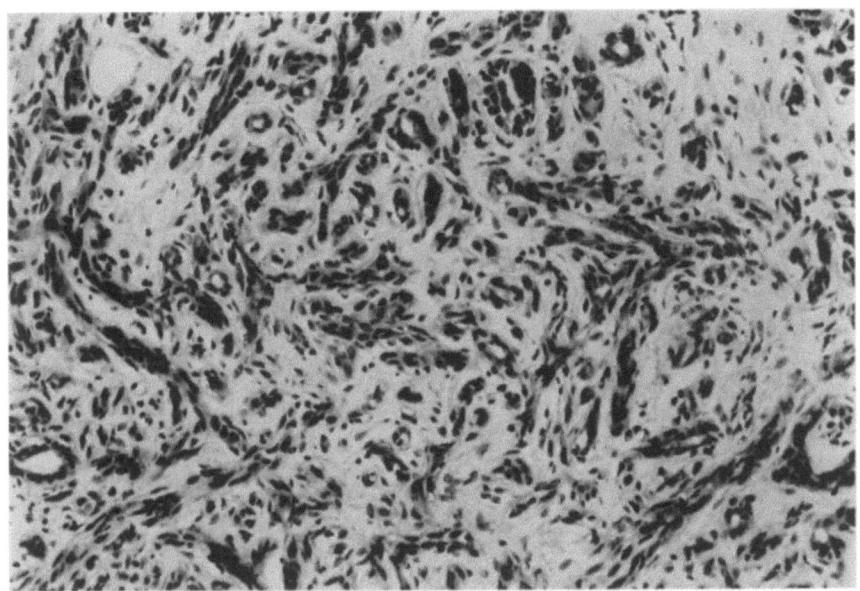

Fig. 14. Fibrosing adenosis. Peripheral tubules, consisting almost entirely of Mt (Gyn. Köln, 927/67). HE 300×

In the transitional stage from fibrosing to *sclerosing adenosis* the changes are basically the same as in the atrophy of the mammary gland. The production of collagen fibres in the center of the focus increases resulting in abundant reticulin structures around the Mt; simultaneously, the epithelial tubuli of the periphery begin to shrink, their Mt, if there are any, survive longer.

6. Intracanalicular Hyperplasia

Sometimes a rather peculiar picture is created by epimyothelial proliferations in an excretory duct of the mammary gland, leading to an almost total obliteration of its lumen (intracanalicular hyperplasia). At the borders of the proliferation the cylindrical epithelium of the duct either remains intact or also proliferates, forming glandular lumina (see Fig. 15a). The Mt obliterating the lumen produce a reticular network, with small hyaline spheres in round lacunae (see Fig. 15b) of punched-out appearance. These myothelial masses and the fibrillar structures produced by them are connected at one or two places with the wall and the basement membrane of the duct. If the intraductal myothelial proliferation is extensive, it will obliterate the duct so completely that remnants of the original epithelial lining will be visible only here and there. The picture is then identical with the one described above (p. 179).

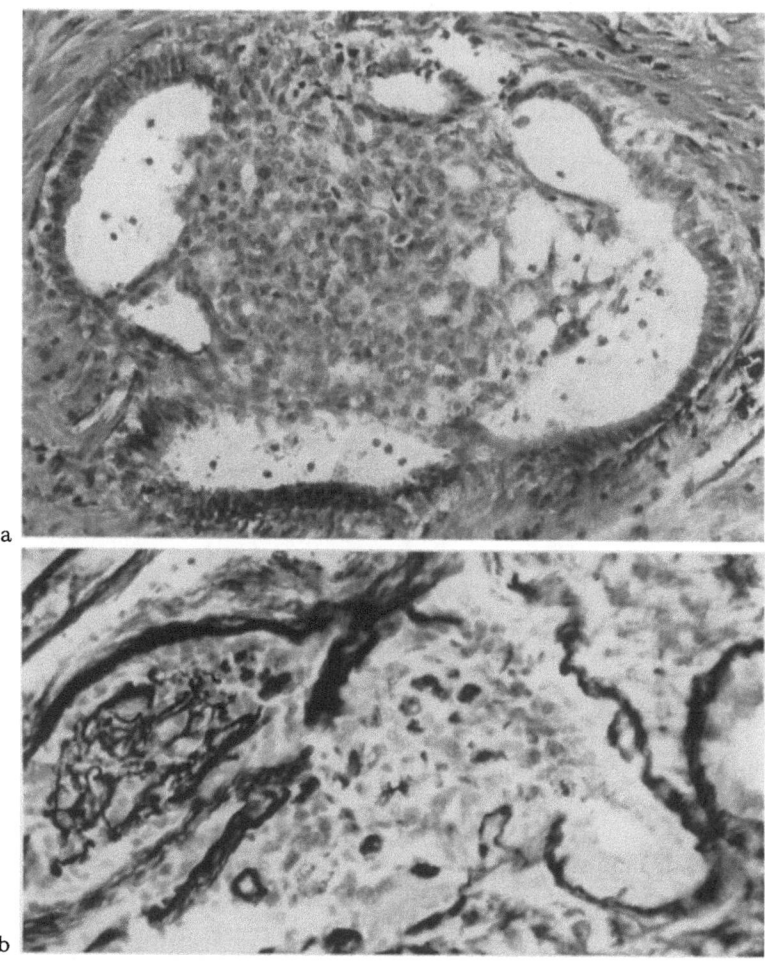

Fig. 15a and b. Intracanalicular hyperplasia of Mt. a (Prag, E 2313/42) He 190×. b With netlike and ovoid inclusions within the hyperplasia (Gyn. Köln, 988/63). Foot. 300×

IV. Benign Tumors Containing Myothelia

Generally speaking, the epithelial tumors of myothelium-containing organs (mammary gland, salivary glands, and sweat glands) may consist wholly of epithelial cells, which are analogous to those of the normal gland, or wholly of Mt (rarely), which resemble the Mt of normal glands, or of a mixture of both cell types (KLEINSASSER, 1969). In the last group the tumors containing Mt may be divided into those that are specific for their epithelial component of one of the organs mentioned above, i.e., tumors that occur solely in that particular organ (1—3), and tumors common to all these organs (4).

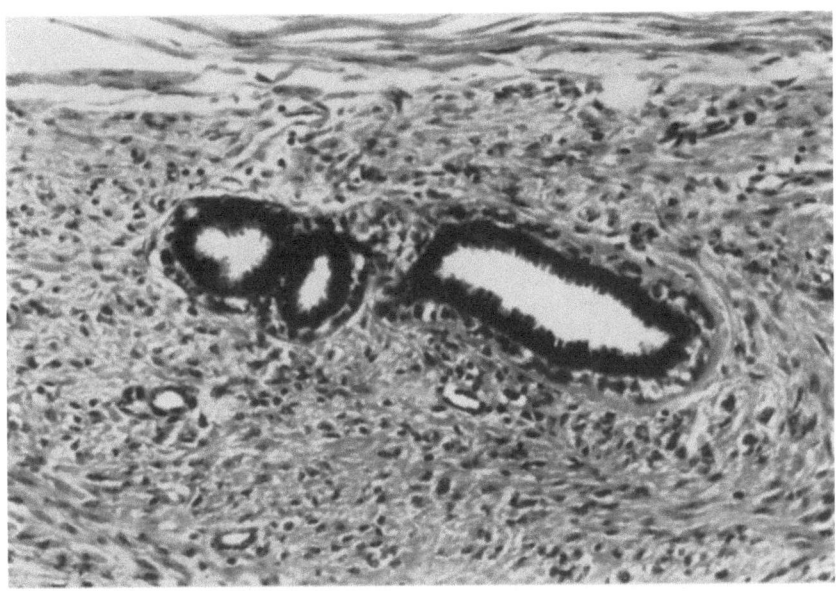

Fig. 16. Adenomyoma of the mammary gland (Marburg, J. 2501/51). HE 190 ×

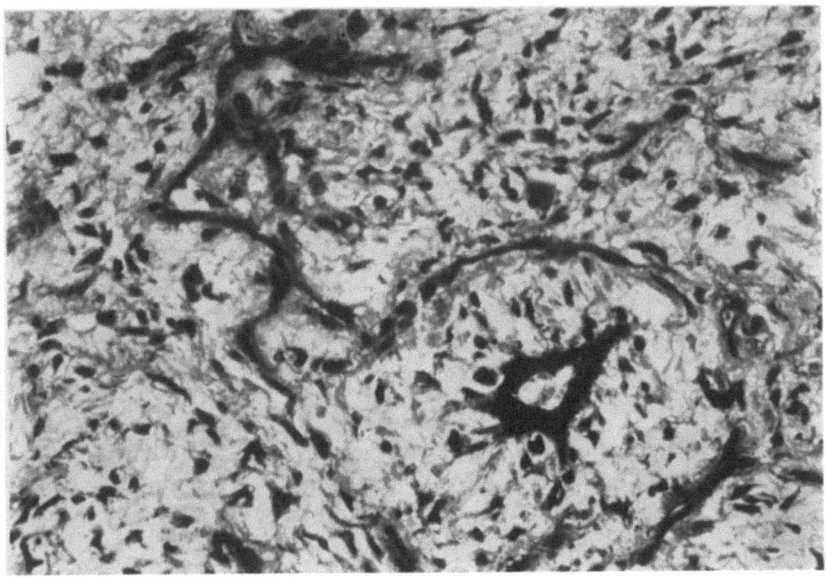

Fig. 17. Sarcoma phyllodes with epithelial cells segregating into the stroma (Wien, S. 628/35). HE 300 ×

1. Benign Tumors Containing Myothelia Occurring only in the Breast

Even in ordinary *fibroadenomas* clear cells may be found, if only in small numbers (BÄSSLER, 1968; ARCHER and OMAR, 1969), between the epithelial layer and the basement membrane. These cells often cause the basement membrane to bulge towards the stroma. They are equivalent to the clear Mt found elsewhere in the mammary gland.

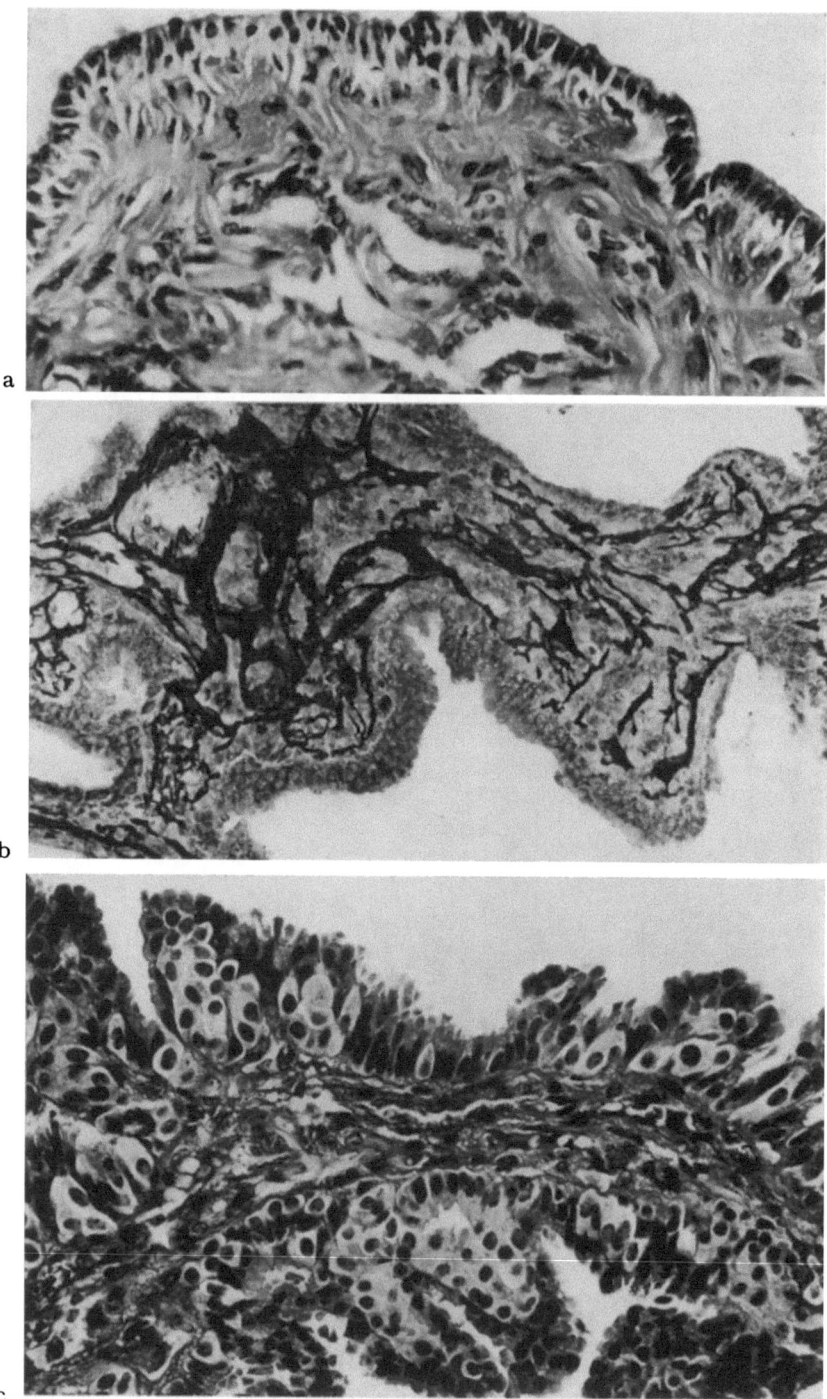

Fig. 18a—c. Intracanalicular papilloma of mammary gland with Mt. a Axial hyperplastic growth of Mt (Marburg, J. 6033/52). HE 300×. b Abundant basement membrane-like structures in between the Mt (Gyn. Köln, 1362/64). Foot silverstain. 190×. c Clear hypoplastic Mt (Bogotá, 1953/63). HE 300×

Adenomas of the nipple also show a characteristic double-layering of the epithelium: one layer of secreting cells covers a layer of basal cuboidal cells characterized by round, dense nuclei and a clear cytoplasm. This arrangement is identical with that in some ducts whose basal layer is formed by Mt.

In a tumor that might be called an *adenofibroma* because of the predominance of mesenchymal elements the sparse ducts also show that characteristic double-layering of the epithelium, the basal layer being formed by Mt. The question arises how to evaluate the long, spindle-shaped cells of the stroma which occasionally develop. With their rod-shaped nuclei and deeply staining cytoplasm they resemble smooth muscle cells, so that some of these tumors ought correctly to be called an *adenofibromyoma* (Fig. 16). ABRAMOW (1901) and MACKENZIE (1968) have described such tumors. It is an open question whether these smooth muscle cells are derived from Mt that have shed their epithelial characteristics in favour of the "myo"-qualities during their neoplastic proliferation and separation from epithelium (see above, p. 183). MELNICK (1932) thought that at least to be a possibility.

Findings in *cystosarcoma phyllodes* also suggest such a possibility. ACKERMAN (1957) described and illustrated in tumors of this kind the occurrence of bundles of what most certainly are smooth muscle fibres. I have been able to confirm that observation several times. Some regions like the one reproduced in Fig. 17 contain glandular lumina and epithelial cords, which imperceptibly radiate into or blend with spindle-shaped stroma cells. One has the impression that at least part of the stroma cells are derived from epithelium or, in other words, that they correspond to proliferated atypical epithelium or myothelial cells that now have assumed a purely mesenchymal shape.

Granting the possibility that proliferated Mt may change into a kind of smooth muscle cell, the question arises whether pure *leiomyomas* of the mammary gland might not also be derived from Mt, a possibility that already PEYRON et al. (1926) have considered.

It is relatively easy to prove the involvement of Mt in the formation of *papillomas of the mammary ducts*. Mt occur in two forms: first, as numerous "typical" Mt that are embedded in the axis of the papilla (see Fig. 18a); these cells are spindle-shaped and irregularly arranged; under the light-microscope they show a fibrillar cytoplasm that stains deeply with eosin, and an oblong, oval nucleus, rich in chromatin; the cells are in close contact with the covering layer of cylindrical epithelium and at the same time produce between them an abundance of reticulin-structures that stain with silver (Fig. 18b). Second, there are well-delimited cuboidal or polygonal cells (see Fig. 18c), which by their clear cytoplasm stand out sharply from the darker cylindrical cells; they are situated immediately above the basement membrane and occur singly or in groups. Also these cells are to be considered as hyperplastic Mt. As proof for that assumption, one can point to pictures where both the clear hyperplastic Mt and the "typical" Mt with fibrillar cytoplasm appear together and seem to blend into each other.

Sometimes an abundance of Mt is found in a particular type of *adenoma* of the mammary gland. These adenomas may occur also as encapsulated nodules, in which a large number of glandular tubuli catch the eye. More detailed observation shows that the glandular tubuli are surrounded by a thick mantle of either polygonal clear cells or spindle-shaped elements (see Fig. 19). The latter predominate in places so much that the glandular structure

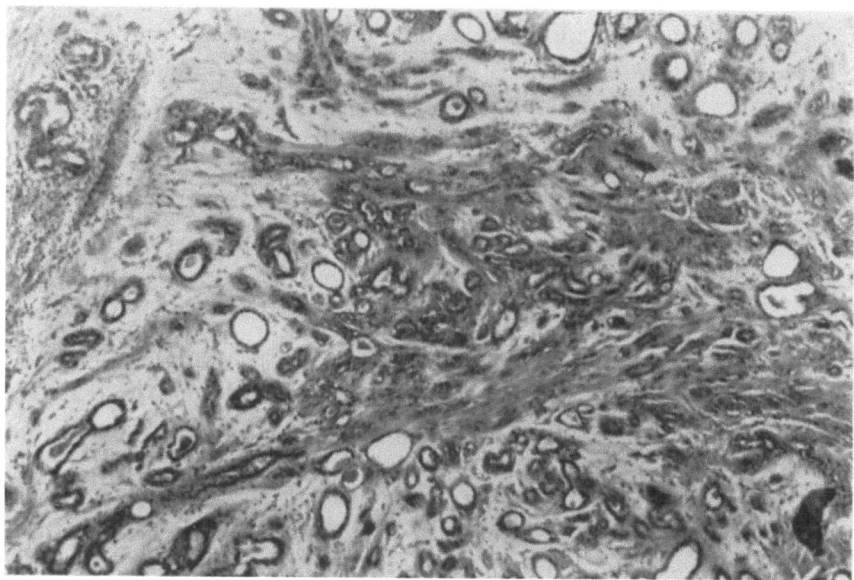

Fig. 19. Adenoma of mammary gland with abundant growth of Mt (Prag, E 8525/43). HE 48×

almost disappears. Silver stains reveal a smooth basement membrane surrounding the purely tubular structures and an incomplete intercellular network between the spindle-shaped cells. In such a tumor both epithelial and myothelial cells are thus represented in a special fashion; one could designate it as an adenoma with a strong myothelial component (myoadenoma?).

2. Benign Tumors Containing Myothelia Occurring only in the Skin

In *syringomas* Mt occasionally will be found beneath the cells lining the lumen. Since they fail to show phosphatase activity they are not regarded as fully developed Mt (LEVER and HASHIMOTO, 1966); LUND (1957) thought that they were only comparable with Mt in a vague sense.

A row of cuboid basal cells in *papillary syringadenomas* or in *papillary hidradenomas of the vulva* may resemble Mt or, at least, may be comparable with them (MAYER, 1941; LEVER, 1948; LUND, 1957).

3. Benign Tumors Containing Myothelia Occurring only in the Salivary Glands

are unknown

4. Tumors Containing Myothelia Occurring in Several Organs

This group of tumors consists of three types, viz., mixed tumors of the salivary gland type, cylindromas (adenoid cystic carcinomas), and a type of tumor for which the term adenomyothelioma seems to be most appropriate. Two facts concerning all three types will be discussed first.

First, although these types of tumors occur in all three organs (mammary gland, salivary glands, sweat glands), they are not necessarily identical: each organ is able to produce its particular variant of a common basic type.

Second, there are transitions between the three types of tumors, in that regions occour in each type that correspond to that of another type. For that reason LEVER (1954) has discussed the question whether all mixed tumors of the skin were in reality myotheliomas. WILLIS (1960) has even refused to accept a subdivision into the three types and consequently proposed to speak simply of pleomorphic adenomas including all three types under this single term. One can however agree with FEYRTER (1961), who rejected such a gross simplification and who pointed out that it was possible to determine and distinguish the three types of tumors from each other in spite of the occurrence of transitional forms, provided the predominant component was kept in mind; in any case they represent clinically well characterized types. More recently, the term "pleomorphic adenoma", proposed by WILLIS (1960), has frequently not been used in the sense intended by WILLIS, i.e., to characterize jointly three or more different types of tumors, but has been applied to mixed tumors of salivary gland type only, whereas the term cylindroma has been replaced by "adenoid cystic carcinoma". There are, thus, several overlapping terms in use for mixed tumors of the salivary gland type and cylindromas, apart from various outmoded terms for mixed tumors. Such a confusion of the nomenclature is particularly great for tumors that I would like to group together as adeno-myotheliomas. These tumors, when arising in the skin, have been given several names by dermatologists, who are — as is well known — enthusiasts for new names. The different terms usually accentuate the preponderance of an individual aspect or a special variety of the one basic form. Similarly, a variety of types of cylindromas are known in dermatology under different names.

There is, thus, on the one hand, tendency to subdivide phenomena by stressing their differences, and, on the other, a tendency to lump everything together by neglecting these differences.

I believe to be steering a middle course by limiting myself to the three basic types mentioned above: mixed tumor, cylindroma (or adenoid cystic carcinoma), and adeno-myothelioma. In principle, that conforms to FEYRTER'S (1961) classification, with the sole difference that instead of FEYRTER'S terms "solid" and "tubular-solid adenoma" the terms "adenomyoepithelioma" or better "adenomyothelioma" are used as introduced by HARTZ (1946) and BAUER and FOX (1952). These terms emphasize correctly the importance of the myothelial component in this type of tumor. One can thus also agree with FEYRTER — who regarded his "clear cell organ" as the source and model for all the three types of tumors, since he considers his "clear cell organ" as identical with the Mt, i.e., the basket cells and the myothelial cells in the organs in question (mammary gland, salivary glands, sweat glands).

a) Mixed Tumor of the Salivary Gland Type

The understanding of this type of tumor has been greatly advanced by two facts that were discovered at about the same time.

First, HEMPLEMANN and WOMACK (1942) pointed out that these tumors contained *two types of mucus*, which were designated as epithelial and mesenchymal (myxomatous). They may be differentiated histologically by their different staining properties with toluidine blue and methylene blue (HEMPLEMANN and WOMACK, 1942; AZZOPARDI and SMITH, 1959) and their different behavior towards hyaluronidase, testicular extract, and extract of leeches (NEGRI and FERRANTE, 1949). Epithelial mucus contains neutral glycoproteins with a small amount of sialuronic acid; mesenchymal mucus contains glycosamine-glycane, composed of hyaluronic acid, chondroitin-4 and/or chondroitin-sulphate (ERICHSEN, 1955; QUINTARELLI and ROBINSON, 1967). The epithelial mucus lies in round lumina, surrounded by cylindrical cells, whereas the mesenchymal mucus lies between spindle and stellate cells in the vicinity of the connective tissue stroma (GRISHMAN, 1952).

Second, PEYRON and his co-workers in a series of brief communications and in a review (1926) analysed the peculiar mixed tumors seen in the mammary glands of dogs and cats. They clearly stressed the important part played by Mt in the development and growth of these tumors and underscored the importance of these findings for the understanding of mixed tumors in human salivary and mammary glands. Their findings in mixed tumors of the mammary gland of dogs have been confirmed repeatedly (HAMPERL, 1939; ALLEN, 1940; COTCHIN, 1952). Later on, SHELDON (1943) stressed the importance of the presence in human mixed tumors of cells he thought to be *myothelia*. That interpretation has been accepted by a good many workers (BAIN et al., 1945; BAUER and BAUER, 1953; BHASKAR and WEINMANN, 1955; AZZOPARDI and SMITH, 1959). It has, furthermore, been supported by recent electron-microscopic investigations: MYLIUS (1960), DAVID and KORTH (1964), and DOYLE et al. (1968) were able to demonstrate typical fibrils 50—60 Å in diameter in these cells. Alcaline phosphatase and adenosintriphosphatase, both characteristic for Mt have been demonstrated not only in mixed tumors but in cylindromas and solid adenomas as well (KAUFMANN and STIEBITZ, 1969).

ENEROTH and WERSÄLL (1966) thought, however, that the fibrils might be related to tonofibrils, but other authors have rejected that interpretation. DEPPISCH and TOKER (1969), on the other hand, were unable to find fibrils in the tumor cells.

It should be noted that ENEROTH and WERSÄLL (1966) and WELSH and MEYER (1968) were able to demonstrate fibrils with the electron-microscope in cells of mixed tumors, which might be considered as myothelial, and in purely epithelial cells too. The latter cells would have no normal prototype and could be considered as a kind of chimera: the differentiations that occur separately in normal tissue would thus take place in one single cell, if only in modified form. These cells are then usually called transitional types (OOTA and TAKAHASHI, 1958).

Attention has repeatedly been drawn to the high content of glycogen of myothelial cells in mixed tumors (e. g., AZZOPARDI and SMITH, 1959). That reminds one of the glycogen content of normal Mt and of their tendency to store glycogen under abnormal conditions.

The fact that mesenchymal mucus occurs in mixed tumors, which are epithelial, has created a number of complicated hypotheses. There has been a tendency to assume that this mesenchymal mucus could only have been supplied by the mesenchymal tissue of the stroma, albeit under the influence of the epithelial or — better — myothelial tumor-cells. AZZOPARDI and SMITH (1959), on the other hand, have simply concluded that the mesenchymal mucus of a mixed tumor is the product of myothelial cells. I agree with that interpretation, since it conforms with the thesis of the duplex nature (i.e., epithelial-mesenchymal) of Mt, as stated earlier. I go even further in that I include the production of chondroid and cartilaginous ground substance among the hidden potentialities of Mt that may become manifest in a tumor. This is complete agreement with CAPONE-BRAGA (1945), who perceived mixed tumors already as "mesenchymoplastic" tumors of the Mt. Mt may even produce true mesenchymal cartilage and may transform themselves into cartilage cells, just as they produce mesenchymal mucus; there is really no need to talk about pseudocartilage. At first glance it may appear incredible that epithelial-ectodermal cells should be able not only to produce mesenchymal intercellular substances but even to change into mesenchymal cells themselves. The assumption may become acceptable, however, if one recalls that Mt in simple hyperplasias are able to produce substances like that of the basement membrane, or that of cylindromas, Hence the production of reticulin and collagen fibres in mixed tumors may now without hesitation be attributed to the myothelial cells. DOYLE et al. (1968) furthermore pointed out that the vacuoles of the myothelial cells in mixed tumors contain a material which is a tropocollagen identical with that surrounding the cells; thus one may assume that the myothelial cells really produce collagenous fibres with a typical periodicity of 640 Å.

It is difficult to accept the fact that epithelial cells of ectodermal origin are able to produce collagen fibres, cartilage and even bone, because the prevailing concept of classification of tissues and tumors is based on the assumption that a strict division can be made between epithelial and mesenchymal tissues and cells. It is, however, "no novel concept that epithelial cells possess the potentiality to develop into tissue of mesodermal appearance" (BIGGS, 1947). MASSON and PEYRON (1914) had in this connection already drawn attention to glia cells and SCHWANN cells.

If this thesis is accepted, then the term "mixed (salivary gland) tumor" should and could be used not because a tumor consists of a mixture of epithelium (whether glandular or squamous) and mesenchymal components as mucus, cartilage and fibrous tissue, but because it presents a particular mixture of epithelium and pluripotent myothelium. The term also implies that it is apparently impossible to specify which cell of the mature gland gives rise to the tumor, be it from a serous acinus or from a part of an excretory duct. Obviously many potentialities lie hidden in all cells of these structures and each potentiality is capable of becoming realized under the conditions of neoplastic proliferation.

These remarks about mixed tumors of the salivary glands are equally valid for the mixed tumors of the *mammary gland* and *skin*. Their identity with those of the salivary glands has repeatedly been confirmed (e. g. BIGGS, 1947: mammary tumors; BÖCK and FEYRTER, 1961: orbit; SIMARD, 1938; NANGLE and SYMMERS, 1950: skin; HIRSCH and HELWIG, 1961: chondroid syringoma of skin) although in individual cases some traits may be accentuated or lacking because of the different realization of the hidden potentialities.

b) Cylindroma (Adenoid Cystic Carcinoma)

As many authors (STILLIANS, 1933; LEVER, 1948a; MYLIUS, 1960; CRAIN and HELWIG, 1961; LEVER and HASHIMOTO, 1966) have pointed out, it is possible to distinguish two types of cells in cylindromas: small basal cells with round nuclei and rich in chromatin, and larger cells with pale nuclei that are situated in the centre of the epithelial masses; these larger cells occasionally surround lumina. LEVER (1948b) mentioned that the formation of the hyaline and mucoid masses, found both on the outer surface of the epithelial masses and in their interior, is always close to the smaller kind of cell, which he interpreted to be myothelial; THACKERAY and LUCAS (1960) and FRIBORSKY (1963) are of the same opinion. To support this interpretation one can point to the myothelial proliferations of the mammary gland showing basement membrane-like deposits between them identical to those seen in cylindromas. FEYRTER (1961b) conceived an impressive schema of their development (see Fig. 20) that fits for both the cylindroma and the hyperplastic proliferations of the Mt in the mammary gland. Processes with identical staining properties extend from the basement membrane surrounding the epithelial masses into the cell masses, which undergo hyaline or mucoid transformation, or may according to FEYRTER be invaded by connective tissue cells, a fact HÜBNER et al. (1969) are rather sceptical about. Moreover, an intercellular substance of reticular arrangement is formed in cylindromas, which STILLIANS (1933) very fittingly compared with the tendrils of vines. This substance is best made evident by staining with silver, and shows connections with the coarser inclusions and the basement membrane.

HÜBNER et al. (1969) supplied strong evidence for the myothelial nature of the basal cell layers in cylindromas of the salivary glands by demonstrating typical fibrils in them with the electron-microscope. Even a cell structure was discovered imitating the normal bipolarity of the Mt, since one-half of these cells was rich in ergastoplasm, while the other contained the myofibrils. Such fibril-containing cells were less common in the so-called Spiegler tumor of the skin.

Basically, the structure of a cylindroma is similar to that of a mixed tumor: an epithelial mass, containing, on the one hand, glandular lumina surrounded

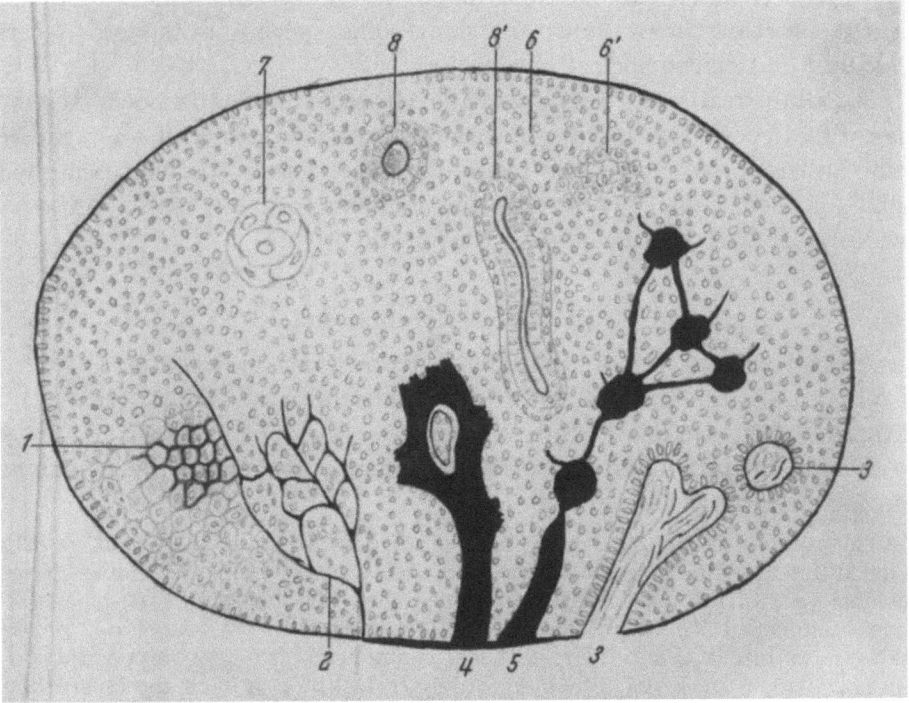

Fig. 20. The intercellular structures in cylindromas (adenocystic carcinomas): *1* amorphous substance; *2* reticular interstitial substance; *3* vascularised interstitial tissue containing cells and collagen fibers. *4* hyalin masses; *5* cylindromatous formations with pearl-like swellings; *6* neoplastic epithelium without and with (*6'*) well developed boundaries of the cells; *7* squamous cell-like neoplastic epithelium; *8* tubular structures. (After FEYRTER, 1961)

by epithelium and, on the other hand, Mt producing ground substance structures like collagen, hyaline and mucus. Even the two types of mucus that occur in mixed tumors can be found in cylindromas (AZZOPARDI and SMITH, 1959). The difference between cylindroma and mixed tumor lies therefore less in the quality than in the quantity and distribution of these structures in both tumor types. In the mixed tumor the diversity of the mesenchymal differentiation prevails, proceeding to the production of cartilage or bone; in the cylindromas the mesenchymal differentiation is more regular and restricted to hyaline and mucoid in specifically arranged masses. Similarly, the "epithelial" differentiations in cylindromas are present only as sparse and small glandular lumina, whereas in mixed tumors various types of cords and tubuli occur. The duplex nature of Mt and the fact that the tissue of origin contains two cell types becomes evident in both types of tumors. It is, therefore, not surprising that mixed-tumor-like areas may occasionally arise in cylindromas, and cylindromatous areas may appear in mixed tumors.

No fundamental difference exists between the cylindromas of the salivary gland, the skin, the sweat glands and the mammary gland (PROPST, 1954), or even of Bartholini's glands (BOSCHBACH, 1969). Certain tumors of the skin, e.g., the turban tumor, however, show some special traits due to certain biological and morphological peculiarities.

For all the reasons already given above it seems futile to associate cylindromas with hypothetical points of origin in special regions of an organ, e.g., acini, different sectors of the excretory duct system, or worse, individual cells. All these cells may possess the hidden (dormant) potentialities that awaken only with the inception of neoplastic growth.

c) Adeno-Myothelioma

A third type of tumor, the adeno-myothelioma also contains two types of cells, viz., epithelium and Mt (GRYNFELTT and AIMES, 1922; KEASBEY and HADLEY, 1954; BHASKAR and WEINMANN, 1955; KERSTING and HELWIG, 1956) and is mainly found in the *skin*, although it may occur in the mammary and salivary glands as well.

The tumors in the skin have been studied most extensively and have been given different names (see WINKELMANN and WOLFF, 1968) depending upon the personal view of the individual who studied their histology and histogenesis. They have been called "myoepitheliomas" (LEVER, 1948; POSTNOV, 1965) or, when taking more into account their epithelial component, as "adenomyoepitheliomas" (HARTZ, 1946; GUBAREWA, 1965). According to LUND (1957) and the illustrations in the original paper by KERSTING and HELWIG (1956) the eccrine spiradenoma, as described by these authors, would belong to this group, although KERSTING and HELWIG felt that their eccrine spiradenoma should be strictly differentiated from myoepithelioma. On the other hand, they admitted that a case of adenomyoepithelioma described by HARTZ (1946) might have been one of eccrine spiradenoma with excessive proliferation of Mt.

LUND (1957) included in the term "nodular hidradenoma" a whole range of tumors of the skin, e.g., myoepithelioma, eccrine spiradenoma, clear-cell epithelioma and solid hidradenoma. Unfortunately, LUND's otherwise recommendable general term cannot be used for similar tumors of the salivary glands and the mammary gland, because it refers directly and solely to the

Fig. 21a—d. Variants of adeno-myotheliomas. a Of the skin (Wien, S. 1736/34). HE 190×. b Of the mammary gland (Bonn, A. 3616/60). HE 150×. c Of the parotid gland with distinct adenomatous part (Prag, E 3344/40). HE 120×. d Of the parotid, representing an almost pure myothelioma (Berlin, 633/39). HE 190×

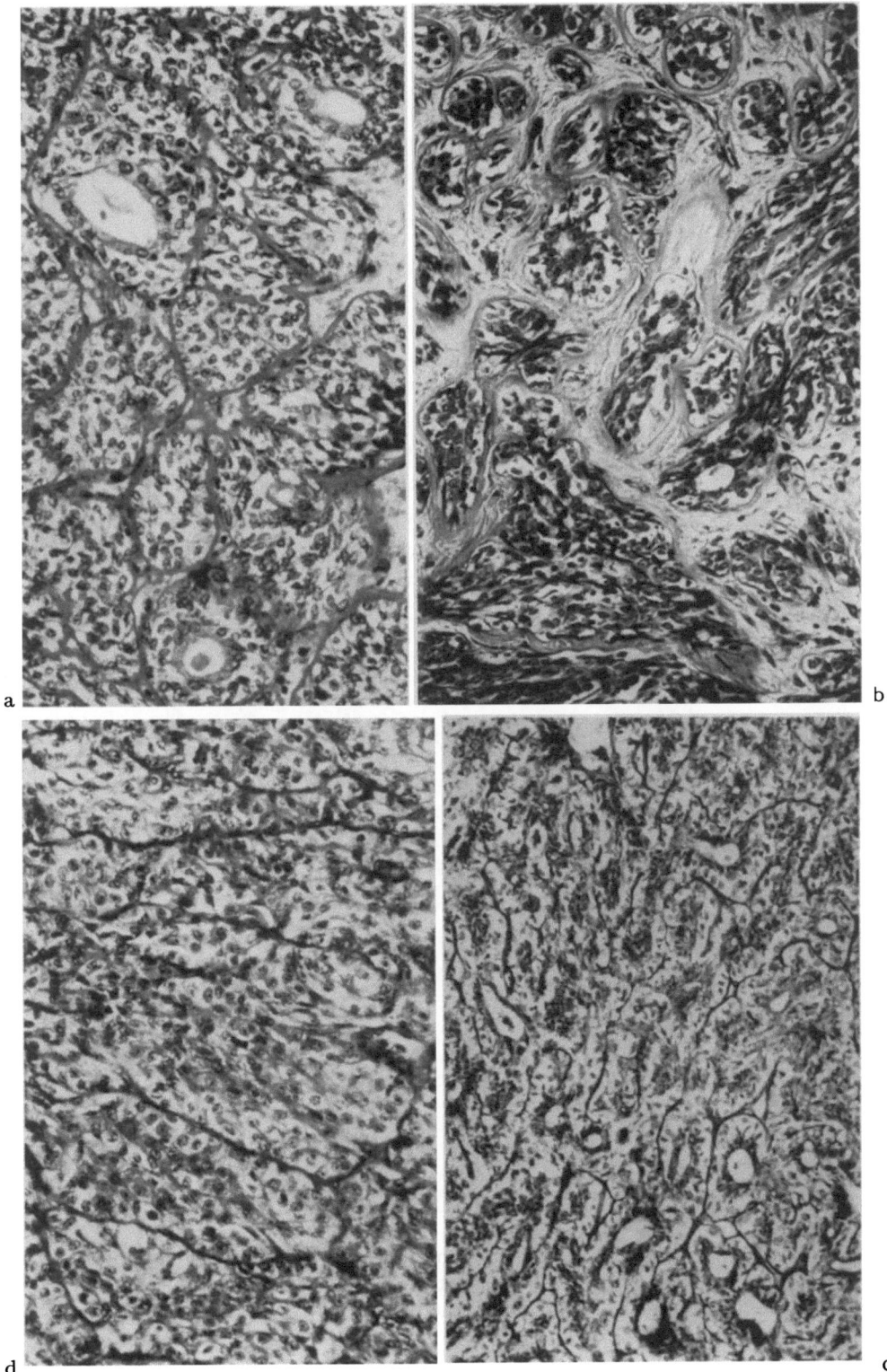

Fig. 21 a-d

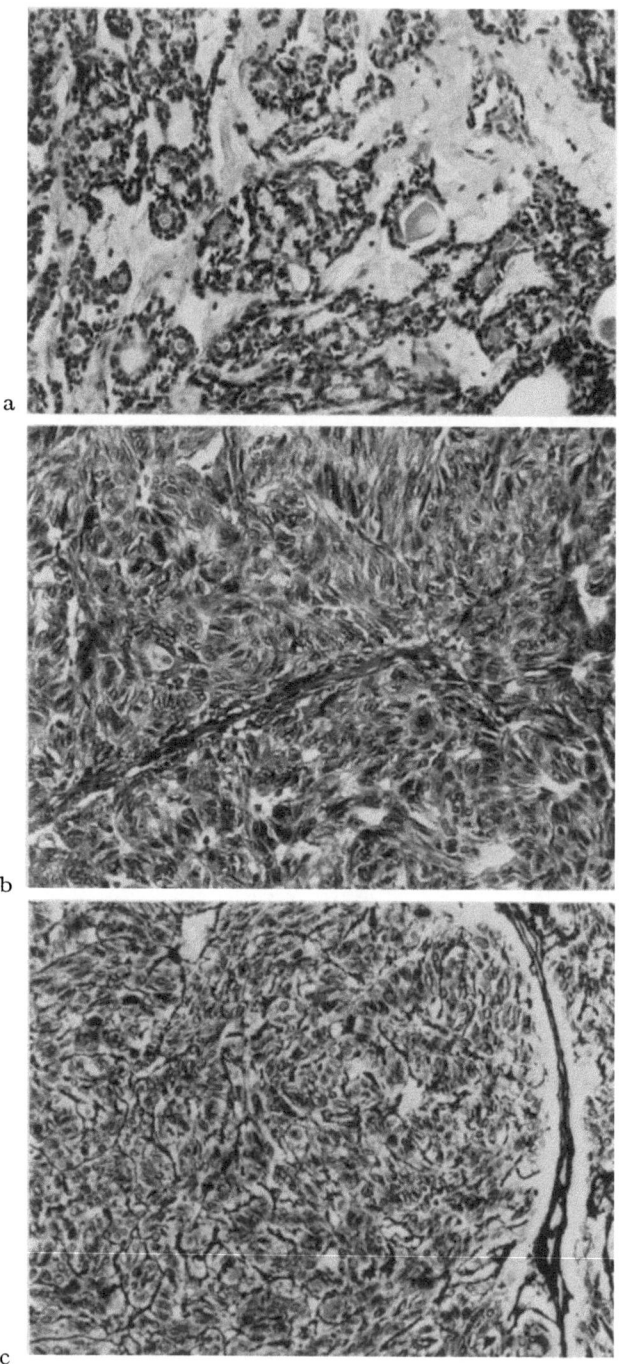

Fig. 22a—c. Different patterns in the same adeno-myothelioma of a salivary gland (Marburg, S 4416/50). a Epithelial structure. HE 120×. b Myomatous structure. HE 150×. c Myomatous structure. Foot silver stain. 150×

sweat glands, so that the comprehensive term "adenomyoepithelioma" or "adenomyothelioma" seems to be preferable as a name applicable to all the tumors belonging to this group. The same arguments apply to the term "solid-cystic hidradenoma" proposed by WINKELMANN and WOLFF (1968), and "eccrine acrospinoma" of JOHNSON and HELWIG (1969).

The basic histological structure of the adeno-myotheliomas is relatively simple (see Figs. 21 and 22). A small, central lumen is surrounded by cuboidal cells. Their cytoplasm is well-stained, but their round nuclei are poor in chromatin. These cells represent the "epithelial" component of the tumor and are surrounded by a layer of loosely arranged stellate or spindle-shaped cells with a small nucleus, rich in chromatin, and a rather pale cytoplasm. These cells are the "mesenchymal" component of the tumor. With the central epithelium these cells may form a single mass, which is surrounded by a basement membrane, or they contain between them reticulin structures connected with the basement membrane, as GRYNFELTT and AIMES (1922) observed.

SHELDON (1941) demonstrated *fibrils*, if only in small numbers, in several of the spindle-shaped cells by light-microscopy, and HASHIMOTO et al. (1966) by electron-microscopy. Others were not able to confirm the presence of fibrils (KERSTING and HELWIG, 1956; BERGHORN et al., 1961; O'HARA et al., 1966), which is not surprising in view of their scarcity. Nevertheless, a number of authors are inclined to regard these cells as myothelial or, at least, as suspect of being of myothelial nature (SHELDON, 1941; MAYER, 1941; LEVER, 1948; EFSKIND and EKER, 1954; HARTZ, 1966). Others repudiate every connection with Mt for lack of evidence (KERSTING and HELWIG, 1956; CRAIN and HELWIG, 1961; KERSTING, 1963; WINKELMANN and WOLFF, 1968); they are not prepared to relate the two types of tumor components to epithelial and myothelial cells, but rather to the two types of secreting cells of the sweat glands; the position of the cells is not thought to be sufficient evidence by itself for their myothelial nature. In view of the proven presence of fibrils and the evident ability of these cells to form intermediate substances the argument against their myothelial nature does not seem very convincing. I am, therefore, inclined to regard them as myothelial or, at least, myothelial-like cells.

BAUER and FOX (1945) and BHASHKAR and WEINMANN (1955) applied the term "adenomyoepithelioma" to similar tumors of the *salivary glands* (see Fig. 21c and d), a term that originally had been suggested by HARTZ (1946) for tumors of the sweat glands. EVANS (1966), too, spoke of an "adenomyoepithelial pattern" of certain tumors of the salivary glands.

The "glycogen-rich reticulated adenoma" of FEYRTER (1963) most probably belongs to this group too. The term "reticulated" refers to the peculiar aspect of the cytoplasm of the tumor-cells after the extraction of the glycogen; FEYRTER traces the tumor to the Mt (basket cells) of the glands.

It had always been emphasized that even cylindromas and mixed tumor of the salivary glands could eventually be included in this group of tumors. This, is, of course, not surprising in view of the above-mentioned close relationship between the three tumor types. I would however prefer to apply the term "adeno-myo-epithelioma" or better "adeno-myothelioma" only for tumors clearly belonging to this group. It covers in a rather general fashion a peculiar type of tumor, occurring in various organs and composed of epi- and myothelial cells in a very special fashion. Any transitions towards mixed tumors or even areas of cartilage (LEVER) and squamous cells may occasionally occour, but these should be considered irrelevant for the classification.

I was able to observe a typical case of adeno-myoepithelioma in the *mammary gland* (see Fig. 21 b). FINCK et al. (1968) described clear-cell myoepitheliomas (see below) in the mammary gland.

In general one has to concede the adeno-myotheliomas some *variability*. Already HARTZ (1946) pointed to the variable involvement of the epithelial cells in his cases (see also Figs. 21a—d and 22a—c). EFSKIND and EKER (1954) drew attention to a similar variability of the involvement of the Mt in some tumors. There are cases where the lumina with their epithelial lining are so obvious that they cannot be missed, and there are others where they have to be looked for. In such cases the histological picture may at first glance be highly confusing, because it may show masses of tumor cells with blurred outlines quite atypical for epithelial structures. If a reticulin network around the cells is demonstrable, either locally or generally in all parts of the tumor, the picture may be quite like that of a myoma (see Fig. 22b) or even of a leiomyosarcoma (SHELDON, 1941). The cells differ, however, from those of pure leiomyomas by their plump spindly shape.

FEYRTER (1961) found *deposits of pigment* in his "solid" and "trabecularsolid" adenomas of the salivary glands, which correspond to our adeno-myotheliomas. The deposits were lipofuscin, which occurs in normal Mt (basket cells) of salivary glands (see above), and ceroid pigment, found in the normal Mt of the mammary gland (see p. 170).

The *clear-cell* myoepithelioma described by LEVER and CASTLEMAN (1952) may very possibly form a special subgroup of the adeno-myotheliomas with absolute predominance of the myothelial cells. It had been explained as such already by BAUER and BAUER (1953), but this concept has been rejected by others (AZZOPARDI, 1958). FINCK et al. (1968) derived the clear-cell hidradenomas in mammary glands from multipotent duct cells, out of which both epithelial and myothelial cells were thought to arise. In my opinion there are two points supporting the thesis of the clear-cell myothelioma as presented by LEVER and CASTLEMAN (1952). First, stress has been laid repeatedly in this paper on the fact that both normal Mt and the myothelial cells of mixed tumors sometimes contain large quantities of glycogen. FEYRTER (1963) even designated a special form of a "glycogen-rich, reticulated adenoma" (s. page 197); Second, LEVER (1954) had pointed out that even in clear-cell myotheliomas two cell types may be distinguished: spindle-shaped cells, which may be transformed into clear cells, and secretory epithelial elements, which are characteristic of epi-myothelial tumors.

V. Malignant Tumors Containing Myothelia

If one admits that Mt, myothelial, or myothelial-like cells occur in benign tumors, then the question arises whether they may occur in malignant tumors too. The difficulties of determining the identity of or the analogy to Mt in benign tumors have been great enough to leave some sceptics unconvinced of their presence, as it has not always been possible to demonstrate all qualities of a myothelial cell (filaments, phosphatase activity, characteristic shape of cell and nucleus, site etc.) in a particular cell under examination. These difficulties apply to an even greater extent to the evaluation and recognition of Mt in malignant tumors. Here we may have to base the assumption that a tumor cell is probably myothelial only by such features as its configuration, spindly shape, deeper staining of its cytoplasm with fuchsin and eosin or PTAH, and by its ability to produce reticulin fibres or ground substance-like masses, and lastly, by the site of the questionable cell and its relation to the basement membrane. These criteria may, in fact, be fulfilled by some malignant tumor cells: occasionally the presence of filaments or fibrils has been demonstrated, although this is not the absolute proof it appears to be, because similar filaments have been observed in other cells too, e.g., monocytes.

When looking for Mt in malignant tumors the investigator will think primarily of malignant variants of the three epi-myothelial tumor types discussed above (p. 189). One of them, the *cylindroma*, may take many years before it metastasizes, hence Anglo-American usage has discarded the old term "cylindroma" and replaced it by the term "adenoid cystic carcinoma". The metastases resemble the primary tumor; what has been said about "benign" cylindromas applies therefore also to metastasizing cylindromas and their metastases.

The situation is different for malignant mixed tumors (1) and malignant myotheliomas (3).

1. Malignant Mixed Tumors of the Salivary Gland Type

Malignant (metastasizing) types of mixed tumors of the *salivary glands* are extremely rare. Malignant transformation of a benign mixed tumor usually occurs as a squamous cell carcinoma or adenocarcinoma. FOOTE and FRAZELL (1954) however describe in detail a few cases of mixed salivary-gland tumors, the metastases of which had retained most of the characteristics of the original mixed tumor, so that the earlier statements concerning the part played by the Mt in mixed tumors apply to them too. The most reliable sign of malignancy may be a polymorphy of the nuclei (GERUGHTY et al., 1969).

In the human *mammary gland* true carcinomas may arise that produce mucoid, chondroid, osteoid or even bony intercellular substances so that "bizarre microscopic configurations" (FOOTE and STEWART, 1940; STEWART, 1950) are created, which resemble those of mixed tumors. FRUHLING et al. (1960) use the term "malignant mixed tumors" for similar tumors. In fact, these tumors contain all varieties of transitional forms between epithelial cells of a typical mammary carcinoma and fibroblasts, chondroblasts and even osteoblasts (CABANNE, 1960). In 1939 I described an analogous tumor producing mucoid and chondroid substances and pointed to its similiarity to myothelial malignant mixed tumors occurring in the mammary gland of dogs; the mucus and cartilage were thought to be truly epithelial. FOOTE and STEWART (1950) also assumed that the cartilage was of epithelial nature, as transitions from epithelial cells via spindle cells to mucoid and chondriod cells could be demonstrated.

Sometimes the picture is dominated by and attention is drawn to the presence of chondroid or osteoid substances. In such cases it is possible to arrive at the wrong diagnosis of chondro-osteoid-sarcoma as STEWART (1950) pointed out. A diagnosis of a malignant epithelial tumor, viz. a malignant mixed tumor, would however be correct because of the pure epithelial portions, no matter how scarce they may be. If there are none whatsoever, no objection can made to a diagnosis of "chondro-osteoid-sarcoma", unless special circumstances prevail (see below).

2. Sarcomas of the Mammary Gland

If the epithelial cells of the mammary gland, the sweat glands and the salivary glands really possess the potentiality to undergo mesenchymal differentiation in benign and malignant tumors, the question seems well founded whether that mesenchymal differentiation might not sometimes dominate the picture so completely that pure benign and malignant mesenchymal tumors result. I have pointed out above (p. 187) that some benign tumors like myomas, especially of the breast, might originate from Mt, or might represent from the histological point of view mesenchymal tumors, although from the histogenetic point of view they might be of epithelial origin. In fact there has been described a *fibrosarcoma of the breast* (CROCKER and MURAD, 1969) whose cells contained fibrils with condensation stripes characteristic under the electronmicroscope for Mt.

Some details found in *chondro-osteoidsarcomas* of the mammary gland may justify the suspicion, that at least some of them are of epithelial-myothelial nature.

One such tumor (A. 2337/60) of a 51 year old woman contained areas which under low magnification would justify the immediate diagnosis of carcinoma (see Fig. 23 a): cords and ducts of deeply stained cells embedded in an abundantly developed, fibrous stroma. The individual elements had a round or angular, chromatin-rich nucleus that lay in a cytoplasm, deeply stained by erythrosin-fuchsin. The distribution of the reticulin fibres (see Fig. 23 b, e) caused some surprise because the cellular cords were not surrounded by a basement membrane, as one might have expected. Not only was this membrane missing, but reticular fibres were to be found between the "epithelial" cells of the cords. They completely ensheathed some of them or surrounded small groups of cells. This reticular structure was very coarse in some parts (see Fig. 23 e), and had almost the appearance of a hyalin substance. There were, indeed, gradual transitions to be observed towards areas where the intercellular ground substance assumed the staining properties of cartilage (see Fig. 23c and d). The tumor cells lay in lacunae, exactly like cartilage cells and showed the effects of shrinkage like normal cartilage

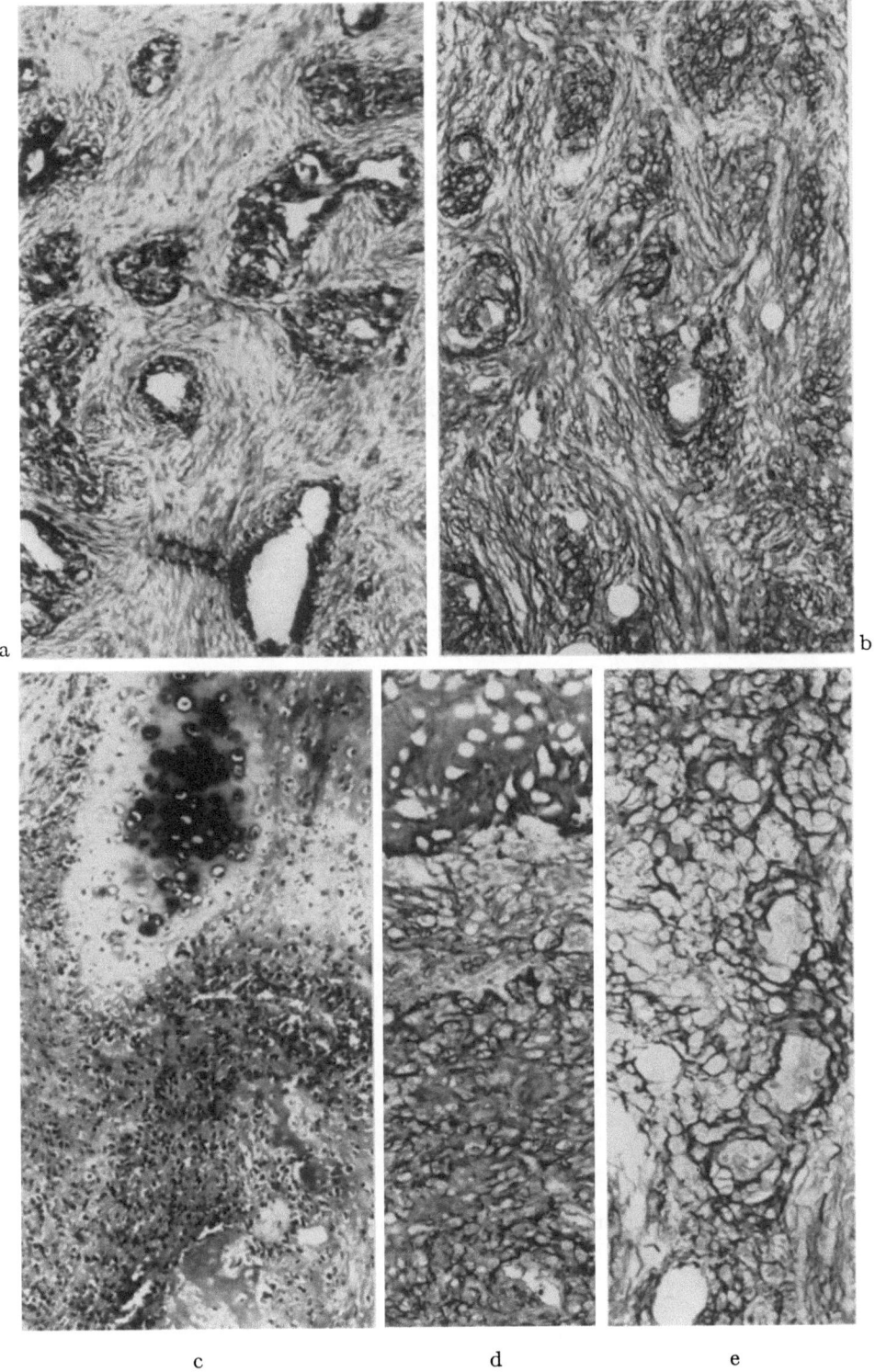

Fig. 23a—e. Chondro-osteoid sarcoma (carcinoma) of the mammary gland (Bonn, A 2337/60). a Epithelial pattern. HE 25×. b Silver stain. 30×. c Formation of cartilage. HE 75×. d Same. Silver stain. 150×. e Coarse reticular network. Silver stain. 150×

cells. Also osteoid substance had developed between the tumor cells which then were enclosed by it and looked like "osteocytes" in immature bone. Even multinuclear giant cells of the osteoclast type were present in such areas.

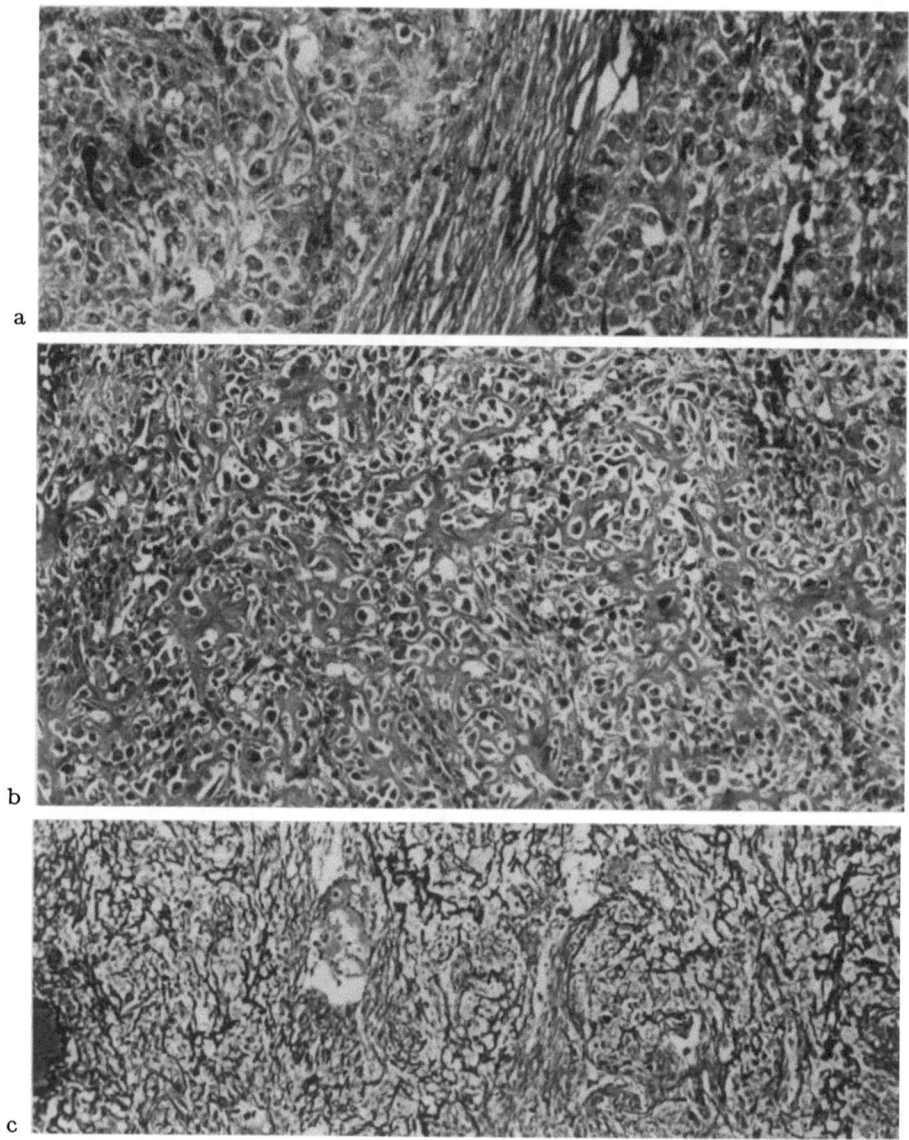

Fig. 24a—c. Osteoid sarcoma (carcinoma) of the mammary gland (Bogotá, 2155/68). a Epithelial pattern. HE 190 ×. b Intercellular deposition of osteoid. HE 150 ×. c Silver stain for reticulin fibers. 75 ×

This is then a tumor with a rudimentary epithelial arrangement of its cells, if only in parts, but behaving like a sarcoma by producing reticular fibres, cartilage and osteoid. Such a tumor ought properly to be called "carcino-chondro-osteoid-sarcoma". The twofold direction of differentiation, which was so pronounced in this tumor, is easily explained if the tissue of origin is traced back to the epithelial and mesenchymal differentiations that take place in the normal epithelium of the mammary gland. I do not propose simply to derive these tumors from myothelia, attractive as such an assumption might appear, because these potentialities may exist in a dormant state in the whole of the mammary tissue.

A second case (A. 2155/68) differs from the previous one only by the arrangement of the tumor cells; the distribution of reticulin fibers about groups of tumor cells and in consequence their epithelial nature is less apparent and is impressive only in places where the connective tissue stroma is more abundant (see Fig. 24a, c). On the other hand, almost everywhere a hyaline-osteoid intercellular substance has developed (see Fig. 24b). The histological diagnosis should therefore be that of a "carcino-osteoid-sarcoma". If in such a tumor the epithelial arrangement of the neoplastic cells were less conspicuous or entirely lacking the word "carcino" might be left out altogether, resulting in a diagnosis of a "osteoid-sarcoma".

Sarcomas of the breast containing osteoid, bones or cartilage have been reported many times in the literature. They are usually thought to originate from the connective tissue portion of fibroadenomas because these have been found frequently with these sarcomas (in 10 of 25 cases — ROTTINO and HOWLEY, 1945; in 16 out of 39 cases — CURRAN and DODGE, 1962). ROBB and McFARLANE (1958) and JERN-STRÖM et al. (1963) have also drawn attention to this peculiar association. On the other hand, ROTTINO and HOWLEY (1945) pointed out that occasionally whole groups of tumor cells are enclosed by reticular fibres, creating the impression of an epithelial arrangement of the tumor cells. Finally, KREIBIG (1925) and BUDD and BRESLIN (1937) have described osteoid-osteosarcomas that were associated with carcinomas. Both types of tumor penetrated one another. Like most other authors they diagnosed the presence of two different tumors, a carcinoma and a sarcoma, which were supposed to have arisen from the epithelial and connective tissue portions of a fibroadenoma simultaneously. If it is granted that the cells of the mammary gland have the power to produce epithelial (carcinomatous) and mesenchymal (sarcomatous) structures, then the somewhat forced assumption that they have a dual origin is no longer necessary. EWING has repeatedly advocated the unitary epithelial origin of these tumors.

GONZALES-LICEA et al. (1967) examined mammary osteoid osteoid-osteosarcomas by electron-microscopy and were not able to demonstrate intracytoplasmatic fibrils. They thought it improbable that these tumors could be related to Mt; even the presence of desmosomes was not regarded as convincing evidence for the original epithelial nature of these tumors. It is remarkable, however, that the authors thought that an epithelial origin of the tumor cells was consistent with their findings. BIGGS (1947) believed it was quite possible that epithelial cartilage might occur in malignant tumors of the breast and also considered the transition of myothelial cells in cartilage as possible.

3. Malignant Adeno-Myotheliomas

Malignant adeno-myotheliomas have been observed mainly in the *skin*. In the literature a few cases of malignant or metastasizing myotheliomas of the sweat glands have been recorded, whereas in the benign variant of this

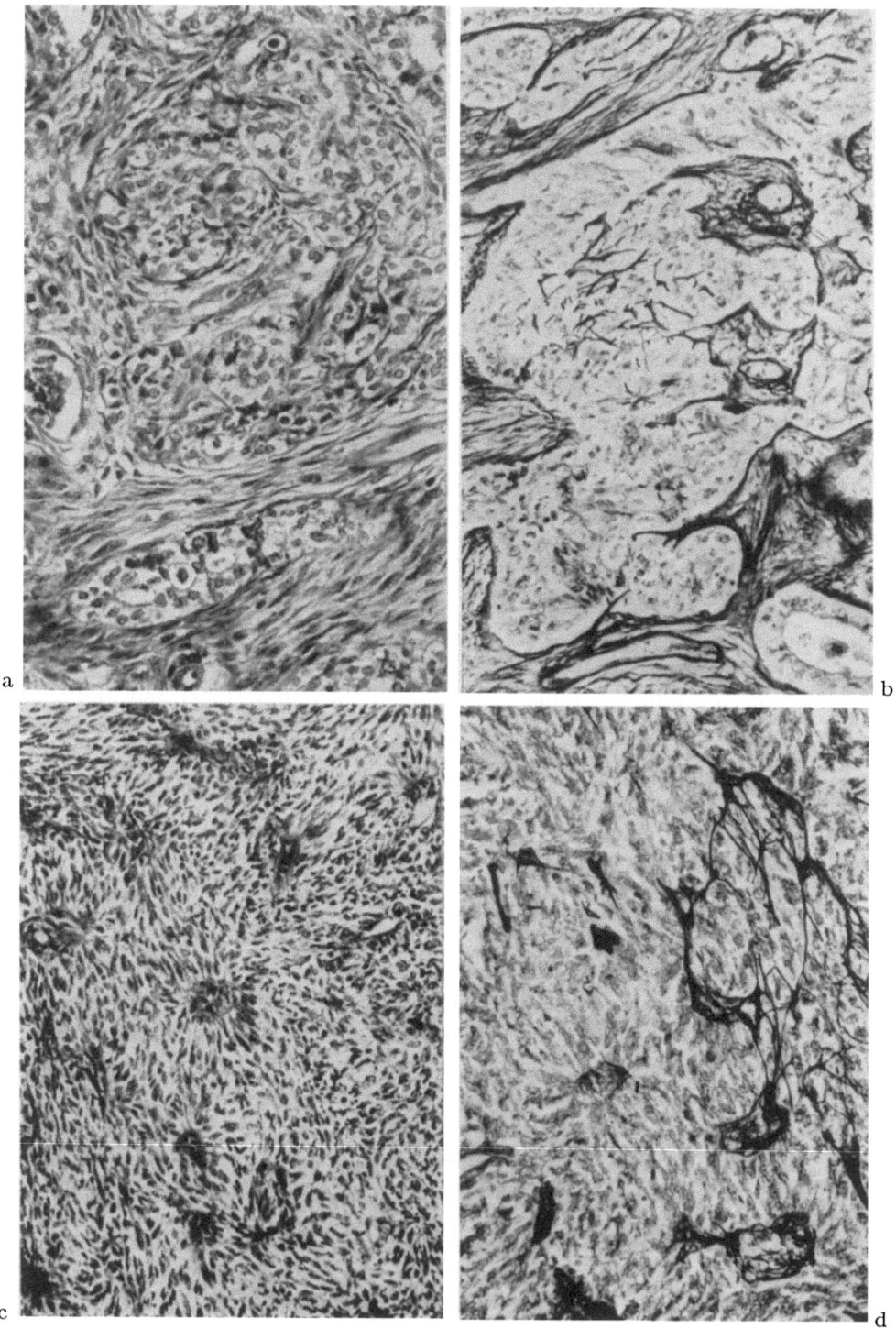

Fig. 25a—d. Malignant adeno-myothelioma of the skin (Bonn, A 84/56). a Primary tumor. HE 190×. b Primary tumor. Foot silver stain. 190×. c Metastasis (Bonn, 9093/57). HE 120×. d Metastasis. Foot silver stain. 120×

tumor myothelial cells or cells likely or suspicious of being Mt have been demonstrated. It is remarkable that most of these cases concern clear-cell myoepitheliomas (KEASBY and HADLEY, 1954; MACKENZIE, 1957; DEVENYI, 1957; SANTLER and EBERHARTINGER, 1965; BERG and McDIVITT, 1968). In DEVENYI'S (1957) case the picture in places was even that of a leiomyomasarcoma.

I have observed a tumor of the skin that evidently arose from the sweat glands and contained myothelial cells.

A man, 57 years of age, had suffered for two years from a tumor of the upper leg, which eventually grew to the size of an egg and was surgically removed (A 84/56). Twenty-two months later metastases of the inguinal lymph glands appeared which were also removed (A. 9093/57). In both lesions the cut surface of the tumor tissue was soft like bone marrow.

Histologically the primary tumor was a mixture of two cell types (see Fig. 25 a and b): there were polygonal cells arranged in clumps and cords.; they showed a pale cytoplasm and oval nuclei, which were moderately rich inchromatin; empty round lumina were seen here and there in between. The other cell type was long and spindle-shaped, with rod-shaped or fusiform nuclei rich in chromatin. Both types of cells intermingled in a variety of ways. The metastasis presented the same picture, except that the spindle-shaped cells were so prevalent in places that the picture resembled a sarcoma (see Fig. 25 c). In addition some spindle-shaped cells had produced a reticulin network in a few places (see Fig. 25 d).

Thus this tumor in its composition of two cell types corresponded to a malignant metastasizing adeno-myothelioma, evidently derived from a sweat gland.

GAUDIER et al. (1931) described a malignant myothelioma of the *mammary gland*, thinking that the proliferated cells of their case had a "potential evolutif" towards Mt, so that the histological picture perhaps resembled that of a carcinosarcoma.

MYLIUS (1960) observed Mt with the light-microscope in malignant myotheliomas of the *salivary glands*.

MEYER et al. (1959) described an invasive *bronchial tumor* of "myoepithelial type".

4. Myothelia in Typical Carcinomas

In the typical solid carcinoma of the *mammary gland* pictures like Fig. 26 are frequently seen. The main mass of the carcinomatous cords consists of pale cells with large, round nuclei, moderately rich in chromatin. Between those and the stroma there is a continous layer of cells with small, round or angular nuclei, rich in chromatin. The cytoplasm of these cells stains deeply with erythrosin and phloxine. Tangential sections show that these cells are long and spindle-shaped (see Figs. 26, 27b) or stellate. Occasionally, these elements reach into the central epithelial mass of a cord, but are easily distinguished from the other cells by their shape, nucleus and the staining of their cytoplasm. The great similarity of these cells with the normal Mt of the excretory ducts of the mammary gland is unmistakable.

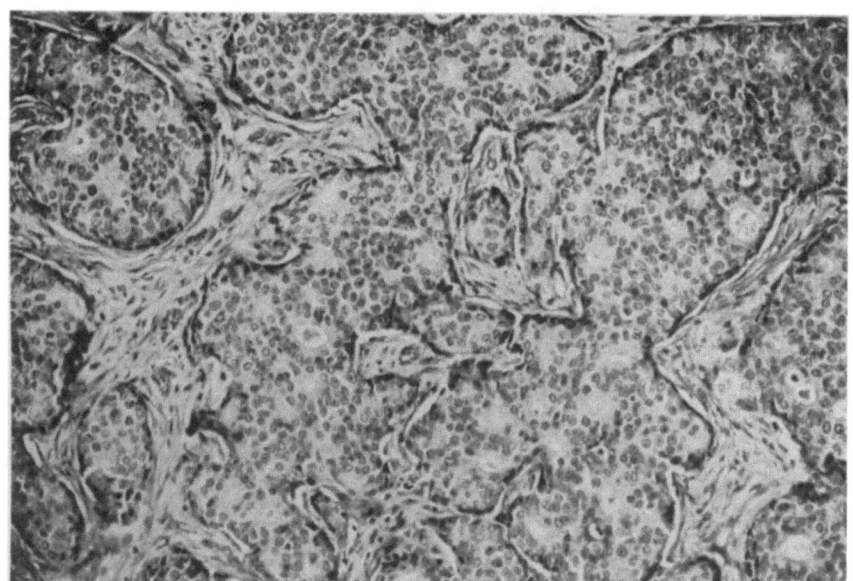

Fig. 26. Myothelial cells surrounding masses of epithelial tumor cells in a carcinoma of the mammary gland (Bogotá, 934/58). HE 120×

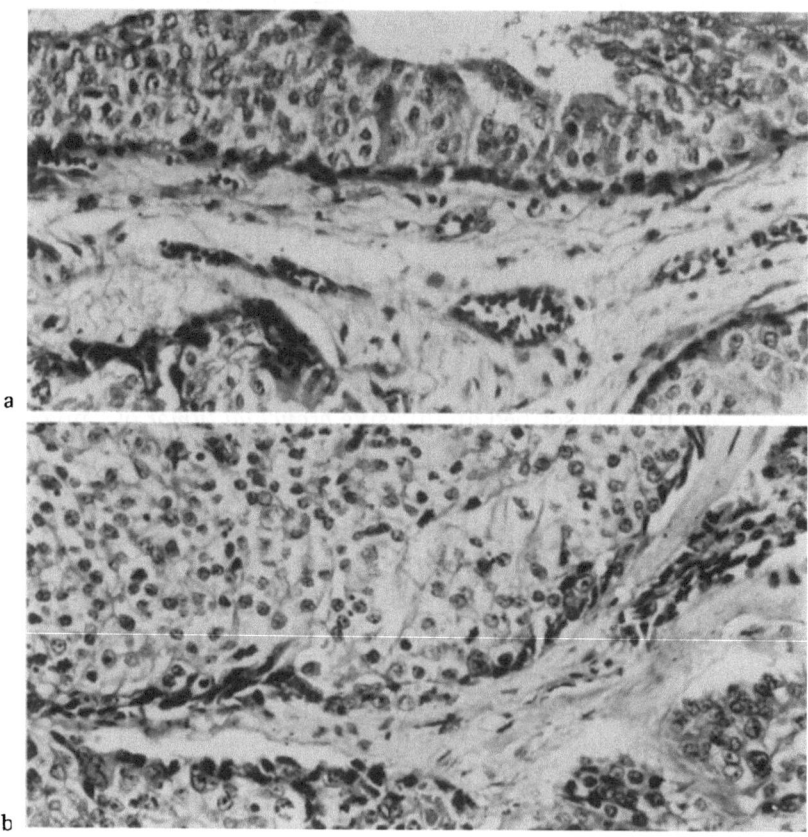

Fig. 27a and b. Myothelial cells surrounding masses of epithelial tumor cells in: a Carcinoma of a salivary gland (Berlin, S 306/38). HE 190×. b Metastasis from a mammary cancer in a lymph node (Bogotá, 637/62). Phloxin-Tartrazin

On the basis of this morphological analogy one should also consider the dark basal cells in carcinomas, described by FEYRTER and HARTMANN (1963) as myothelial elements. Indeed, SARKAR and KALLENBACH (1966) have been able to distinguish such spindle-shaped elements as Mt by selectively staining them with tannin-phosphotungstic-acid-amido-black (TPA), according to PUCHTLER and LEBLOND.

LEE et al. (1933) have described cells of the myothelial type in carcinomas of the mammary gland that were arranged in the periphery of the tumor masses like a comb. As these carcinomas always proliferated intracanalicularly,

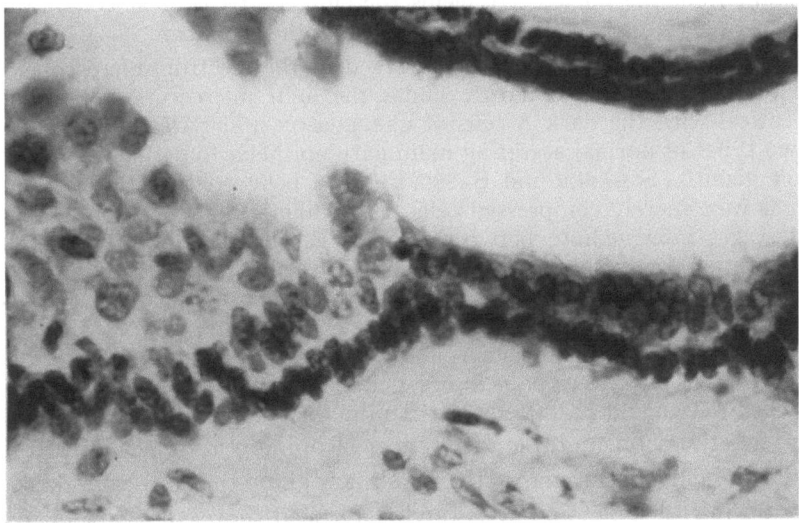

Fig. 28. Intraductal growth of a mammary carcinoma replacing only the surface epithelium, over the remaining normal Mt (Bogotá, 2511/58). HE 480×

the authors could not exclude with certainty that residual normal Mt were present. Indeed, a somewhat similar picture may be seen when a carcinoma invades a mammary duct (see Fig. 28): here, too, the pale carcinoma cells stand out clearly from a basal cell layer, which merges so obviously into the normal myothelial layer as to leave no doubt that it belongs to the normal myothelium and not to the carcinoma. It is however not surprising that the Mt remain in place, even though the covering cylindrical epithelium is replaced by carcinoma cells because of the strong bonds between the basal Mt and the basement membrane. In the case illustrated by Fig. 28 the spindle-shaped basal cells cannot represent residual normal Mt but are instead newly formed tumor cells, because a similar myothelial differentiation of tumor cells may also be found in lymph node metastases, as already observed by SARKAR and KALLENBACH (1966).

Light-microscopy thus allows a fairly accurate evaluation of the peculiar peripheral cells in carcinomas. There are considerable differences of opinion, however, as regards the electron-microscopic assessment of cells thought to be of myothelial nature in carcinomas.

There is agreement only about the occurrence of fibrils in the cells of mammary carcinomas. The thickness of these myofibrils is similar to those of normal Mt: 50 Å (WELLINGS and ROBERTS, 1963), 50—60 Å (SCHÄFER and BÄSSLER, 1969), 50—80 Å (BUSCH and MERKER, 1968). MURAD and SCARPELLI (1967) went so far as to relate scirrhous carcinomas to Mt, because the Mt produce substances of the basement membrane type as well as fibrils. This view is almost identical with that of FEYRTER and HARTMANN (1963), who traced the gelatinous mammary carcinoma back to the so-called clear-cell-organ of the mammary gland, i.e., the Mt. Fibrils may be demonstrated, however, in more centrally situated cells by electron microscopy, even in the vicinity of the nuclei, whereas in normal Mt they are seen mainly more distant from the nucleus. It seems therefore that the clear cells, rather than the more peripheral dark cells, could be of a myothelial nature.

HAGUENAU and ARNOULT (1959) observed in the electron-microscope the cells thought to be of myothelial nature under the light microscope. They considered them identical with the dark A-cells of CASPERSSON and SANTESSON and with one of the two types of normal secreting mammary epithelia (not the Mt of the normal mammary gland!). SCHÄFER and BÄSSLER (1969) believed that the dark A-cells of carcinomas were merely compressed cells. They, like MURAD and VON HAAM (1968), detected stages intermediate between A- and B-cells (BERGER, 1964). The basal dark cells were also thought to be degenerating elements (MURAD and SCARPELLI, 1967) or cells shrunk by loss of water, or even invading histiocytes. WELLINGS and ROBERTS (1963), WAUGH and VAN DER HOEVEN (1962), and MURAD and SCARPELLI (1962) were not able to distinguish A- and B-cells at all. BUSCH and MERKER (1968) differentiated cells that were poor in organelles, equivalent to B-cells, and cells rich in organelles that could be differentiated into clear and dark structural elements.

There are thus considerable differences of opinion about the understanding of the cells found in carcinomas of the mammary gland that appear "dark" under the electron-microscope. The cells obviously need more and careful investigations.

Under the light-microscope well-stained cells, resembling myothelial cells by their shape and position, can also be found in solid *carcinomas of the salivary glands* (see Fig. 27b), the picture being identical with the corresponding one in mammary carcinomas.

MYLIUS (1960) observed them also in all adenocarcinomas of the salivary glands except in clear-cell carcinomas. KLEINSASSER et al. (1968) and HÜBNER et al. (1969) found with the electron microscope that Mt participated in the formation of carcinomas of the salivary ducts: the Mt contained fibrils, glycogen and lipofuscin granules, such as are normally found in the basket cells. The development of two cell types, epithelial and myothelial, in these tumors makes them very similar to malignant adeno-myotheliomas.

5. Carcino-Sarcomas

In an earlier paper (1939) I used a specific tumor of the human mammary gland as a model, to explain how the duplex nature of the Mt might help to understand carcino-sarcomas. Since then I have been able to observe a number of such pertinent tumors of the *mammary gland*. They had in common a clear-cut epithelial portion embedded in a sarcomatous appearing stroma. When the reticular fibres were stained, transitional stages became recognizable here and there as the epithelial portions seemed to merge with the sarcomatous ones. These were not simply carcinomas with areas of epithelial spindle cells as JONES (1969) thought, since the cells of the purely epithelial portion were surrounded in typical fashion by reticulin fibres, whereas the spindly cells of the sarcomatous portions were embedded individually in a rich reticular network and proliferated on their own. Neither were these neoplasms just composed of two fundamentally different tumor types, for example, a carcinoma and a sarcoma, as already has been explained above (p. 200).

Once more the duplex nature of the Mt seems to become visible with the tendency of that type of tumor to proliferate at the same time in epithelial and mesenchymal forms. This does not imply, of course, that these tumors are directly derived from Mt or that the spindle-shaped cells are true myothelial cells. These tumors merely seem to represent a manifestation in the most primitive form of epithelial and mesenchymal potentialities of the epithelium of some glands.

VI. Final Considerations

In conclusion, when we examine the findings, opinions, and assumptions about Mt (especially their presence in hypoplasias and tumors), we find that they all relate to the problem of morphological differentiation in normal tissue and in tumors arising from them. It is customary and one of the daily tasks of the diagnostician in the field of pathological histology to infer the genesis of a tumor from the various differentiations he sees in it, viz. to draw conclusions on the origin of a tumor from its metastases. In the present communication I have, in a sense, taken the opposite approach by starting with the differentiations in normal tissue, i.e., of a certain cell-type like the Mt, then proceeded by looking at its various forms in different tumors. This route has produced such surprising results, that it seemed at times to have led us astray.

Obviously, a tumor cell need not resemble exactly the normal cell from which it arises. But in what limits may a tumor cell deviate from the normal cell with its range of differentiation and still be recognized as arising from that cell? If we define a normal cell by its essential morphological characteristics, then the tumor cell obviously takes great liberties. The complete and essential characteristics of normal cells are hardly ever reproduced in the tumors. Often one has to be content with only a few characteristics, sometimes with only a single one, when we are required to trace a tumor cell back to the parent cell from which it arose. In these circumstances it is not surprising that critical authors describe the presence of Mt in tumors as only the presence of analogues to normal Mt. Also in this paper "myothelial" cells or cells of a "myothelial nature" have been mentioned only all too often.

The problem of establishing analogies between tumor cells and normal cells has become even more difficult for further reasons: the tumor cell we relate with a normal cell may have few characteristics possessed by the normal cell, and some of characteristics may even be those of other cells in the same organ. Morphological qualities normally localized in different cells of the mother organ may thus occur together in one and the same cell in tumors of this organ: the cells become a kind of chimera. Furthermore, the differentiation of tumor cells may lead to morphological and functional qualities of tissues that are related only embryologically to the organ in which the tumor arose: the differentiation into squamous epithelium occurring in tumors of the salivary or the mammary glands may serve as an example. This recourse to a — however distantly — related tissue is intelligible because the glands as well as squamous epithelium are derived from the ectoderm.

The position of the Mt in this system is a special one, because they inherently possess both epithelial and mesenchymal characteristics. Although from the embryonal point of view Mt may be considered as ectodermal, it is not surprising that the mesenchymal part of the cell also gives rise to various differentiations in tumors. After all, even mesenchyme and ectoderm originate from the same source, the pluripotent cell of the egg. The development of ectodermal epithelium and mesenchymal fibrous tissue takes place only by suppression of certain potentialities of the originally pluripotent cell. Further suppression of potentialities leads to the differentiation into epidermis and glands, on the one hand, and of collagenous fibres, cartilage, etc., on the other hand. We should, however, not forget that even the well-differentiated cell of an organ carries the complete genetic information of the individual in a partly suppressed state. It appears that this "repression" of developmental potentialities associated with organogeny and differentiation may be abolished to a varying extent in the tumor cell. The rules by which this "derepression" operates are not yet clear.

The myothelial or myothelial-like cells in tumors seem able to revert to the earliest developmental stages and to produce ectodermal epithelium and mesenchymal structures as well.

The numerous possible differentiations open to tumor cells may extend far beyond a single organ and call for the greatest restraint in making statements about the starting point of a tumor. Even if a certain cell-type predominates in a tumor, even if it is named after this cell type, it is merely an assumption when we say the tumor has originated from that and no other type of cell. Nobody has ever witnessed that origin. It is surprising to see with what conviction a tumor at times is related to a certain cell type, for example, a part of a duct system, from which, on the basis of a single cellular characteristic, it is said to originate. The fallacy of such a procedure is particularly obvious in the tumors composed of Mt and epithelium. MASSON has summarized this succinctly: "Just because a tumor has certain morphological characteristics, which are reminiscent of one or the other sector (of a gland), it has not necessarily originated from this and no other sector".

The thesis derived from the Mt, viz., that ectodermal, epithelial cells are able in certain circumstances to produce mesenchymal structures, introduces a factor of uncertainty into the accepted classification of tumors, according to which epithelial tumors are named adenomas and carcinomas, and mesenchymal tumors are named chondromas, myomas, and sarcomas, etc. If epithelial, ectodermal cells were really able to produce cartilage and muscle fibres, then epithelial chondromas and myomas, even chondro- and myocarcinomas could exist. This may conceivably be true for certain sarcomas of the mammary gland (s. above), perhaps even more likely for fibromas and myomas of organs that contain Mt. Yet, however, likely as it may appear, it seems inappropriate to invalidate a classification of tumors that has proved its value many times over. The exceptional and borderline case presented here may only point to the fact that all classifications of natural phenomena, including those of tumors, are the work of man and thus have limits that anybody with a feeling for scientific orderliness will find inconvenient and disturbing — but refreshing on the other hand as providing material for new thoughts and considerations.

VII. Summary

I. (p. 162) Myothelium (Mt) comprises: the basket cells of the salivary glands and mammary gland, the spindle-shaped cells of the excretory ducts and sweat glands, and the basal cell layer of some excretory ducts. Mt are characterized by the presence of contractile myofibrils and by their close relationship to the ground substance of the basement membrane, characteristics which they share with mesenchymal smooth muscle fibres. On the other hand, the Mt behave like epithelial cells with the neighboring cells lining the lumen. This duplex function is matched by prospective duplex potentialities.

II. (p. 167) Oedematous swelling may occur in Mt independent of the covering epithelial cells; Mt may store glycogen, fat, and pigments (lipofuscin and ceroid). When glands atrophy, Mt usually survive longer than the epithelial cells.

III. (p. 176) Sometimes Mt will proliferate without the epithelium taking part. It may proliferate in foci (see Fig. 29d), as rosettes (see Fig. 29f), or diffusely (see Fig. 29e). Mt together with proliferating epithelium form epimyothelial cell islands in salivary glands and in the mammary gland. They also play a part in fibrosing adenosis and intracanalicular cell proliferations in the mammary gland.

IV. (p. 184) Mt are involved in numerous benign tumors, specific for the mammary gland, skin, and salivary glands. They play a determining role in the development of mixed tumors of the salivary gland-type (see Fig. 29j), cylindromas, adeno-myotheliomas (see Fig. 29h), and myotheliomas which occur in basically similar forms in the mammary gland, the salivary glands, and the skin (sweat glands). The mesenchymal potentialities of the Mt are manifested by the production of collagenous, hyaline, mucoid, and cartilaginous substances.

V. (p. 199) Myothelial cells may be demonstrated in malignant variants of mixed tumors and adeno-myotheliomas. Certain chondro-osteoid sarcomas (see Fig. 29l) of the mammary gland may probably be best conceived of as

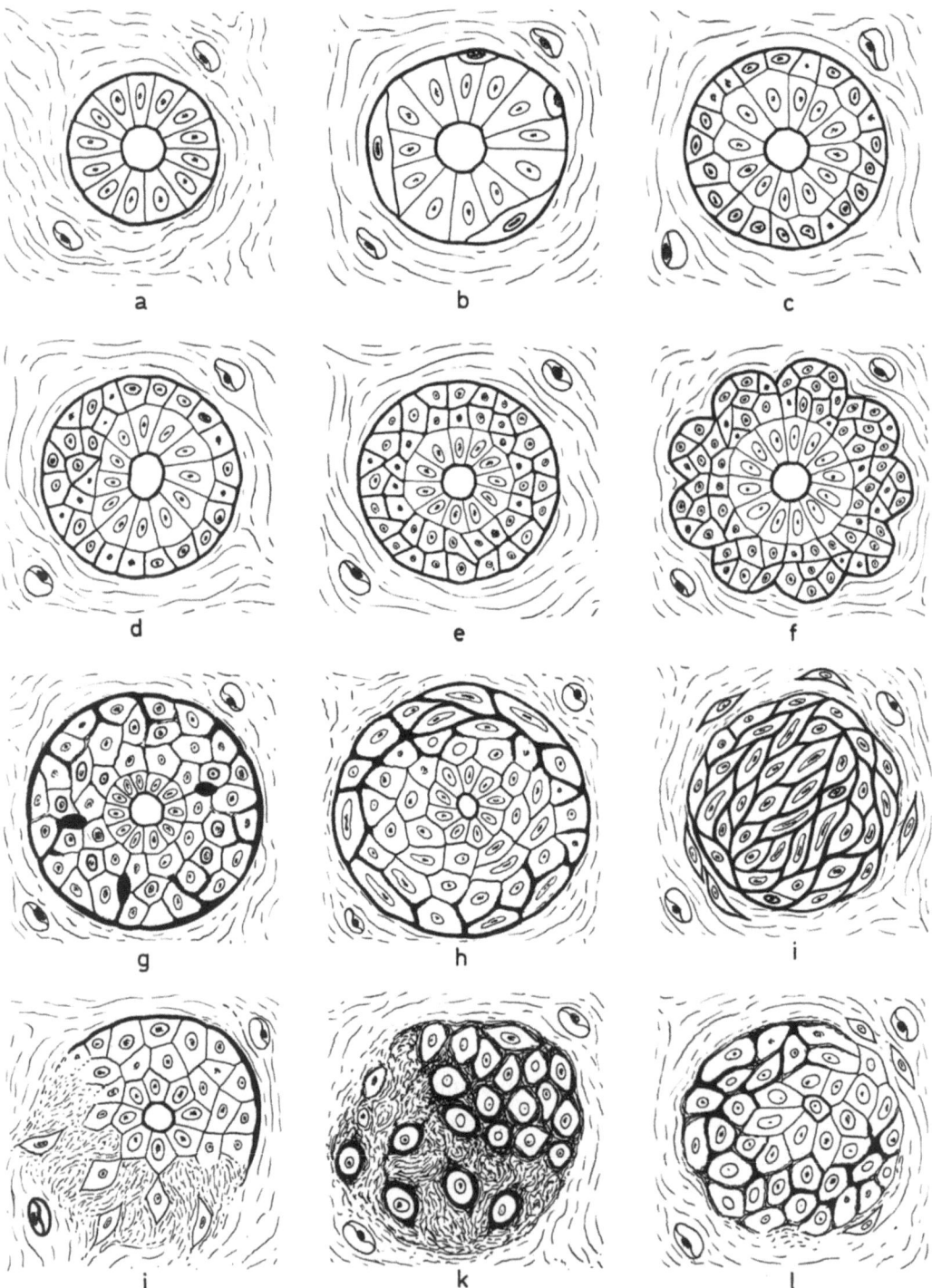

Fig. 29a–l. Schematic presentation of the Mt in different conditions. a no Mt present (e.g. pancreas); b single Mt present (in transverse and longitudinal section); c water containing Mt forming a basal layer (compare with Fig. 2); d localized hyperplasia of Mt (compare with Fig. 9a); e diffuse hyperplasia of Mt (compare with Fig. 9c); f rosette-

malignant myotheliomas with one-sided differentiation of cartilaginous or osteoid intermediary substance. Myothelial cells may differentiate at the borders of epithelial complexes in typical solid carcinomas of the mammary gland and salivary glands. Some carcino-sarcomas of these organs may best be conceived of as malignant epi-myothelial neoplasms.

References

ABRAMOW, S. S.: Ein Fall von Adenomyoma der Brustdrüse. Cbl. allg. Path. path. Anat. **12**, 926 (1901).
ACKERMAN, L. V.: Seminar on lesions of the breast. Amer. Soc. of clinical Path. 1957.
ALLEN, A. C.: So-called mixed tumours of the mammary gland of dog and man (with special reference to the general problem of cartilage and bone formation). Arch. Path. **29**, 589—642 (1940).
ARCHER, F., OMAR, M.: The fine structure of fibro-adenoma of human breast. J. Path. Bact. **99**, 113—117 (1969).
— — Pink cell (oncocytic) metaplasia in a fibroadenoma of the human breast: electron-microscopic observations. J. Path. Bact. **99**, 119—124 (1969).
ARCHER, F. L., KAO, V. C. Y.: Immunohistochemical identification of actomyosin in myothelium of human tissues. Lab. Invest. **18**, 669—674 (1968).
AZZOPARDI, J. G.: Clear-cell hidradenoma. J. Path. Bact. **76**, 379—382 (1958).
— SMITH, A. D.: Salivary gland tumours and their mucins. J. Path. Bact. **77**, 131—140 (1959).
BÄSSLER, R.: Neuere Aspekte der normalen und pathologischen Feinstruktur der Mamma. Hippokrates (Stuttg.) **39**, 237—244 (1968).
— BRETHFELD, V.: Enzymhistochemische Studien an der Milchdrüse. Gravidität, Laktation, Involution und experimentelle Stauung mit besonderer Berücksichtigung myoepithelialer Zellen. Histochemie **15**, 270—286 (1968).
— SCHÄFER, A.: Elektronenmikroskopische Cytomorphologie der Gynäkomastie. Virchows Arch. Abt. A Path. Anat. **348**, 356—373 (1969).
— — PAEK, S.: Elektronenmikroskopische und histochemische Untersuchungen zur Morphologie und Funktion myoepithelialer Zellen. Verh. dtsch. Ges. Path. **1967**, 301—308.
BAIN, G. O., KOWALEWSKI, K. P., MACGREGOR, J. W.: Mixed tumors (pleomorphic adenomas) of the salivary glands. Acta gastro-ent. belg. **19**, 70—81 (1956).
BARTON, A.: An electron microscope study of human breast cells in fibroadenosis and carcinoma. Brit. J. Cancer **18**, 682—685 (1964).
BAUER, W. H., BAUER, J. D.: Classification of glandular tumours of salivary glands (Study of one hundred and forty-three cases). Arch. Path. **55**, 328—346 (1953).
— FOX, R. A.: Adenomyoepithelioma (cylindroma) of platal mucous glands. Arch. Path. **39**, 96—102 (1945).
BERG, J. W., MCDIVITT, R. W.: Pathology of sweat gland carcinoma. Pathology annual **3**, 124—144 (1968).

shaped hyperplasia of Mt (compare with Fig. 9b, 12d); g septa and ovoid bodies within the layer of hyperplastic Mt (compare with Fig. 12a); h proliferation of Mt with the production of an intercellular reticular network e.g. in an adeno-myothelioma (compare with Fig. 21d); i proliferation of Mt mimicking smooth muscle fibers, g. e,. in a myothelioma (compare with Fig. 22b, c); j mixed tumor with Mt splitting of and production of mucus; k carcino-sarcoma with production of mucus and osteoid (compare with Fig. 23); l osteoid sarcoma (compare with Fig. 24)

BERGER, H.: Beitrag zur elektronenoptischen Zelldifferenzierung des soliden Mammacarcinoms und der Mastopathia cystica des Menschen. Z. Krebsforsch. 66, 73—86 (1964).
BERGHORN, B. M., BRYCE, B. L., HELWIG, E. B.: Eccrine spiradenome: a pharmacologic study. Arch. Derm. 84, 434—438 (1961).
BERTKAU, F.: Ein Beitrag zur Anatomie und Physiologie der Milchdrüse. Anat. Anz. 30, 161—180 (1907).
BHASKAR, S. N., WEINMANN, J. P.: Tumors of the minor salivary glands. Oral Surg. 8, 1278—1297 (1955).
BIGGS, R.: The myoepithelium in certain tumours of the breast. J. Path. Bact. 59, 437—444 (1947).
BÖCK, J., FEYRTER, F.: Über die benignen epithelialen Geschwülste der menschlichen Orbita. I. Das Cylindrom. Albrecht v. Graefes Arch. Ophthal. 163, 25—62 (1961).
— — Über die benignen epithelialen Geschwülste der menschlichen Orbita. II. Der benigne vulgäre sog. Mischtumor. Albrecht v. Graefes Arch. Ophthal. 163, 63—87 (1961).
BOGART, B. I.: The fine structural localization of alcaline and acid phosphatase activity in the rat submandibular gland. J. Histochem. Cytochem., 16, 572—581 (1968).
BOSCHBACH, F. W.: Adenoid-zystisches Karzinom der Bartholinischen Drüse. Geburtsh. u. Frauenheilk. 29, 474—477 (1969).
BUDD, J. W., BRESLIN, FR. J.: Carcino-osteogenetic sarcoma. Amer. J. Cancer 31, 207—211 (1937).
BUNTING, H.: Cytochemical properties of apocrine sweat glands normally present in the human mammary gland. Anat. Rec. 101, 5—12 (1948).
— WISLOCKI, G. B., DEMPSEY, E. W.: The chemical histology of the human eccrine and apocrine sweat glands. Anat. Rec. 100, 61—78 (1948).
BUSCH, W., MERKER, H. J.: Elektronenmikroskopische Untersuchungen an menschlichen Mammacarcinomen. Virchows Arch. Abt. A. Path. Anat. 344, 456—371 (1968).
CABANNE, F.: Les sarcomes osteogeniques des parties molles et visceres. Arch. Anat. path. 8 A, 131—147 (1960).
CAPONE BRAGA, M.: Una nuova interpretazione genetica dei tumori misti delle ghiandole salivari in base allo studio dei mioepiteli. Arch. De Vecchi Anat. pat. 7, 563—582 (1945).
CASPERSSON, T., SANTESSON, L.: Studies on protein metabolism in the cells of epithelial tumours. Acta radiol. (Stockh.), Suppl. 46, 1 (1942).
COTCHIN, E.: Mammary neoplasms of the bitch. J. comp. Path. 68, 1—16 (1958).
CRAIN, R. C., HELWIG, E. B.: Dermal cylindroma (dermal eccrine cylindroma). Amer. J. clin. Path. 35, 504—515 (1961).
CROCKER, D. J., MURAD, T. M.: Ultrastructure of fibrosarcoma in a male breast. Cancer 23, 891—899 (1969).
CRUICKSHANK, A. H.: Benign lymphoepithelial salivary lesion to be distinguished from adenolymphoma. J. clin. Path. 18, 391—400 (1965).
CURRAN, R. C., DODGE, O. G.: Sarcoma of the breast, with particular reference to its origin from fibroadenoma. J. clin. Path. 15, 1—16 (1962).
DAVID, H., KORTH, I.: Submikroskopische Untersuchungen an Mischtumoren. Zbl. allg. Path. path. Anat. 106, 78—85 (1964).
DEMPSEY, E. W., BUNTING, H., WISLOCKI, G. B.: Observations on the chemical cytology of the mammary gland. Amer. J. Anat. 81, 309—341 (1947).
DEPETRIS, S., KARLSBAD, G., PERNIS, B.: Filamentous structures in the cytoplasm of normal mononuclear phagocytes. J. Ultrastruct. Res. 7, 39 (1962).

Deppisch, L. M., Toker, C.: Mixed tumours of the parotid gland. An ultrastructural study. Cancer (Philad.) 24, 174—184 (1969).
Devenyi, I.: Malignes Schweißdrüsen-Myoepitheliom. Zbl. allg. Path. path. Anat. 96, 469—473 (1957).
Dewey, M. M.: A histochemical and biochemical study of the parotid gland in normal and hypophysectomized rats. Amer. J. Anat. 102, 243—271 (1958).
Dietz, H.: Das Verhalten der großen Kopfspeicheldrüsen des Kaninchens nach Unterbindung ihres Ausführungsganges und nach Transplantation. Frankfurt. Z. Path. 66, 416—425 (1955).
Doyle, L. E., Lynn, L. A., Panopio, I. T., Crass, G.: Ultrastructure of the chondroid regions of benign mixed tumor of salivary gland. Cancer (Philad.) 22, 225—233 (1968).
Dyx, W.: Über argentaffine, makrophage Körnchenzellen. Inaug.-Diss. Danzig 1941.
Efskind, J., Eker, R.: Myo-epitheliomas of the skin. Acta derm.-venereol. (Stockh.) 34, 279—283 (1954).
Ellis, R. A.: Fine structure of the myoepithelium of the eccrine sweat glands of man. J. Cell Biol. 27, 551—563 (1965).
Eneroth, C. M., Wersäll, J.: Fine structure of the epithelial cells in mixed tumors of the parotid gland. Ann. Otol. (St. Louis) 75, 95—102 (1966).
Erichsen, S.: A histochemical study in mixed tumours of the canine mammary gland. Acta path. microbiol. scand. 36, 491—502 (1955b).
Ericson, S.: The parotid gland in subjects with and without rheumatoid arthritis. A sialographic and physiologic study. Acta radiol. (Stockh.), Suppl. 275, 167 (1968).
Evans, R. W.: Histological appearances of tumors. Edinbourgh-London: Livingstone 1966.
Feyrter, F.: Über das solide (tubulär-solide) Adenom der Schleim- und Speicheldrüsen. Frankfurt. Z. Path. 71, 300—326 (1961).
— Zur Frage der Endokrinie des sogenannten Speicheldrüsenmischtumors. Dtsch. med. Wschr. 86, 335—339 (1961).
— Über das glykogenreiche retikulierte Adenom der Speicheldrüsen. Z. Krebsforsch. 65, 446—(1963).
— Gottron, H., Nikolowski, W. N.: Über das Cylindrom der Haut. Arch. klin. exp. Derm. 214, 54—104 (1961/62).
— Hartmann, G.: Über die carcinoide Wuchsform des Carcinoms mammae, insbesondere das Carcinoma solidum (gelatinosum) mammae. Frankfurt. Z. Path. 73, 24—39 (1963).
Finck, F. M., Schwinn, C. P., Keasbey, L. E.: Clear cell hidradenome of the breast. Cancer (Philad.) 22, 125—135 (1968).
Foote, Fr. W., Frazell, E. L.: Tumors of the salivary glands. Atlas of tumor pathology, sect. IV, fasc. 11. Washington: AFIP 1954.
— Stewart, F. W.: A histologic classification of carcinoma of the breast. Amer. J. Cancer 40, 74—99 (1940).
Friborsky, V.: Adenoid cystic carcinoma of salivary glands. Path. et Microbiol. (Basel) 26, 17—28 (1963).
Fruhling, L., Batzenschlager, A., Blum, E.: Epitheliosarcomes vrais (tumeurs mixtes maligne) et cancers doubles didermiques de la vessie. Ann. Anat. path., N.S. 4, 5—42 (1959).
Gaudier, Grandclaude, Lambret, M.: Tumeur maligne du sein à type myo-épithélial. Ann. Anat. path. 8, 68—70 (1931).
Gedigk, P., Fischer, R.: Über die Entstehung von Lipopigmenten in Muskelfasern. Untersuchungen beim experimentellen Vitamin-E-Mangel der Ratte und an Organen des Menschen. Virch. Arch. path. Anat. 332, 431—468 (1959).

GERUGHTY, R. M., SCOFIELD, H. H., BROWN, F. M., HENNIGAR, G. R.: Malignant mixed tumors of salivary gland origin. Cancer (Philad.) 24, 471—486 (1969).
GODWIN, J. T.: Benign lymphoepithelial lesion of the parotid gland. Cancer (Philad.) 5, 1089—1103 (1952).
GOLDSTEIN, D. J.: On the origin and morphology of myoepithelial cells of apocrine sweat glands. J. invest. Derm. 37, 301—310 (1961).
GONZALES-LICEA, A., YARDLEY, J. H., HARTMANN, W. H.: Malignant tumor of the breast with bone formation. Studies by light and electron microscopy. Cancer (Philad.) 20, 1234—1247 (1967).
GRISHMAN, EDITH: Histochemical analysis of mucopolysaccharide soccurring in mucus-producing tumours. Cancer (Philad.) 5, 700—707 (1952).
GRYNFELTT, E., AIMES, A.: Etude histologique de deux tumeurs des glandes sudoripares. Bull. Ass. franç. Cancer 11, 91—109 (1922).
GUBAREWA, A. V.: Adenomyoepitheliomas of the skin. Arch. Path. 1965/2, 32—37 [russisch].
GÜNTHER, R.: Myoepitheliale Wucherungen in der Brustdrüse. Virchows Arch. path. Anat. 300, 450—455 (1937).
HAGUENAU, F.: Les myofilaments de la cellule myoépithéliale. Etude au microscope electronique. C. R. Acad. Sci. (Paris) 249, 182—184 (1959).
— ARNOULT, J.: Le cancer du sein chez la femme. Etude comparative au microscope electronique et au microscope optique. Bull. Ass. franç. Cancer 46, 177—211 (1959).
HAMPERL, H.: Beiträge zur normalen und pathologischen Histologie menschlicher Speicheldrüsen. Z. mikr.-anat. Forsch. 27, 1—55 (1931).
— Die Fluorescenzmikroskopie menschlicher Gewebe. Virchows Arch. path. Anat. 292, 1—51 (1934).
— Über die Myothelien (myo-epithelialen Elemente) der Brustdrüse. Virchows Arch. path. Anat. 305, 171—215 (1939).
— Über fluorescierende Körnchenzellen (Fluorocyten). Virchows Arch. path. Anat. 318, 32—47 (1950).
— Über fluorescierende Mesenchymzellen (Fluorocyten). Leitz-Mitt. Wissenschaft u. Technik 4, 243—246 (1969).
HARTROFT, W. S.: In vitro and in vivo production of a ceroidlike substance from erythrocytes and certain lipids. Science 113, 673—674 (1951).
— PORTA, E. A.: Ceroid. Amer. J. med. Sci. 250, 324—345 (1965).
HARTZ, PH. H.: Adenomyoepithelioma of sweat gland. Report of a case. Amer. J. clin. Path. 16, 385—389 (1946).
HASHIMOTO, K., GROSS, B. G., NELSON, R. G., LEVER, W. F.: Eccrine spiradenoma. Histochemical and electron microscopic studies. J. invest. Derm. 46, 347—365 (1966).
— — LEVER, W. F.: The ultrastructure of human embryo skin. II. The formation of intradermal portion of the eccrine sweat duct and of the secretory segment during the first half of embryonic life. J. invest. Derm. 46, 513—529 (1966).
HEMPLEMANN, L. H., WOMACK, N. A.: The pathogenesis of mixed tumors of the salivary gland type. Ann. Surg. 116, 34—42 (1942).
HIBBS, R. G.: The fine structure of human eccrine sweat glands. Amer. J. Anat. 103, 201 (1958).
HIRSCH, P., HELWIG, E. B.: Chondroid Syringoma. Arch. Derm. 84, 835—847 (1961).
HOLLMANN, K. H.: L'ultrastructure de la glande mammaire de la souris en lactation. J. Ultrastruct. Res. 2, 423—443 (1959).
HÜBNER, G., KLEINSASSER, O., KLEIN, H. J.: Zur Feinstruktur der Speichelgangcarcinome. Ein Beitrag zur Rolle der Myoepithelzellen in Speicheldrüsengeschwülsten. Virchows Arch. Abt. A. Path. Anat. 346, 1—14 (1969).

HÜBNER, G., KLEINSASSER, O., KLEIN, H. J.: Zur Feinstruktur und Genese der Cylindrome der Speicheldrüsen. Weitere Untersuchungen zur Rolle myoepithelial differenzierter Zellen der Speicheldrüsengeschwülste. Virchows Arch. Abt. A Path. Anat. 347, 296—315 (1969).

HURLEY, H. J., SHELLEY, W. B.: The role of the myoepithelium of the human apocrine sweat gland. J. invest. Derm. 22, 143—156 (1954).

JERNSTRÖM, P., LINDBERG, A. L., MELAND, O. N.: Osteogenic sarcoma of the mammary gland. Amer. J. clin. Path. 40, 521—526 (1963).

JOHNSON, B. L., HELWIG, B. B.: Eccrine acrospinoma. A clinopathologic study. Cancer 23, 641—657 (1969).

JONES, E. L.: Primary squamous-cell carcinoma of the breast with pseudosarcomatous stroma. J. Path. Bact. 97, 383—385 (1969).

KARNAUCHOW, P. N.: Myo-epithelium in gynecomastia. Amer. J. Path. 30, 1169—1179 (1954).

KAUFMANN, F., STIEBITZ, R.: Zur Enzymhistochemie der Speicheldrüsen. Acta histochem. (Jena) 32, 221—243 (1969).

KEASBEY, L. E., HADLEY, G. G.: Clear-cell hidradenoma. Report of three cases with widespread metastases. Cancer (Philad.) 7, 934—952 (1954).

KERSTING, D. W.: Clear cell hidradenoma and hidradenocarcinoma. Arch. Derm. 87, 323—333 (1963).

— HELWIG, E. B.: Eccrine spiradenoma. Arch. Derm. 73, 199—227 (1956).

KLEINSASSER, O.: Einteilung, Morphologie und Verhalten der epithelialen Speicheldrüsen. H.N.O. 17, 197—211 (1969).

— KLEIN, H. J., HÜBNER, G.: Speichelgangcarcinome. Eine den Milchgangcarcinomen der Brustdrüse analoge Gruppe von Speicheldrüsentumoren. Arch. klin. exp. Ohr.-, Nas.- u. Kehlk.-Heilk. 192, 100—115 (1968).

KOPF, A. W.: The distribution of alkaline phosphatase in normal and pathologic human skin. Arch. Derm. 75, 1—37 (1957).

KREIBIG, W.: Zur Kenntnis seltener Geschwulstformen der weiblichen Brustdrüse. Virchows Arch. path. Anat. 256, 649—665 (1925).

KUZMA, J. F.: Myoepithelial proliferations in the human breast. Amer. J. Path. 19, 473—489 (1943).

LANGER, E., HUHN, S.: Der submikroskopische Bau der Myoepithelzelle. Z. Zellforsch. 47, 507—516 (1958).

LEE, B. J., PACK, G. T., SCHARNAGEL, I.: Sweat gland cancer of the breast. Surg. Gynec. Obstet. 56, 975—996 (1933).

LEESON, C. G.: The histochemical identification of myoepithelium with particular reference to the Harderian and extraorbital lacrimal glands. Acta anat. (Basel) 40, 87 (1960).

LENNOX, B., PEARSE, A. G. E., RICHARDS, H. G. H.: Mucin-secreting tumours of the skin: with special reference to the so-called mixed-salivary tumour of the skin and its relation to hidradenoma. J. Path. Bact. 64, 865—880 (1952).

LEVER, W. F.: Pathogenesis of benigne tumours of cutaneous appendages and of basal cell epithelioma. Arch. Derm. Syph. (Chic.) 57, 679—724 (1948a).

— Myoepithelial sweat gland tumor: Myoepithelioma. Report of three cases with a review of the literature. Arch. Derm. Syph. (Chic.) 57, 332—347 (1948b).

— Histology of the skin. Philadelphia-London-Montreal: J. B. Lippincott Comp. 1954.

— CASTLEMAN, B.: Clear-cell myo-epithelioma of the skin. Amer. J. Path. 28, 691—699 (1952).

— HASHIMOTO, K.: Die Histogenese einiger Hautanhangstumoren im Lichte histochemischer und elektronenmikroskopischer Befunde. (Ekkrines Porom, Ekkrines Spiradenom, Syringom, Cylindrom, verkalkendes Epitheliom.) Hautarzt 17, 161—173 (1966).

LINZELL, J. L.: The silver staining of myoepithelial cells, particuliarly in the mammary gland and their relation to the ejection of milk. J. Anat. (Lond.) **86**, 49—57 (1952).
— Some observations on the contractile tissue of the mammary glands. J. Physiol. (Lond.) **130**, 257—267 (1955).
LÖWENSTEIN, C.: Über atypische Epithelwucherungen und Tumoren der Speicheldrüsen, besonders der Parotis. Frankfurt. Z. Path. **4**, 187—202 (1910).
LUND, H. J.: Tumors of the skin. Atlas of tumor pathology, vol. I/2. Washington 1957.
MACKENZIE, D. H.: A clear cell hidradenocarcinoma with metastases. Cancer (Philad.) **10**, 1021—1023 (1957).
— A fibro-adenoma of the breast with smooth muscle. J. Path. Bact. **96**, 231—232 (1968).
MAEDA, R.: The origin and characteristics of ceroid. Acta path. jap. **17**, 439—456 (1968).
MASSON, P.: Tumeurs humaines, 2. ed. Paris: Maloine 1956.
MASSON, PEYRON: A propos des tumeurs mixtes des glandes salivaires. Specifité cellulaire et tumeurs mixtes. Ass. Franc. Etude Cancer **7**, 219—263 (1914).
MAYER, I.: Zur Histologie der Hidradenome. Frankfurt. Z. Path. **55**, 548—580 (1941)
MELNICK, P. J.: Fibromyoma of the breast. Arch. Path. **14**, 794—798 (1932).
MEYER, A., DELARUE, J., PEUTEUIL, G., LIOT, F.: Sur un cas de tumeur a cellules myo-epitheliales localisé a la region juxta-scissurale du poumon gauche. J. franç. Méd. Chir. thor. **8**, 310—316 (1954).
MORGAN, W. S., CASTLEMAN, B.: A clinicopathologic study of "Mikulicz's disease". Amer. J. Path. **29**, 471—503 (1953).
MÜLLER, H. B.: Die postnatale Entwicklung der Harderschen Drüse der weißen Ratte. II. Fermenthistochemische Befunde. Histochemie **20**, 181—196 (1969).
MURAD, M. T., v. HAAM, E.: Transformation of myothelial cells into epithelial cells in pregnancy. Proc. 25th Ann. Meeting E. M. Soc. of Amer. 62—63 (1967).
— — The ultrastructure of fibrocystic disease of the breast. Cancer (Philad.) **22**, 587—600 (1968a).
— — Ultrastructure of myoepithelial cells in human mammary gland tumors. Cancer (Philad.) **21**, 1137—1149 (1968b).
— SCARPELLI, D. G.: The ultrastructure of medullary and scirrhous mammary duct carcinoma. Amer. J. Path. **50**, 335—360 (1967).
MYLIUS, E. A.: The identification and the role of the myoepithelial cell in salivary gland tumours. Acta path. microbiol. scand., Suppl. **139**, 1—59 (1960).
NANGLE, E. J., SYMMERS, W. ST. C.: Pleomorphic sweat-gland adenoma of the foot. J. Bone Jt. Surg. **32 B**, 70—73 (1950).
NEGRI, L., FERRANTE, R.: Orientamenti istogenetici e adeguamenti classificativi della malignita nelle ghiandole salivari (con applicazione delle mesomucinasi allo studio delle componenti stromali). Arch. De Vecchi Anat. pat. **12**, 373—440 (1949).
NEWMAN, W., FEIGIN, I., WOLF, A., KABAT, E.: Histochemical studies of tissue enzymes: IV. Distribution of some enzyme systems which liberate phosphate at pH 9.2 as determined with various substrates and inhibitors; Demonstration of 3 groups of enzymes. Amer. J. Path. **26**, 257—306 (1950).
NOBACK, C. R., MONTAGNA, W.: Histochemical studies of the basophilia, lipase and phosphatases in the mammalian pancreas and salivary glands. Amer. J. Anat. **81**, 343—367 (1947).
O'HARA, J. M., BENSCH, K., IOANNIDES, G., KLAUS, S. N.: Eccrine sweat gland adenoma, clear cell type. A histochemical study. Cancer (Philad.) **19**, 1438—1450 (1966).
OOTA, K., TAKAHASHI, N.: Electron microscopic studies on the so-called benign mixed tumour of the salivary gland. Gann **49**, 234—235 (1958).

Peyron, A., Corsy, F., Surmont, J.: Sur la pathologie comparée des tumeurs de la mamelle. Bull. Ass. franç. Cancer 15, 21—62 (1926).
Pirilä, V., Eränkö, O.: Distribution of histochemically demonstrable alkaline phosphatase in normal and pathologic human skin. Acta path. microbiol. scand. 27, 650—660 (1950).
Postnov, Yu. V.: Myoepithelioma of the sweat glands. Arch. Path. 1965, 38—43 [Russisch].
Propst, A.: Zur Morphologie der Cylindrome. Frankfurt. Z. Path. 65, 97—110 (1954).
Quintarelli, G., Robinson, L.: The glycosaminoglycans of salivary gland tumors. Amer. J. Path. 51, 19—37 (1967).
Richardson, K. G.: Contractile tissues in the mammary gland, with special reference to myothelium in the goat. Proc. roy Soc. B 136, 30—45 (1949).
Robb, P. M., McFarlane, A.: Two rare breast tumors. J. Path. Bact. 75, 293—298 (1958).
Rottino, A., Howley, C. P.: Osteoid sarcoma of the breast a complication of fibroadenoma. Arch. Path. 40, 44—50 (1945).
Rowlatt, C., Franks, L. M.: Myoepithelium in mouse prostate. Nature (Lond.) 202, 707 (1964).
Saar, Freiherr v. G.: Über Cystadenoma mammae und Mastitis chronica cystica. Langenbecks Arch. klin. Chir. 84, 223—279 (1907).
Santler, R., Eberhartinger, C.: Malignes Klarzellen-Myoepitheliom. Dermatologica (Basel) 130, 340—347 (1965).
Sarkar, K., Kallenbach, E.: Myoepithelial cells in carcinoma of human breast. Amer. J. Path. 49, 301—307 (1966).
Schäfer, A., Bässler, R.: Vergleichende elektronenmikroskopische Untersuchungen am Drüsenepithel und am sog. lobulären Carcinom der Mamma. Virchows Arch. Abt. A Path. Anat. 346, 269—286 (1969).
Schultz, A.: Pathologische Anatomie der Brustdrüse. In: Henke-Lubarsch, Bd. VII/2. 1—208, 1933.
Scott, B. L., Pease, D. C.: Electron microscopy of the salivary and lacrimal glands of the rat. Amer. J. Anat. 104, 115—161 (1959).
Seifert, G., Geiler, G.: Vergleichende Untersuchungen der Kopfspeichel- und Tränendrüsen zur Pathogenese des Sjörgen-Syndroms und der Mikulicz-Krankheit. Virchows Arch. path. Anat. 330, 402—424 (1957).
Shear, M.: Histochemical localisation of alkaline phosphatase and adenosine triphosphatase in myoepithelial cells of the rat salivary glands. Nature (Lond.) 203, 770 (1964).
Sheldon, W. H.: The myoepithelium in sweat gland tumours. Distribution, histology, embryology and function. Arch. Path. 31, 326—337 (1941).
— So-called mixed tumours of the salivary glands. Arch. Path. 35, 1—20 (1943).
Shelley, H. B., Mescon, H.: Histochemical demonstration of secretory activity in human eccrine sweat glands. J. invest. Derm. 18, 289—301 (1952).
Simard, L. C.: Tumour of the palm having the structure of a mixed tumour of the salivary glands. Amer. J. Cancer 33, 182—195 (1938).
Silver, I. A.: Myoepithelial cells in the mammary and parotid gland. J. Physiol. (Lond.) 125, Proceed. of the Physiol. Soc. 8 P (1954).
Skorpil, F.: Über das Speicheldrüsenadenom. Virchows Arch. path. Anat. 306, 714—736 (1940).
— Über das benigne Lymphom der Ohrspeicheldrüse. Frankfurt. Z. Path. 56, 514—533 (1942).
— Über das Vorkommen von sog. hellen Zellen (Lamprozyten) in der Milchdrüse. Beitr. path. Anat. 108, 378—393 (1943).
Stewart, F. W.: Tumors of the breast. Atlas of tumor pathology, Sect. IX Fasc. 34. Washington: AFIP 1950.

STILLIANS, A. W.: Naevo-epithelioma adenoides (cylindroma) of the scalp. Arch. Derm. Syph. (Chic.) **27**, 481 (1933).

TAMARIN, A.: Myoepithelium of the rat submaxillary gland. J. Cell Biol. **23**, 93 A abstract (1964).

— Myoepithelium of the rat submaxillary gland. J. Ultrastruct. Res. **16**, 320—338 (1966).

TANDLER, B.: Ultrastructure of the human submaxillary gland. III. Myoepithelium. Z. Zellforsch. **68**, 852—863 (1965).

TANNENBAUM, M., WEISS, M., MARX, A.: Ultrastructure of the human mammary ductule. Cancer (Philad.) **23**, 958—978 (1969).

THACKERAY, A. C., LUCAS, R. B.: The histology of cylindrome of mucous gland origin. Brit. J. Cancer **14**, 612—620 (1960).

WAUGH, D., HOEVEN, E. VAN DER: Fine structure of the human adult female breast. Lab. Invest. **11**, 220—228 (1962).

WEBER, H. W.: Über anatomische Befunde bei männlicher Brustdrüsenvergrößerung. Frankfurt. Z. Path. **61**, 547—556 (1949/50).

WEISS, P.: Submikroskopische Charakteristika und Reaktionsformen der glatten Muskelzelle unter besonderer Berücksichtigung der Gefäßwandmuskelzelle. Z. mikr.-anat. Forsch. **78**, 305—331 (1968).

WELLINGS, S. R., ROBERTS, P.: Electron microscopy of sclerosing adenosis and infiltrating duct carcinoma of the human mammary gland. J. nat. Cancer Inst. **30**, 269—287 (1963).

WELSH, R. A., MEYER, A. T.: Mixed tumors of human salivary gland: Histogenesis. Arch. Path. **85**, 433—447 (1968).

WILLIS, R. A.: Pathology of tumours, 3. ed. London: Butterworth 1960.

WINKELMANN, R. K., WOLFF, K.: Solid-cystic hidradenoma of the skin. Arch. Derm. Syph. (Chic.) **97**, 651—661 (1968).

ZIMMERMANN, K. W.: Speicheldrüsen der Mundhöhle und die Bauchspeicheldrüse. In: Handbuch der mikroskopischen Anatomie, Bd. V, S. 1. Berlin: Springer 1927.

Author Index

Page numbers in *italics* refer to bibliography

Abdel-Latif, A. A., Brody, J., Ramahi, H. 95, *148*
— see Ling, C. V. M. 95, *155*
Abramow, S. S. 187, *213*
Ackerman, L. V. 187, *213*
Adachi, M. 148
— Aronson, S. M. 102, 111, 137, *148*
— Volk, B. W. 102, 111, 127, 129, 143, *148*
— Wallace, B. J., Schneck, L., Volk, B.W. 94, 102, 111, 125, 127, 142, 143, *149*
Adair, F. E. 61, *67*
— see Urban, J. A. 59, *88*
Adams, C. W. M. 133, 140, *149*
Adams, R. D. *149*
— Foley, J. M. 133, *149*
— see Victor, M. 133, *160*
Agranoff, B. W., see Foote, J. L. 134, 145, 146, *152*
Aguilar, M. J., see Kamoshita, S. 102, 143, *154*
— see Sacks, O. 102, 114, 128, 147, *158*
Ahrén, K. 17, 19, 23, 24, 26, 52, 57, *67*
— Etienne, M. 24, 26, 51, 52, 57, *67*
— Hamberger, L. 51, *67*
— Jacobsohn, D. 24, 26, 49, 50, 57, *67*
— see Hamberger, L. 51, *77*
Ahumada, I. C., Del Castillo, E. B. *67*

Aimes, A., see Grynfeltt, E. 194, 197, *216*
Alberici, M., see De Robertis, E. 94, 95, 137, *151*, *152*
— see Rodriguez de Lores Arnaiz, G. 95, *158*
Albers, R. W., Rodriguez de Lores Arnaiz, G., de Robertis, E. 95, *149*
Albores Culebro, C. 66, *67*
Albright, F., see Forbes, A. P. 65, 66, *74*
Aldridge, W. N. 140, *149*
Aleu, F. P., Katzman, R., Terry, R. T. 94, 135, 136, 140, *149*
— Samuels, S., Ransohoff, J. 94, 96, 139, 143, *149*
— see Katzman, R. 136, 140, *154*
Alivisatos, J. G., see McCullagh, E. 66, *81*
Allen, A. C. 190, *213*
Allen, E., see Chamberlin, T. L. 20, *71*
Allen, R. J., see Foote, J. L. 134, 145, 146, *152*
Alpers, B. J. 92, *149*
Altegoer, E. 134, *149*
Altmann, H. W. 8, *67*
Alvord, E. C., Jr., Stevenson, L. D., Vogel, St., Egle, L. R. 133, 145, *149*
Ametani, T., see Tani, E. 95, 140, *159*
Anderson, J. M. 99, 134, 135, 142, 145, *149*

Anderson, R. R., Brookreson, A. D., Turner, C. W. 24, *67*
Anton, E., see Brandes, D. 30, *70*
Appel, S. H. 145, *149*
Appicciutoli, L., see Bignami, A. 137, *150*
Archer, F., Omar, M. 174, 185, *213*
Archer, F. L., Kao, V. C. Y. 164, *213*
Argonz, J., Del Castillo, E. B. 65, *67*
Arhelger, St. W., Husely, R. A. 53, *68*
Aristoteles 67, *68*
Arnoult, J., see Haguenau, F. 13, *76*, 164, 178, 208, *216*
Aronson, B. E., see Aronson, S. M. 102, *149*
Aronson, S. M., Aronson, B. E. 102, *149*
— Lewitan, A., Rabiner, A. M., Epstein, N., Volk, B. W. 128, *149*
— Volk, B. W. 104, *149*
— see Adachi, M. 102, 111, 137, *148*
— see Kanoff, A. 128, *154*
Asboe-Hansen, G. 29, *68*
Ashbury, A. K., see Pant, S. S. 94, *157*
Asperger, H. 148
Astwood, E. B., Geschickter, C. F. 17, 23, 24, *68*
— — Rausch, E. O. 17, 23, 51, *68*

Auchincloss, H., see
  Frantz, V. K.   64, 75
Aurebeck, G., see
  Nelson, E.   102, 124, 156
Austin, J., McAfee, D.,
  Shearer, L.   129, 149
Averbach, M. M.   65, 68
Averill, R. L. W.   44, 68
— Ray, E. W., Lyons,
  W. R.   44, 68
Averill, S. C., see
  Ray, E. W.   44, 84
Axelrod, J., see
  Eisenfeld, A. J.   38, 73
Azzopardi, J. G.   198, 213
— Smith, A. D.   190, 191, 193, 213

Bässler, R.   48, 60, 61, 63, 68, 163, 185, 213
— Brethfeld, V.   14, 30, 32, 46, 68, 165, 166, 167, 175, 213
— Flörchinger, J.   8, 10, 68
— Forssmann, W.   13, 37, 43, 68
— Paek, S.   30, 64, 68
— Schäfer, A.   12, 13, 21, 64, 68, 166, 176, 213
— Schäfer, A., Paek, S.   14, 46, 68, 165, 213
— Schulze, G.,
  Schriever, D.   29, 69
— see Brandt, G.   56, 70
— see Lani, K.   44, 79
— see Schäfer, A.   85, 208, 219
Baethmann, A., see
  Reulen, H. J.   95, 157
Bain, G. O., Kowalewski,
  K. P., MacGregor, J. W.   190, 213
Bakay, L., Lee, J. C.   95, 136, 149
— see Lee, J. C.   94, 135, 155
Baldwin, R. L.,
  Martin, R. J.   8, 69
Balinsky, B. I.   4, 69
Banerjee, M. R.,
  Walker, R. J.   9, 69

Banker, B. Q., Robertson,
  J. T., Victor, M.   100, 104, 143, 149
Barbieri, G., see Olivi, M.   27, 83
Bardin, C. W., Liebelt,
  A. G., Liebelt, R. A.   40, 69
Bargeton, E., see
  Habib, R.   134, 153
Bargmann, W., Fleisch-
  hauer, K., Knoop, A.   43, 69
Barlow, R. M., Dickinson,
  A. G.   135, 150
— see Cancilla, P. A.   135, 151
— see Dickinson, A. G.   135, 152
Barnard, S., see
  Brandes, D.   30, 70
Barnes, J. M., see
  Magee, P. N.   136, 156
Barrnett, R. J., see
  Torack, R. M.   95, 160
Barton, A.   213
Bartuska, D. G., see
  Eskin, B. A.   54, 73
Batzenschlager, A., see
  Fruhling, L.   199, 215
Bates, R. W., see
  Riddle, O.   41, 85
Bauer, J. D., see Bauer,
  W. H.   190, 198, 213
Bauer, W. H., Bauer, J. D.   190, 198, 213
— Fox, R. A.   190, 197, 213
Beato, M., Dienstbach, F.   37, 69
Bechar, M., Bornstein, B.,
  Elian, M., Sandbank, U.   133, 150
Beck, W. C.   148
Benda, C. E.   133, 150
Benecke, G., see
  Schmidt, G. W.   134, 158
Bengtsson, B., Norgren, A.   53, 69
Bensch, K., see O'Hara,
  J. M.   166, 197, 218
Bensch, K. G., see
  Herman, M. M.   132, 153

Benson, G. K., Cowie, A. T.,
  Cox, C. P., Flux, D. S.,
  Folley, S. J.   21, 26, 27, 69
— — — Folley, S. J.,
  Hosking, Z. D.   26, 69
— — — Goldzweig, S. A.   7, 20, 23, 24, 26, 27, 69
— — Folley, S. J.,
  Tindal, J. S.   21, 24, 44, 49, 57, 69
— Folley, S. J.   48, 49, 69
Berde, B.   46, 69
— Cerletti, A.   46, 69
Berg, J. W., McDivitt,
  R. W.   205, 213
Bergenstal, D. M., see
  Levine, H. J.   67, 80
Berger, H.   13, 69, 178, 208, 214
Berghorn, B. M., Bryce,
  B. L., Helwig, E. B.   197, 214
Berk, F.   3, 69
Berka, F.   27, 60, 63, 70
Bern, H. A., see
  Soemarwoto, J. N.   26, 86
Bernheimer, H.   129, 150
Berswordt-Wallrabe, R. v.   7, 70
— see Elger, W.   6, 73
— see Neumann, F.   7, 83
— Turner, C. W.   26, 56, 70
Bertrand, I., see
  Bogaert, L. van   91, 98, 99, 100, 128, 138, 139, 150
Bertkau, F.   164, 214
Besezny   163
Best, C. H., see Salter, J.   57, 85
Betz, E., see Schlote, W.   94, 137, 158
Bhaskar, S. N., Wein-
  mann, J. P.   190, 194, 197, 214
Biedermann, K.   17, 70
Bielschowsky, M.   92, 150
Biggs, R.   192, 203, 214

Bignami, A., Marinacci, F., Zappella, M., Tingey, A. H.   131, *150*
— Palladini, G.   136, *150*
— — Appicciutoli, L., Maccagnani, F.   137, *150*
Birkle, K., see Boemke, F.   64, *70*
Bittorf, A.   66, *70*
Blackwood, W., Buxton, P. H., Cumings, J. N., Robertson, J., Tucker, S. M.   92, *150*
— Cumings, J. N.   92, 100, 138, 144, *150*
Bloch, K.   64, *70*
Blond, D., see Whittam, R.   142, *160*
Blum, E., see Fruhling, L.   199, *215*
Böck, J., Feyrter, F.   192, *214*
Böhming, R.   59, 60, 63, 64, *70*
Boemke, F., Birkle, K.   64, *70*
Bogaert, L. van   91, 98, 100, 104, 128, 138, *150*
— Bertrand, I.   91, 98, 99, 100, 128, 138, 139, *150*
— see Hooft, C.   *154*
— see Ishino, H.   93, *154*
— see Martin, J. J.   134, *156*
— see Poser, C. M.   133, 145, *157*
— see De Vries, E.   100, *152*
Bogart, B. I.   167, *214*
Bohle, A.   63, *70*
Bond, P. R., see Gerstl, B.   134, 144, *153*
Bonting, S. L.   95, *150*
Bornstein, B., see Bechar, M.   133, *150*
Borowicz, K., see Zelman, I. B.   133, *160*
Boschbach, F. W.   194, *214*
Bottomley, A. C., Folley, S. J.   53, *70*
Boyd, R. W., see Weichert, C. K.   16, *89*

Bradley, T. R., Clark, P. M.   43, *70*
— Cowie, A. T.   44, *70*
Brady, see Moore   140
Brady, R. O., see Percy, A. K.   129, *157*
Brandes, D., Anton, E., Barnard, S.   30, *70*
Brandt, G.   56, *70*
— Bässler, R.   56, *70*
Braucher, P. F., see Riddle, O.   41, *85*
Braumühl, A. von   93, *150*
Braverman, L. B., see Smith, Th. C.   19, 50, *86*
Bredt, H.   64, *70*
Bresciani, F.   9, *70*
Breslin, Fr. J., see Budd, J. W.   203, *214*
Brethfeld, V., see Bässler, R.   14, 30, 32, 46, 68, 165, 166, 167, 175, *213*
Breustedt, H.-J., see Kracht, J.   65, *79*
Brissaud, H. E., see Habib, R.   134, *153*
Brody, J., see Abdel-Latif, A. A.   95, *148*
Broman, J.   3, *70*
Bromberg, Y. M., see Zondek, B.   89
Brookreson, A. D., see Anderson, R. R.   24, *67*
Brouha, H.   3, *70*
Brown, F. M., see Gerughty, R. M.   199, *216*
Brown, W. J., see Sacks, O.   102, 114, 128, 147, *158*
Browne, J. S. L., see Selye, H.   23, *86*
Browning, H. C., White, W. D.   41, *70*
— — Gibbs, W.   41, *71*
Brucher, J. M., Dom, R., Robin, A.   102, 108, 132, 143, *150*
Brumby, P. J., see Hancock, J.   26, *77*
Bryce, B. L., see Berghorn, B. M.   197, *214*

Bubis, J. J., Luse, S. A.   *150*
Buchanan, D. S., Davis, R. L.   102, 104, *150*
Budd, J. W., Breslin, Fr. J.   203, *214*
Budzilovich, G., see Feigin, I.   102, 134, 138, *152*
Bues, F., see Suchenwirth, R.   66, *87*
Bunge, R. P.   140, *150*
Bunting, H.   27, *71*, 164, 166, *214*
— Wislocki, B., Dempsey, E. W.   166, *214*
— see Dempsey, E. W.   27, 30, 46, *73*, 164, 165, 166, 167, *214*
— see Duran-Reynals, F.   29, 63, *73*
Burrows, H.   65, *71*
Busch, J. P. zum   66, *71*
Busch, W., Merker, H.-J.   13, *71*, 208, *214*
Buxton, P.-H., see Blackwood, W.   92, *150*
Byrnes, E. W., see Geschickter, C. F.   23, *75*

Cabanne, F.   200, *214*
Cabrera, M., see Ledeen, R.   144, *155*
Cairy, C. F., see Reinecke, E. P.   21, *84*
Calov, W. L., Whyte, H. M.   64, *71*
Canavan, M.   91, 98, 100, 129, *151*
Cancilla, P. A., Barlow, R. M.   135, *151*
Candiani, M. A., see Veronesi, U.   27, *88*
Canivenc, R., Mayer, G.   44, *71*
Capone Braga, M.   191, *214*
Carlson, D. M., see Hansen, R. G.   30, *77*
Carlson, K. L., see Spellacy, W. N.   66, *86*

Carlton, W. W.   136, 141, *151*
— Kreutzberg, G.   136, *151*
Carr, S., see Prensky, A. L.   133, 134, 145, 146, *157*
Caspersson, T.   12, *71*
— Santesson, L.   166, 208, *214*
Castaigne, P., see Ribadeau-Dumas, J. L.   135, *157*
Castleman, B., see Lever, W. F.   198, *217*
— see Morgan, W. Z.   181, *218*
Catchpole, H. R., Lyons, W. R.   43, *71*
— — Regan, W. M.   43, *71*
— see Lyons, W. R.   43, *80*
Cavanagh, J. B., see Laurence, K. M.   92, *155*
Centeno, J., see Luchsingen, Y.   61, *80*
Cerletti, A., see Berde, B.   46, *69*
Chadwick, A., see Forsyth, J. A.   45, *75*
Chain, E., Duthie, E. S.   29, 63, *71*
Chalkley, H. W.   7, *71*
Chamberlin, T. L., Gardner, W. U., Allen, E.   20, *71*
Chamorro, A.   23, *71*
Chaudhury, R. R., Walker, J. M.   46, *71*
Cheatle, G. L., Cutler, M.   64, *71*
Chen, G. C., see Suzuki, K.   144, *159*
Chen, Th. T., Johnson, R. E., Lyons, W. R., Li, C. H., Cole. D. R.   53, *71*
Chentsov, S., see Suetina, J. A.   37, *87*
Chentsov, Y., Chentsov, S.   37, *71*
— see Suetina, J. A.   37, *87*

Chiquoine, A. D.   48, *71*
Chou, S. M.   141, *151*
— Waisman, H. A.   133, 134, *151*
Christensen, E., Hojgaard, K.   *151*
— Krabbe, K. H.   92, *151*
Ciacco, E. I., see Nelson, W. O.   10, *83*
Clark, B. G., Shapiro, S., Monroe, R. G.   66, *71*
Clark, P. M., see Bradley, T. R.   43, *70*
Clasen, R. A., Pandolfi, S., Russell, J., Stuart, D., Hass, G. M.   136, 137, *151*
Clifton, K. H., Furth, J.   41, *71*
Clotten, R., see Sander, C.   134, *158*
Cohen, R. S., see Weichert, C. K.   16, *89*
Cole, D. R., see Chen, Th. T.   53, *71*
Cole, J. D., see Kaye, G. I.   140, *154*
Cole, M., see Victor, M.   133, *160*
Cole, R., Hopkins, T. R.   44, *71*
Cole, R. D., see Lyons, W. R.   19, *80*
Collip, J. B., see McEuen, C. S.   17, 50, 51, *81*
— see Noble, R. L.   *83*
— see Selye, H.   23, 51, *86*
Colmant, J. H.   99, 135, *151*
Consolandi, G.   27, *71*
Cooke, J. V.   66, *72*
Copeland, M. M.   63, *72*
Corner, G. W.   23, *72*
Cornog, J. L., Jr., Gonatas, N. K., Feierman, J. R.   94, 137, *151*
Corsy, F., see Peyron, A.   187, 190, *219*
Cotchin, E.   190, *214*
Cote, L. J., see Fahn, S.   95. *152*
Courtecuisse, V., see Fiske, S. W. C.   37, *74*

Cowan, D. M., see King, R. J. B.   37, *78*
Cowie, A. T.   7, 20, 24, 26, 57, *72*
— Folley, S. J.   43, 50, 54, *72*
— — Cross, B. A., Harris, G. W., Jacobsohn, D., Richardson, K. C.   45, *72*
— — Malpress, F. H., Richardson, K. C.   21, 26, *72*
— Lyons, W. R.   39, *72*
— Tindal, J. S., Yokoyama, A.   26, *72*
— see Benson, G. K.   7, 20, 21, 23, 24, 26, 27, 44, 49, 57, *69*
— see Bradley, T. R.   44, *70*
— see Kon, S. K.   2, *79*
Cox, C. P., see Benson, G. K.   7, 20, 21, 23, 24, 26, 27, *69*
Crain, R. C., Helwig, E. B.   192, 197, *214*
Crass, G., see Doyle, L. E.   190, 191, *215*
Crocker, A. C.   127
Crocker, D. J., Murad, T. M.   200, *214*
Crome, L.   133, *151*
— Dutton, G., Ross, C. F.   133, 134, *151*
— Pare, C. M. B.   *151*
— Tymms, V., Woolf, L. I.   133, 145, *151*
Crompton, M. R.   93, *151*
Cross, B. A., see Cowie, A. T.   45, *72*
Cruickshank, A. H.   181, 182, *214*
Cumings, J. N.   99, *151*
— Grundt, I. K., Yanagihara, T.   134, 145, 146, *151*
— see Blackwood, W.   92, 100, 138, 144, *150*
— see Yanagihara, T.   144, *160*
Curran, R. C., Dodge, O. G.   203, *214*
Curtiss, C.   17, 23, 24, *72*

Cutler, M. 2, 61, 64, *72*
— see Cheatle, G. L. 64, *71*
Czochanska-Kruk, J., see Zelman, I. B. 133, *160*

Daane, Th. A., Lyons, W. R. 19, 23, 24, *72*
Dabelow, A. 2, 4, 11, 27, 61, *72*
Dalla Pria, S., see Mahesh, V. B. 66, *80*
Dambska, M., Szelozynska, K., Kamraj-Mazurkiewicz, K. 134, *151*
Damm, H. C., Turner, C. W. 40, *72*
Dancis, J., Levitz, M., Westall, R. G. 134, *151*
— see Silverman, J. 134, *159*
Danowski, T. S. 65, 66, *72*
David, H., Korth, I. 190, *214*
Davis, R. L., see Buchanan, D. S. 102, 104, *150*
Davison, A. N. 146, *151*
— Dobbing, J. 145, *151*
Davson, H. 142, *151*
Dawson, E. K. 60, *72*
Delarue, J., see Meyer, A. 205, *218*
Del Castillo, E. B., see Ahumada, I. C. *67*
— see Argonz, J. 65, *67*
Dellweg, H. 37, *72*
De Lores Arnaiz, G. R., see De Robertis, E. 94, 95, 137, *151*, *152*
Dempsey, E. W., Bunting, H., Wislocki, G. B. 27, 30, 46, *73*, 164, 165, 166, 167, *214*
— see Bunting, H. 166, *214*
De Petris, S., Karlsbad, G., Pernis, B. *214*
Deppisch, L. M., Toker, C. 191, *215*

De Robertis, E. 141, *151*
— Alberici, M., de Lores Arnaiz, G. R. 95, *151*
— Sellinger, O. Z., de Lores Arnaiz, G. R., Alberici, M., Ziehrer, L. M. 94, 137, *152*
— see Albers, R. W. 95, *149*
— see Rodriguez de Lores Arnaiz, G. 95, *158*
De Robertis, E. D. P., see Zadunaisky, J. A. 95, *160*
Desclin, L. 48, *73*
Devenyi, I. 205, *215*
De Vries, E., Bogaert, L. van, Edgar, G. W. F. 100, *152*
Dewey, M. M. 167, *215*
Dichgans, J., see Klein, H. 92, *155*
Dickinson, A. G., Barlow, R. M. 135, *152*
— see Barlow, R. M. 135, *150*
Diczfalusy, E., Tillinger, K. G., Westman, A. 63, *73*
Dieckmann, H. 27, 61, *73*
Dienstbach, F., see Beato, M. 37, *69*
Dietz, H. 181, *215*
Diezel, P. B., Martin, K. 134, *152*
Diniz, C. R., see Jervell, K. J. 9, *78*
Djojosoebagio, S., Turner, C. W. 56, *73*
Dobbing, J., see Davison, A. N. 145, *151*
Dodge, O. G., see Curran, R. C. 203, *214*
Dom, R., see Brucher, J. M. 102, 108, 132, 143, *150*
Don, A., see Kaye, G. I. 140, *154*
Donohue, W. L. 99, 133, 134, 145, *152*
Donovan, B. T., Jacobsohn, D. 52, 54, *73*
Dorfman, R. I., Shipley, R. A. 53, *73*

Doyle, L. E., Lynn, L. A., Panopio, I. T., Crass, G. 190, 191, *215*
Dratman, M. D., see Eskin, B. A. 54, *73*
Dreifuss, F. E., Netsky, M. G. 92, *152*
Dubois, J. 7, *73*
Dufty, M. L., see Torack, R. M. 95, *160*
Dumont, J. N. 43, *73*
Dunn, M. R., see Eskin, B. A. 54, *73*
Duran-Reynals, F., Bunting, H., Wagenen, G. van 29, 63, *73*
Duthie, E. S., see Chain, E. 29, 63, *71*
Dutton, G., see Crome, L. 133, 134, *151*
Dykshorn, S. W., see Riddle, O. 41, *85*
Dyx, W. 173, *215*

Earle, K. M., see Lampert, P. W. 94, *155*
— see Schochet, S. S., Jr. 129, *158*
Eberhartinger, C., see Santler, R. 205, *219*
Edgar, G. W. F., see De Vries, E. 100, *152*
Effkemann, G., see Herold, L. 17, *77*
Efskind, J., Eker, R. 197, 198, *215*
Eggeling, H. von 3, 11, *73*
Egle, L. R., see Alvord, E. C., Jr., 133, 145, *149*
Eickman, P. L., see Zu Rhein, G. M. 100, 138, 147, *160*
Eiselsberg, F. 98, 100, *152*
Eisen, M. J. 19, 65, *73*
Eisenfeld, A. J., Axelrod, J. 38, *73*
Eker, R., see Efskind, J. 197, 198, *215*
Elger, W., Berswordt-Wallrabe, R. von, Neumann, F. 6, *73*
— Neumann, F. 5, *73*

Elger, W., see Neumann, F. 5, 6, 7, *83*
Elian, M., see Bechar, M. 133, *150*
Ellis, R. 48, 73, 164, 165, 166, *215*
Emge, L. A. 17, *73*
Eneroth, C. M., Wersäll, J. 191, *215*
Eng, L. F., see Gerstl, B. 134, 145, 146, *153*
Epstein, N., see Aronson, S. M. 128, *149*
Eränkö, O., see Pirilä, V. 166, *219*
Erbslöh, F. 93, 133, *152*
Erichsen, S. 190, *215*
Ericson, S. 181, *215*
Ericsson, L. E., see Helminen, H. J. 30, *77*
Escourolle, R., see Ribadeau-Dumas, J. L. 135, *157*
Eskin, B. A., Bartuska, D. G., Dunn, M. R., Jacob, G., Dratman, M. D. 54, *73*
Etienne, M., see Ahrén, K. 24, 26, 51, 52, 57, *67*
Evans, J. P., see Raimondi, A. J. 139, *157*
Evans, R. W. 197, *215*
Ewing 203

Fahn, S., Cote, L. J. 95. *152*
Farquhar, M. D., Hartmann, J. F. 141, *152*
Fauvet, E. 17, 24, *73*
Federlin, K., see Sandritter, W. 9, *85*
Feierman, J. R., see Cornog, J. L., Jr. 94, 137, *151*
Feigin, I., Budzilovich, G. 138, *152*
— Pena, C. E., Budzilovich, G. 102, 134, 138, *152*
— see Silverman, J. 134, *159*
— see Newman, W. 166, *218*
Ferguson, D. J. 20
— Visscher, M. B. 20, 53, *73*

Ferrante, R., see Negri, L. 190, *218*
Ferreri, F. L., Griffith, D. R. 50, *74*
Feyrter, F. 164, 167, 176, 179, 189, 190, 192, 193, 197, 198, *215*
— Gottron, H., Nikolowski, W. N. *215*
— Hartmann, G. 176, 207, 208, *215*
— s. Böck, J. 192, *214*
Finck, F. M., Schwinn, C. P., Keasbey, L. E. 198, *215*
Fiol, R. E., see Menkes, J. H. 134, 146, *156*
Fischer, O. 92, 94, *152*
Fischer, R., Schaefer, H. E. 32, *74*
— see Gedigk, P. 170, *215*
— see Schaefer, H. E. 32, *85*
Fiske, S. W. C., Courtecuisse, V., Haguenau, F. 37, *74*
Fleischhauser, K., see Bargmann, W. 43, *69*
Flörchinger, J., see Bässler, R. 8, 10, *68*
Fluhmann, C. F., see Laqueur, G. L. 50, *79*
Flux, D. S. 39, 49, 53, *74*
— Munford, R. E. 7, 40, *74*
— see Benson, G. K. 21, 26, 27, *69*
Folch-Pi, J., see Lees, M. B. 127, *155*
Foley, J. M., see Adams, R. D. 133, *149*
Folley, S. J. 2, 7, 16, 21, 24, 43, 45, 53, *74*
— Greenbaum, A. L. *74*
— Gutkelch, A. N., Zuckerman, S. 7, 20, 53, *74*
— McNaught, M. L. 30, *74*
— Young, F. G. 43, *74*
— see Benson, G. K. 21, 24, 26, 27, 44, 48, 49, 57, *69*

Folley, S. J., see Bottomley, A. C. 53, *70*
— see Cowie, A. T. 21, 26, 43, 45, 50, 54, *72*
— see Forsyth, J. A. 45, *75*
— see Heuverswyn, J. van 7, 53, *77*
— see Wagenen, G. van 53, *89*
Foncin, J. F. 94, 135, *152*
— Gaches, J., Le Beau, J. *152*
Foote, F. W., Frazell, E. L. 199, *215*
— Stewart, F. W. 59, 60, 63, 74, 199, 200, *215*
Foote, J. L., Allen, R. J., Agranoff, B. W. 134, 145, 146, *152*
Forbes, A. P., Henneman, P. H., Griswold, G. C., Albright, F. 65, 66, *74*
Forbes, Th. R. 50, *74*
Ford, F. R., Livingston, S., Pryles, C. V. 131, *152*
Forssmann, W. 43, *74*
— see Bässler, R. 13, 37, 43, *68*
Forsyth, J. A., Folley, S. J., Chadwick, A. 45, *75*
Fox, J., see Lampert, P. W. 94, *155*
Fox, R. A., see Bauer, W. H. 190, 197, *213*
Fox, R. R., see O'Leary, J. L. 94, *157*
Franks, L. M., see Rowlatt, C. 163, *219*
Frantz, V. K., Pickren, J. W., Melcher, G. W., Auchincloss, H. 64, *75*
Frazell, E. L., see Foote, Fr. W. 198, 199, *215*
Frazier, C. N., Mu, J. W. 20, *75*
French, L. E., see Long, D. M. 94, 96, 139, 143, *155*
Friborsky, V. 192, *215*
Friede, R. L. 141, 147, *152*

Author Index

Friede, R. L., Jong, R. de 97, *152*
Frilley, M., see Raynaud, A. 5, *84*
Fruhling, L., Batzenschlager, A., Blum, E. 199, *215*
Furth, J., see Clifton, K. H. 41, *71*

Gaburro, D., Martin, J. J., Scarpa, P., Volpone, S. 102, *152*
Gaches, J., see Foncin, J. F. *152*
Gahres, E. E., see Rosen, S. W. 67, *85*
Gajdusek, D. C., see Lampert, P. W. 94, *155*
Gambetti, P., Mellmann, W. J., Gonatas, N. K. 94, 102, 124, 126, 141, 143, 148, *152*
Gardner, W. U. 19, 20, 21, 23, 24, 50, *75*
— Smith, G. M., Strong, L. C. 19, *75*
— Strong, L. C. 7, *75*
— Turner, C. W. 43, *75*
— White, A. 20, *75*
— see Chamberlin, T. L. 20, *71*
— see Heuverswyn, J. van 7, 53, *77*
Garrett, F. A., Talmage, R. V. 20, *75*
Gaudier, Grandclaude, Lambret, M. 205, *215*
Gedigk, P., Fischer, R. 170, *215*
Geiler, G., see Seifert, G. 181, *219*
Gerken, H., see Henn, R. 102, *153*
Gerstl, B., Malamud, N., Eng, L. F., Hayman, R. B. 134, 145, 146, *153*
— — Hayman, R. B., Bond, P. R. 134, 144, *153*
Gerughty, R. M., Scofield, H. H., Brown, F. M., Hennigar, G. R. 199, *216*

Geschickter, C. F. 3, 63, 64, *75*
— Byrnes, E. W. 23, *75*
— Hartman, C. G. 21, *75*
— Speert, H. 20, *75*
— see Astwood, E. B. 17, 23, 24, 51, *68*
Gibbs, C. J. Jr., see Lampert, P. W. 94, *155*
Gibbs, W., see Browning, H. C. 41, *71*
Giordano, G. G., see Morcaldi, L. 102, *156*
Girardie, J., Wolff, E. 30, *75*
Globus, J. H., Strauss, I. 98, 100, *153*
Glock, G. E., McLean, P. 8, 31, *75*
Godwin, J. T. 181, *216*
Gögl, H., Lang, F. J. 2, *75*
Gössner, W. 46, *75*
Goldenberg, V. E., Wiegenstein, L., Mottet, N. K. 64, *75*
Goldstein, D. J. 164, 165, 166, *216*
Goldzweig, S. A., see Benson, G. K. 7, 20, 23, 24, 26, 27, *69*
Gomez, E. T., Turner, C. W. 40, 54, *75*
— see Lewis, A. A. 40, *80*
— see Turner, C. W. 20, *88*
Gonatas, J., see Korey, S. R. 128, *155*
Gonatas, N. K. 148
— Terry, R. D., Weiss, M. 94, 135, 139, *153*
— Zimmerman, H. M., Levine, S. 94, *153*
— see Cornog, J. L., Jr., 94, 137, *151*
— see Gambetti, P. 94, 102, 124, 126, 141, 143, 148, *152*
Gonzales-Licea, A., Yardley, J. H., Hartmann, W. H. 203, *216*
Gordon, J., see King, R. J. B. 37, *78*

Gordon, J. S., see Torack, R. M. 95, *160*
Gordon, S., see Vigneaud, P. G. du 45, *88*
Gorski, J., Noteboom, W. D., Nicolette, J. A. 38, *76*
Gottron, H., see Feyrter, F. *215*
Grandclaude, see Gaudier 205, *215*
Graumann, W. 3, 4, 12, *76*
Green, J. D., Harris, G. W. 49, *76*
Greenbaum, A. L., Slater, T. F. 10, *76*
— see Folley, S. J. *74*
Greenblatt, R. B., see Mahesh, V. B. 66, *80*
Greenhouse, A. H., Neuburger, K. T. 92, *153*
Gregg, W. I. 67, *76*
Griffith, D. R., Turner, C. W. 10, 53, *76*
— see Ferreri, F. L. 50, *74*
— see Moon, R. C. 10, 24, *82*
Grishman, E. 190, *216*
Griswold, G. C., see Forbes, A. P. 65, 66, *74*
Gross, B. G., see Hashimoto, K. 164, 197, *216*
Grosvenor, C. E., Turner, C. W. 49, *76*
Gruber, G. B. 27, 61, *76*
Grueter, F., see Stricker, P. 40, 41, *87*
Grumbach, M. M., see Wyk, J. J. v. *89*
Grumbrecht, P. 17, 65, *76*
Grundt, I. K., see Cumings, J. N. 134, 145, 146, *151*
Gruner, J. E. 135, *153*
Grynfeltt, E., Aimes, A. 194, 197, *216*
Guazzi, G. C., see Hooft, C. *154*
— see Ishino, H. 93, *154*
— see Martin, J. J. 134, *156*

Guazzi, G. C., see Morcaldi, L. 102, *156*
Gubarewa, A. V. 194, *216*
Günther, R. 176, *216*
Gutkelch, A. N., see Folley, S. J. 7, 20, 53, 74

Haagensen, C. D. 2, *76*
Haam, E. v., see Murad, T. M. 48, *82*, 166, 183, 208, *218*
Habbe, K. 64, *76*
Habib, R., Bargeton, E., Brissaud, H. E., Raynaud, J., Le Ball, J. C. 134, *153*
Hachmeister, M., see Kracht, J. 65, *79*
Hadfield, D. 39, *76*
— Young, S. 39, *76*
Hadley, G. G., see Keasbey, L. E. 194, 205, *217*
Haenel, H. 66, *76*
Hager, H. 95, 147, *153*
Haguenau, F. 13, 14, 48, *76*, 164, *216*
— Arnoult, J. 13, *76*, 164, 178, 208, *216*
— see Fiske, S. W. C. 37, *74*
Haland, M. 161
Hallervorden, J. 130, *153*
Hamada, H., Neumann, F., Junkmann, K. 6, *76*
Hamberger, L., Ahrén, K. 51, *77*
— see Ahrén, K. 51, *67*
Hamperl, H. 14, 46, 59, *77*, 170, 182, 190, *216*
Hancock, J., Brumby, P. J., Turner, C. W. 26, *77*
Handa, H., see Tani, E. 95, 140, *159*
Hanenberger 67
Hansen, R. G., Carlson, D. M. 30, *77*
Harder 48
Hardy, M. H. 4, *77*
Harreveld, A. van 95, 142, *153*
— Khattab, F. I. 95, 139, *153*

Harris, A. B., see O'Leary, J. L. 94, *157*
Harris, B. 94, 137, *153*
Harris, G. W., see Cowie, A. T. 45, *72*
— see Green, J. D. 49, *76*
Hartman, C. G., see Geschickter, C. F. 21, *75*
Hartmann, G., see Feyrter, F. 176, 207, 208, *215*
Hartmann, J. F. 142, *153*
— see Farquhar, M. D. 141, *152*
— see Long, D. M. 94, 96, 139, 143, *155*
Hartmann, M. 58, *77*
Hartmann, W. H., see Gonzales-Licea, A. 203, *216*
Hartroft, W. S. 171, *216*
— Porta, E. A. 171, *216*
Hartz, Ph. H. 190, 194, 197, 198, *216*
Hashimoto, K., Gross, B. G., Nelson, R. G., Lever, W. F. 164, 197, *216*
— — Lever, W. F. 164, 197, *216*
— see Lever, W. F. 188, 192, *217*
Hass, G. M., see Clasen, R. A. 136, 137, *151*
Hauser, G. A., see Neimeier, R. 66, *82*
Hayashida, T. 45, *77*
Hayman, R. B., see Gerstl, B. 134, 144, 145, 146, *153*
Helminen, H. J., Ericsson, L. E., Orrenius, S. 30, *77*
Helwig, E. B., see Berghorn, B. M. 197, *214*
— see Crain, R. C. 192, 197, *214*
— see Hirsch, P. 192, *216*
— see Johnson, B. L. 197, *217*
— see Kersting, D. W. 194, 197, *217*

Hemplemann, L. H., Womack, N. A. 190, *216*
Henn, R., Gerken, H., Wiedemann, H.-R. 102, *153*
Henneman, P. H., see Forbes, A. P. 65, 66, *74*
Hennigar, G. R., see Gerughty, R. M. 199, *216*
Herman, M. M., Huttenlocher, P. R., Bensch, K. G. 132, *153*
Herold, L., Effkemann, G. 17, *77*
Herpol, J., see Hooft, C. *154*
Herzog, I., see Scheinberg, L. C. 94, 140, *158*
Heuverswyn, J. van, Folley, S. J., Gardner, W. U. 7, 53, *77*
Heytler, P. G., see Nelson, W. O. 10, *83*
Hibbs, R. G. 48, *77*, 166, *216*
Higashi, K. *77*
Higuchi, K. 29, 44, *77*
Hirano, A., Levine, S., Zimmerman, H. M. 94, 95, 96, 143, 147, *153*
— Zimmerman, H. M., Levine, S. 94, 95, 96, 136, 139, 147, *153*
Hirner, A. 94, 97, *154*
Hirsch, P., Helwig, E. B. 192, *216*
Hjac, T., see Zarzycki, L. 30, *89*
Höhn, E. O. 20, 49, *77*
Hoeven, E. van der, see Waugh, D. 13, *89*, 165, 208, *220*
Hoffmann, F. 65, *77*
Hogan, G. R., Richardson, E. P., Jr. 100, 102, *154*
Hojgaard, K., see Christensen, E. *151*
Hollmann, K. H. 164, 166, *216*

Hollmann, K. H., see
 Verley, J. M. 37, *88*
Holmes, R. 30, *77*
Holzner, J. H., Kaufmann, F. 30, *77*
Hooft, C., Valcke, R., Herpol, J., Bogaert, L. van, Guazzi, G. C. *154*
Hopkins, T. R., see Cole, R. 44, *71*
Hoshino, K. 6, *77*
Hosking, Z. D., see Benson, G. K. 26, *69*
Howley, C. P., see Rottino, A. 203, *219*
Hübner, G., Kleinsasser, O., Klein, H. J. 192, 193, 208, *216, 217*
— see Kleinsasser, O. 208, *217*
Huffman, D. F., see Reinecke, E. P. 21, *84*
Hughes, E. S. R. 4, *77*
Hughes, L. E., Kershaw, G. F., Shaw, I. G. 135, *154*
Huhn, S., see Langer, E. 14, 48, *79*, 164, *217*
Humboldt, A. v. 67, *77*
Humphrey, L. J., Swedlow, M. 54, *77*
Hunter, J. 41, *77*
Hurley, H. J., Shelley, W. B. 165, *217*
Husely, R. A., see Arhelger, St. W. 53, *68*
Huttenlocher, P. R., see Herman, M. M. 132, *153*
Hyden, H. 97, *154*

Ihnen, M., Perez-Tamayo, R. 27, *77*
Ingleby, H. 65, *77*
Inman, D. R., see King, R. J. B. 37, *78*
Ioannides, G., see O'Hara, J. M. 166, 197, *218*
Ishino, H., Guazzi, G. C., Bogaert, L. van 93, *154*

Jacob, G., see Eskin, B. A. 54, *73*
Jacobsohn, D. 17, 20, 52, 54, 57, *78*
— Norgren, A. 51, *78*
— see Ahrén, K. 24, 26, 49, 50, 57, *67*
— see Cowie, A. T. 45, *72*
— see Donovan, B. T. 52, 54, *73*
Jacobsohn, H. J., see Jensen, E. V. 37, *78*
Jakobovits, A. 67, *78*
Jeffers, K. R. 8, *78*
Jellinger, K. 92, 97, 132, 139, *154*
— Seitelberger, F. 92, 97, 102, 108, 129, 132, 143, *154*
— see Seitelberger, F. *158*
Jensen, E. V., Jacobson, H. J. 37, *78*
Jernström, P., Lindberg, A. L., Meland, O. N. 203, *217*
Jervell, K. J., Diniz, C. R., Mueller, G. C. 9, *78*
Jervis, G. A. 98, 100, 142, *154*
Johnson, A. B. 127, 142, 148, *154*
Johnson, B. L., Helwig, E. B. 197, *217*
Johnson, R. E., see Chen, Th. T. 53, *71*
— see Lyons, W. R. 19, 38, 39, 53, *80*
— see Ray, E. W. 44, *84*
Johnson, R. M. *78*
— Meites, J. 40, 49, 50, *78*
Jones, D. B. 60, *78*
Jones, E. L. 209, *217*
Jong, R. de, see Friede, R. L. 97, *152*
Jongh, S. E. de, see Laqueur, E. 16, *79*
Josimovich, J. B., McLaren, J. A. 44, *78*
Junkmann, K. 41, *78*
— Neumann, F. 6, *78*
— see Hamada, H. 6, *76*

Kabat, E., see Newman, W. 166, *218*
Kallenbach, E., see Sarkar, K. 207, *219*
Kamoshita, S., Rapin, I., Suzuki, K., Suzuki, K. 102, 127, 128, 137, 143, 144, 145, 146, *154*
— Reed, G. B., Jr., Aguilar, M. J. 102, 143, *154*
— see Suzuki, K. 144, *159*
Kamraj-Mazurkiewicz, K., see Dambska, M. 134, *151*
Kanoff, A., Aronson, S. M., Volk, B. W. 128, *154*
Kao, V. C. Y., see Archer, F. L. 164, *213*
Kaplan, W. D., see Knudson, A. G., Jr. 104, *155*
Karlsbad, G., see De Petris, S. *214*
Karlson, P. 37, *78*
Karnauchow, P. N. 175, 176, *217*
Karsner, H. T. 64, *78*
Katsoyamis, P. G., see Vigneaud, P. G. du 45, *88*
Katzman, R. 136, 142, *154*
— Aleu, F., Wilson, C. 136, 140, *154*
— see Aleu, F. P. 94, 135, 136, 140, *149*
— see Scheinberg, L. C. 94, *158*
Kaufmann, F., Stiebitz, R. 190, *217*
— see Holzner, J. H. 30, *77*
Kaye, G. I., Cole, J. D., Don, A. 140, *154*
Keasbey, L. E., Hadley, G. G. 194, 205, *217*
— see Finck, F. M. 198, *215*
Keller, M., see Neimeier, R. 66, *82*
Kershaw, G. F., see Hughes, L. E. 135, *154*

Kersting, D. W. 197, *217*
— Helwig, E. B. 194, 197, *217*
Khattab, F. I., see Harreveld, A. van 95, 139, *153*
Kidd, M. 94, 135, *155*
Kikkawa, Y., see Suzuki, K. 95, 136, 147, *159*
King, R. J. B., Gordon, J., Inman, D. R. 37, *78*
— — Cowan, D. M., Inman, D. R. 37, *78*
Kirkham, W. R., Turner, C. W. 7, 10, 24, 27, *78*
Kitchell, R. L., see Weber, A. T. 8, *89*
Klatzo, I. 94, 95, 139, 148, *155*
— Seitelberger, F. 95, *155*
Klaus, S. N., see O'Hara, J. M. 166, 197, *218*
Klebanoff, S., see Ross, R. 13, *85*
Klein, H., Dichgans, J. 92, *155*
Klein, H. J., see Hübner, G. 192, 193, 208, *216*, *217*
— see Kleinsasser, O. 208, *217*
Klein, M., see Mayer, G. 2, *81*
Kleinsasser, O. 184, *217*
— Klein, H. J., Hübner, G. 208, *217*
— see Hübner, G. 192, 193, 208, *216*, *217*
Klubinska, B., see Zarzycki, L. 30, *89*
Knebel, U., see Schlote, W. 94, 137, *158*
Knoop, A., see Bargmann, W. 43, *69*
Knudson, A. G., Jr., Kaplan, W. D. 104, *155*
Kochakian, C. D. 38, *79*
Koelliker, A. 3, *79*
Kolkmann, F.-W., see Rein, H. 94, 137, *157*

Kolkmann, F.-W., see Ule, G. 94, 95, *160*
— see Wegener, K. 136, *160*
Kolkmann, W. 142, *155*
— Ule, G. 94, 135, *155*
— Völzke, E. 102, 114, 137, *155*
Kon, S. K., Cowie, A. T. 2, *79*
Konjetzny, G. E. 64, *79*
Kopf, A. W. 166, *217*
Korey, S. R., Gonatas, J. 128, *155*
Korth, I., see David, H. 190, *214*
Koskinas, G., see Sträussler, E. 92, *159*
Kowalewski, K. P., see Bain, G. O. 190, *213*
Krabbe, K. H., see Christensen, E. 92, *151*
Kracht, J., Hachmeister, M., Breustedt, H.-J., Zimmermann, H.-D. 65, *79*
Kraus, E. J. 66, *79*
Kreibig, W. 203, *217*
Kreutzberg, G., see Carlton, W. W. 136, *151*
Kruger, L., see Maxwell, D. E. 94, *156*
Kueckens, H. 61, *79*
Kunert, J. 17, 64, *79*
Kuru, H. 27, *79*
Kuzma, J. F. 14, 46, *79*, 182, *217*

Labhardt, F., see Neimeier, R. 66, *82*
Labhart, A. 66, *79*
Lahl, R. 133, *155*
Lake, B. D. 129, *155*
Lambret, M., see Gaudier 205, *215*
Lampert, P. W., Earle, K. M., Gibbs, C. J., Jr., Gajdusek, D. C. 94, *155*
— Fox, J., Earle, K. 94, *155*

Lampert, P. W., Schochet, S. S., Jr. 94, 95, 136, 137, 140, 141, *155*
— see Schochet, S. S., Jr. 129, *158*
Landing, B. H. 148
— see Nakai, H. 100, 132, *156*
Lang, F. J., see Gögl, H. 2, *75*
Langer, E., Huhn, S. 14, 48, *79*, 164, *217*
Lani, K. 30, 44, *79*
— Bässler, R. 44, *79*
Laqueur, E., de Jongh, S. E. 16, *79*
Laqueur, G. L. 16, 50, *79*
— Fluhmann, C. F. 50, *79*
Laurence, K. M., Cavanagh, J. B. 92, *155*
Lauritzen, C. 37, *79*
Lawler, H. C., see Vigneaud, V. du 45, *88*
Leathem, J. H., see Reece, R. P. 17, *84*
Le Ball, J. C., see Habib, R. 134, *153*
Le Beau, J., see Foncin, J. F. 152
Leblond 207
Ledeen, R., Salsman, K., Cabrera, M. 144, *155*
Lee, B. J., Pack, G. T., Scharnagel, I. 207, *217*
Lee, J. C., Bakay, L. 94, 135, *155*
— see Bakay, L. 95, 136, *149*
Lees, M. B., Folch-Pi, J. 127, *155*
Leeson, C. G. 167, *217*
Leeson, R. 46, 48, *79*
Leigh, D. 92, 97, 138, *155*
Leninger, A. L. 141, *155*
Lennox, B., Pearse, A. G. E., Richards, H. G. H. 163, *217*
Leonard, S. L. 23, 51, *79*
— Reece, R. P. 17, 19, 50, 51, 53, *79*
— see Reece, R. P. 52, *84*

Leonard, S. L., see Smithcors, J. F. 23, 26, 50, 86
Letterer, E. 58, 79
Leuschner, U. 29, 30, 79
Lever, W. F. 188, 189, 192, 194, 197, 198, 217
— Castleman, B. 198, 217
— Hashimoto, K. 188, 192, 217
— see Hashimoto, K. 164, 197, 216
Levine, H. J., Bergenstal, D. M., Thomas, L. B. 67, 80
Levine, S., see Gonatas, N. K. 94, 153
— see Hirano, A. 94, 95, 96, 136, 139, 143, 147, 153
Levitz, M., see Dancis, J. 134, 151
Lewis, A. A., Gomez, E. T., Turner, C. W. 40, 80
— Turner, C. W. 17, 20, 80
Lewitan, A., see Aronson, S. M. 128, 149
Li, C. H., see Chen, Th. T. 53, 71
— see Lyons, W. R. 19, 38, 39, 53, 80
Liebelt, R. A., see Bardin, C. W. 40, 69
Lieser, H. 17, 23, 80
Lindberg, A. L., see Jernström, P. 203, 217
Ling, C. V. M., Abdel-Latif, A. A. 95, 155
Linneweh, F., Solcher, H. 145, 155
Linzell, J. L. 14, 24, 46, 80, 164, 165, 218
Liot, F., see Meyer, A. 205, 218
Litten, L. 61, 80
Litwer, G. 41, 80
Livingston, S., see Ford, F. R. 131, 152
Löwenstein, C. 181, 218
Long, D. M., Hartmann, J. F., French, L. E. 94, 96, 139, 143, 155

Lores Arnaiz, G. R. de, see De Robertis, E. 94, 95, 137, 151, 152
Lucas, R. B., see Thackeray, A. C. 192, 220
Luchsinger, Y., Centeno, J. 61, 80
Lüers, Th., Spatz, H. 93, 156
Lund, H. J. 188, 194, 218
Luse, S. A., see Bubis, J. J. 150
Lustig, H. 3, 80
Lynn, L. A., see Doyle, L. E. 190, 191, 215
Lyons, W. R. 17, 23, 24, 26, 43, 63, 80
— Catchpole, H. R. 43, 80
— Johnson, R. E., Cole, R. D., Li, C. H. 19, 80
— Li, C. H., Johnson, R. E. 19, 38, 39, 53, 80
— McGinty, D. A. 26, 27, 80
— see Averill, R. L. W. 44, 68
— see Catchpole, H. R. 43, 71
— see Chen, Th. T. 53, 71
— see Cowie, A. T. 39, 72
— see Daane, Th. A. 19, 23, 24, 72
— see Ray, E. W. 44, 84
— see Scharf, G. 20, 26, 27, 85

Maccagnani, F., see Bignami, A. 137, 150
Mac Gregor, J. W., see Bain, G. O. 190, 213
Mackenzie, D. H. 187, 205, 218
Maeda, R. 171, 218
Maeder, L. M. A. 8, 80
Magee, P. N., Stoner, H. B., Barnes, J. M. 136, 156
Mahesh, V. B., Dalla Pria, S., Greenblatt, R. B. 66, 80

Malamud, N. 133, 145, 156
— see Gerstl, B. 134, 144, 145, 146, 153
Malpress, F. H., see Cowie, A. T. 21, 26, 72
Mandell, S., see Scheinberg, L. C. 140, 158
Marin, O., Vial, J. D. 94, 135, 156
Marinacci, F., see Bignami, A. 131, 150
Marshall, J. R., see Wider, J. A. 66, 89
Martin, J. J., Bogaert, L. van, Guazzi, G. C. 134, 156
— see Gaburro, D. 102, 152
Martin, K., see Diezel, P. B. 134, 152
Marti, R. J., see Baldwin, R. L. 8, 69
Marx, A., see Tannenbaum, M. 166, 220
Masshoff, W. 61, 80
Masson, P. 170, 182, 183, 210, 218
Masson, Peyron 163, 192, 218
Matuschka, M. 161
Maxwell, D. E., Kruger, L. 94, 156
May, W. W. 135, 156
Mayer, G., Klein, M. 2, 81
— see Canivenc, R. 44, 71
Mayer, I. 188, 197, 218
McAdams, A. J., see Passarge, E. 134, 157
McAfee, D., see Austin, J. 129, 149
McCullagh, E., Alivisatos, J. G., Schaffenburg, C. A. 66, 81
McDivitt, R. W., see Berg, J. W. 205, 213
McDonald, G. J., Reece, R. P. 17, 24, 27, 81
McEuen, C. S. 81
— Selye, H., Collip, J. B. 17, 50, 51, 81

McEuen, C. S., see Noble, R. L. *83*
— see Selye, H. 51, *86*
McFarlane, A., see Robb, P. M. 203, *219*
McGinty, D. A., see Lyons, W. R. 26, 27, *80*
McIlwain, H. 140, *156*
McLaren, J. A., see Josimovich, J. B. 44, *78*
McLean, P., see Glock, G. E. 8, 31, *75*
McNaught, M. L., see Folley, S. J. 30, *74*
Meier-Ruge, W. 30, *81*
Meites, J. 17, 19, 21, 24, 39, 53, *81*
— Sgouris, J. T. 44, *81*
— Turner, C. W. 43, *81*
— see Johnson, R. M. 40, 49, 50, *78*
— see Nicoll, C. S. 54, *83*
— see Reinecke, E. P. 21, *84*
— see Talwalker, P. K. 39, 41, 50, *87*
Meland, O. N., see Jernström, P. 203, *217*
Melcher, G. W., see Frantz, V. K. 64, *75*
Mellmann, W. J., see Gambetti, P. 94, 102, 124, 126, 141, 143, 148, *152*
Melnick, P. J. 187, *218*
Menkes, J. H. 133, 134, 144, 145, *156*
— Phillippart, H., Fiol, R. E. 134, 146, *156*
Menozzi, C., Scarlato, G. 135, *156*
Merckel, C. G., see Nelson, W. O. 51, *83*
Merker, H. J., see Busch, W. 13, *71*, 208, *214*
Merz, W. 63, *81*
Mescon, H., see Shelley, H. B. 166, *219*
Meyer, A., Delarue, J., Peuteuil, G., Liot, F. 205, *218*

Meyer, A. T., see Welsh, R. A. 191, *220*
Meyer, H. 51, *81*
Meyer, J. E. 100, 138, 139, *156*
Meyer, W. 67
Mixner, J. P. *81*
— Turner, C. W. 20, 21, 23, 24, 27, 40, 54, *81*
— see Reece, R. P. 51, *84*
Möbius, G., Nizze, H. 64, *82*
Monroe, R. G., see Clark, B. G. 66, *71*
Montagna, W., see Noback, C. R. 166, *218*
Moon, R. C. 10, 54, *82*
— Griffith, D. R., Turner, C. W. 10, 24, *82*
— Turner, C. W. 17, 53, *82*
Moore, Brady 140
Morcaldi, L., Salvati, G., Giordano, G. G., Guazzi, G. C. 102, *156*
Morgan, W. Z., Castleman, B. 181, *218*
Morse, W. I. 130, *156*
Moser, H. W., see Prensky, A. L. 133, 134, 145, 146, *157*
Mosimann, W. 8, 56, *82*
Mossakowski, M. J. 133, *156*
Mostafi, F. K., see Suzuki, T. 141, *159*
Mottet, N. K., see Goldenberg, V. E. 64, *75*
Mu, J. W., see Frazier, C. N. 20, *75*
Mühlbrock, O. 20, *82*
Mueller, G. C., see Jervell, K. J. 9, *78*
Müller, H. B. 167, *218*
Müllerheim, R. 64, *82*
Mugnaini, E., Walberg, F. 141, *156*
Mullan, S., see Raimondi, A. J. 139, *157*

Munford, R. E. 10, 30, 49, *82*
— see Flux, D. S. 7, 40, *74*
Munger, B. L. 48, *82*
Munson, P. L. 55, *82*
Murad, T. M., Haam, E. v. 48, *82*, 166, 183, 208, *218*
— Scarpelli, D. G. 208, *218*
— see Crocker, D. J. 200, *214*
Mylius, E. A. 48, *82*, 190, 192, 205, 208, *218*

Nakai, H., Landing, B. H., Schubert, W. K. 100, 132, *156*
Nandi, S. 7, 37, 39, 43, *82*
— see Wellings, S. R. 37, *89*
Nangle, E. J., Symmers, W. St. C. 192, *218*
Nara, S., Yasunor, K. T. 141, *156*
Neame, K. D. 145, *156*
Needham, D. M., Shoenberg, C. F. 48, *82*
Negri, L., Ferrante, R. 190, *218*
Neimeier, R., Hauser, G. A., Keller, M., Labhardt, F., Wenner, R., Stampfli, V. 66, *82*
Nelson, E., Aurebeck, G. 102, 124, *156*
Nelson, R. G., see Hashimoto, K. 164, 197, *216*
Nelson, W. O. 20, 23, 24, 39, *82*
— Heytler, P. G., Ciacco, E. I. 10, *83*
— Merckel, C. G. 51, *83*
Netsky, M. G., see Dreifuss, F. E. 92, *152*
Neuberger, K. T., see Greenhouse, A. H. 92, *153*
Neumann, F., Elger, W. 5, 6, *83*

Neumann, F., Elger, W., Berswordt-Walrabe, R. von 7, *83*
— see Elger, W. 5, 6, *73*
— see Hamada, H. 6, *76*
— see Junkmann, K. 6, *78*
Neumann, H. O., Oing, M. 3, *83*
Newman, W. 60, *83*
— Feigin, I., Wolf, A., Kabat, E. 166, *218*
Nguyen-Duong, H., see Schlote, W. 94, 137, *158*
Nicolette, J. A., see Gorski, J. 38, *76*
Nicoll, C. S. 8, *83*
— Meites, J. 54, *83*
— see Talwalker, P. K. 50, *87*
Nikolowski, W. N., see Feyrter, F. *215*
Nizze, H., see Möbius, G. 64, *82*
Noback, C. R., Montagna, W. 166, *218*
Noble, R. L., McEuen, C. S., Collip, J. B. *83*
Noel, P. R., see Palmer, A. C. 136, *157*
Noetzel, H., see Sander, C. 134, *158*
Nordmann, M. 64, *83*
Norgren, A. 20, 24, 26, *83*
— see Bengtsson, B. 53, *69*
— see Jacobsohn, D. 51, *78*
Norton, W. R., Poduslo, S. E., Suzuki, K. 144, *156*
Norton, W. T., see Suzuki, K. 144, *159*
Noteboom, W. D., see Gorski, J. 38, *76*
Nyirjesy, I. 66, *83*

O'Brien, J. S. 144, *157*
— Sampson, E. L. 146, *157*
Oesterreich, R., Slawyk 66, *83*

O'Hara, J. M., Bensch, K., Ioannides, G., Klaus, S. N. 166, 197, *218*
Oing, M., see Neumann, H. O. 3, *83*
O'Leary, J. L., Harris, A. B., Fox, R. R., Smith, J. M., Tidwell, M. 94, *157*
Olivi, M., Barbieri, G. 27, *83*
Olsson, Y., see Sourander, P. 129, *159*
Omar, M., see Archer, F. 174, 185, *213*
Oota, K., Takahashi, N. 191, *218*
Orrenius, S., see Helminen, H. J. 30, *77*
Ouchterlony 45
Overzier, C. 64, *83*
Ozzello, L., Speer, F. D. 29, 63, *83*

Pack, G. T., see Lee, B. J. 207, *217*
Paek, S. 30, 32, *83*
— see Bässler, R. 14, 30, 46, *68*, 165, *213*
Palladini, G., see Bignami, A. 136, 137, *150*
Palmer, A. C., Noel, P. R. 136, *157*
Pandolfi, S., see Clasen, R. A. 136, 137, *151*
Panopio, I. T., see Doyle, L. E. 190, 191, *215*
Pant, S. S., Ashbury, A. K., Richardson, E. P., Jr. 94, *157*
Pare, C. M. B., see Crome, L. *151*
Passarge, E., McAdams, A. J. 134, *157*
Pearse, A. G. E., see Lennox, B. 163, *217*
Pease, D. C., see Scott, B. L. 163, 165, *219*
Peiffer, J. 131, *157*
— Solcher, H. 133, 134, *157*

Peiffer, J., see Schmidt, G. W. 134, *158*
Pena, C. E., see Feigin, I. 102, 134, 138, *152*
Percy, A. K., Brady, R. O. 129, *157*
Perez-Tamayo, R., see Ihnen, M. 27, *77*
Pernis, B., see De Petris, S. *214*
Perrini, F. 30, *83*
Peryt, A., see Zarzycki, L. 30, *89*
Peters, A. 136, *157*
Peters, G. 148
Petsche, H., Seitelberger, F. 136, *157*
Peuteuil, G., see Meyer, A. 205, *218*
Peyron, A., Corsy, F., Surmont, J. 187, 190, *219*
Pfeiffer, E. F., see Sandritter, W. 9, *85*
Philipp, E. 63, *83*
Phillippart, H., see Menkes, J. H. 134, 146, *156*
Philp, J. R., see Wellings, S. R. 37, *89*
Pickren, J. W., see Frantz, V. K. 64, *75*
Pilz, H. 146, *157*
Pirilä, V., Eränkö, O. 166, *219*
Poduslo, J. F., see Suzuki, K. 144, *159*
Poduslo, S. E., see Norton, W. R. 144, *156*
— see Suzuki, K. 144, *159*
Popenoe, E. A., see Vigneaud, V. du 45, *88*
Porta, E. A., see Hartroft, W. S. 171, *216*
Poser, C. M., Bogaert, L. van 133, 145, *157*
Postnov, Yu. V. 194, *219*
Prensky, A. L., Carr, S., Moser, H. W. 133, 134, 145, 146, *157*

Prensky, A. L., Moser, H. W. 134, 145, *157*
Price, D., Williams-Ashman, H. G. 44, *83*
Propst, A. 194, *219*
Pryles, C. V., see Ford, F. R. 131, *152*
Puchtler 207
Puletti, F., see Zu Rhein, G. M. 100, 138, 147, *160*

Quinn, D. J., see Samson, F. E., Jr. 95, *158*
Quintarelli, G., Robinson, L. 190, *219*

Rabiner, A. M., see Aronson, S. M. 128, *149*
Raimondi, A. J., Evans, J. P., Mullan, S. 139, *157*
Ramahi, H., see Abdel-Latif, A. A. 95, *148*
Ransohoff, J., see Aleu, F. 94, 96, 139, 143, *149*
Rapin, I., Suzuki, K., Suzuki, K. *157*
— see Kamoshita, S. 102, 127, 128, 137, 143, 144, 145, 146, *154*
Rapoport, S. M. 8, *83*
Ratzenhofer, M. 27, *83*
— Schauenstein, E. 27, 29, *83, 84*
Rausch, E. O., see Astwood, E. B. 17, 23, 51, *68*
Ray, E. W., Averill, S. C., Lyons, W. R., Johnson, R. E. 44, *84*
— see Averill, E. L. W. 44, *68*
Raynaud, A. 4, 5, 6, *84*
— Frilley, M. 5, *84*
— Raynaud, J. 5, 6, *84*
Raynaud, J., see Habib, R. 134, *153*
— see Raynaud, A. 5, 6, *84*
Reece, R. P., Leathem, J. H. 17, *84*

Reece, R. P., Leonard, S. L. 52, *84*
— Mixner, J. P. 51, *84*
— see Leonard, S. L. 17, 19, 50, 51, 53, *79*
— see McDonald, G. J. 17, 24, 27, *81*
— see Tucker, H. A. 10, *88*
Reed, G. B., Jr., see Kamoshita, S., 102, 143, *154*
Regan, W. M., see Catchpole, H. R. 43, *71*
Rein, G. 3, *84*
Rein, H., Kolkmann, F.-W., Sil, R., Ule, G. 94, 137, *157*
— see Wegener, K. 136, *160*
Reinecke, E. P., Meites, J., Cairy, C. F., Huffman, D. F. 21, *84*
Ressler, C., see Vigneaud, P. G. du 45, *88*
Rett, A. 134, 148, *157*
Reulen, H. J., Baethmann, A. 95, *157*
Ribadeau-Dumas, J. L., Escourolle, R., Castaigne, P. 135, *157*
Richards, H. G. H., see Lennox, B. 163, *217*
Richardson, E. P. 98
Richardson, E. P., Jr., see Hogan, G. R. 100, 102, *154*
— see Pant, S. S. 94, *157*
Richardson, K. C. 7, 14, 46, *85*
— see Cowie, A. T. 21, 26, 45, *72*
Richardson, K. G. 163, 164, 165, *219*
Richterich, B., see Smith, Th. C. 20, 24, *86*
Riddle, O. 44, 45, *85*
— Bates, R. W., Dykshorn, S. W. 41, *85*
— Braucher, P. F. 41, *85*
Riedel, G. 63, *85*
Roback, H. M., Scherer, H. J. 142, *158*

Robb, P. M., McFarlane, A. 203, *219*
Robertis, E. de, see Albers, R. W. 95, *149*
— see De Robertis, E. *151*
Roberts, C. W., see Vigneaud, P. G. du 45, *88*
Roberts, P., see Wellings, S. R. 208, *220*
Robertson, D. M., Wasan, S. M., Skinner, D. B. 94, *158*
Robertson, J., see Blackwood, W. 92, *150*
Robertson, J. T., see Banker, B. Q. 100, 104, 143, *149*
Robin, A., see Brucher, J. M. 102, 108, 132, 143, *150*
Robinson, L., see Quintarelli, G. 190, *219*
Robinson, N. 97, *158*
Rodriguez de Lores Arnaiz, G., Alverici, M., De Robertis, E. 95, *158*
— see Albers, R. W. 95, *149*
Rosen, S. W., Gahres, E. E. 67, *85*
Rosenburg, A. 61, *85*
Ross, C. F., see Crome, L. 133, 134, *151*
Ross, G. T., see Wider, J. A. 66, *89*
Ross, R., Klebanoff, S. 13, *85*
Rottino, A., Howley, C. P. 203, *219*
Rowlatt, C., Franks, L. M. 163, *219*
Rozin, S., see Zondek, B. *89*
Ruppert, H. L., see Turner, C. W. 26, *88*
Rushton, D. I. 134, 145, *158*
Russell, J., see Clasen, R. A. 136, 137, *151*

Saameli, K. 46, *85*
Saar, v. G. 173, 174, *219*

Sacks, O., Brown, W. J., Aguilar, M. J. 102, 114, 128, 147, *158*
Salsman, K., see Ledeen, R. 144, *155*
Salter, J., Best, C. H. 57, *85*
Salvati, G., see Morcaldi, L. 102, *156*
Samaha, F. J. 95, *158*
Samoilov, W. J., see Suetina, J. A. 37, *87*
Sampson, E. L., see O'Brien, J. S. 146, *157*
Samson, F. E., Jr., Quinn, D. J. 95, *158*
Samuels, S., see Aleu, F. 94, 96, 139, 143, *149*
Sandbank, U., see Bechar, M. 133, *150*
Sander, C., Clotten, R., Noetzel, H., Wehinger, H. 134, *158*
Sandritter, W., Federlin, K., Pfeiffer, E. F. 9, *85*
Santesson, L., see Caspersson, T. 166, 208, *214*
Santler, R., Eberhartinger, C. 205, *219*
Sarkar, K., Kallenbach, E. 207, *219*
Sastry, P. S., Stancer, H. C. 129, *158*
Sautter, I. H., see Weber, A. T. 8, *89*
Scarlato, G., see Menozzi, C. 135, *156*
Scarpa, P., see Gaburro, D. 102, *152*
Scarpelli, D. G., see Murad, T. M. 208, *218*
Schachner, S. H. 67, *85*
Schade, S. L., see Spellacy, W. N. 66, *86*
Schäfer, A., Bässler, R. 85, 208, *219*
— see Bässler, R. 12, 13, 14, 21, 46, 64, 68, 165, 166, 176, *213*
Schaefer, H. E., Fischer, R. 32, *85*
— see Fischer, R. 32, *74*

Schaffenburg, C. A., see McCullagh, E. 66, *81*
Schairer, E. 8, *85*
Schaltenbrand, G. 66, *85*
Scharf, G., Lyons, W. R. 20, 26, 27, *85*
Scharnagel, I., see Lee, B. J. 207, *217*
Schauenstein, E., see Ratzenhofer, M. 27, 29, *83*, *84*
Scheinberg, L. C., Herzog, I., Taylor, J. M., Katzman, R. 94, *158*
— Taylor, J. M., Herzog, I., Mandell, S. 140, *158*
Scher, W., see Segal, S. J. 38, *86*
Scherer, H. J., see Roback, H. M. 142, *158*
Schimmelbusch, C. 64, *85*
Schipp, R. 13, *85*
Schlote, W., Betz, E., Knebel, U., Nguyen-Duong, H. 94, 137, *158*
Schmidt, G. W., Benecke, G., Peiffer, J. 134, *158*
Schmidt, Hugo 3, *85*
Schmitt, Heinrich 3, *85*
Schneck, L., see Adachi, M. 94, 102, 111, 125, 127, 142, 143, *149*
Schnurbusch, F. 64, *85*
Schochet, S. S., Jr., Lampert, P. W., Earle, K. M. 129, *158*
— see Lampert, P. W. 94, 95, 136, 137, 140, 141, *155*
Scholz, W. 145, *158*
Schriever, D. 63, *85*
— see Bässler, R. 29, *69*
Schröder, J. M., Wechsler, W. 94, 95, 96, 139, 143, *158*
Schubert, W. K., see Nakai, H. 100, 132, *156*
Schultz, A. 2, 11, 27, *85*, 173, 174, *219*

Schulze, G. 29, *86*
— see Bässler, R. 29, *69*
Schwinn, C. P., see Finck, F. M. 198, *215*
Scofield, H. H., see Gerughty, R. M. 199, *216*
Scott, B. L., Pease, D. C. 163, 165, *219*
Segal, S. J., Scher, W. 38, *86*
Seifert, G. 61, *86*
— Geiler, G. 181, *219*
Seitelberger, F. 93, 94, 97, 100, 108, 129, 131, 132, *158*
— Jellinger, K. *158*
— Weingarten, K. *159*
— see Jellinger, K. 92, 97, 102, 108, 129, 132, 143, *154*
— see Klatzo, I. 95, *155*
— see Petsche, H. 136, *157*
— see Sluga, E. 94, 135, *159*
Sellinger, O. Z., see De Robertis, E. 94, 137, *152*
Selye, H. 23, 40, 48, 49, *86*
— Browne, J. S. L., Collip, J. B. 23, *86*
— McEuen, C. S., Collip, J. B. 51, *86*
— see McEuen, C. S. 17, 50, 51, *81*
Semb, C. 64, *86*
Sgouris, J. T., see Meites, J. 44, *81*
Shapiro, S., see Clark, B. G. 66, *71*
Shaw, I. G., Winkler, C. E., Terlecki, S. 135, *159*
— see Hughes, L. E. 135, *154*
Shear, M. 167, *219*
Shearer, L., see Austin, J. 129, *149*
Sheldon, W. H. 190, 197, 198, *219*
Shelley, H. B., Mescon, H. 166, *219*

Shelley, W. B., see Hurley, H. J. 165, *217*
Shipley, R. A., see Dorfman, R. I. 53, *73*
Shoenberg, C. F., see Needham, D. M. 48, *82*
Short, R. H. D. 7, *86*
Sil, R., see Rein, H. 94, 137, *157*
Silver, I. A. 30, 46, *86*, 163, 167, *219*
Silverman, J., Dancis, J., Feigin, I. 134, *159*
Simard, L. C. 192, *219*
Skinner, D. B., see Robertson, D. M. 94, *158*
Skorpil, F. 168, 169, 181, *219*
Skou, J. C. 95, 142, *159*
Slater, T. F. 10
— see Greenbaum, A. L. 10, *76*
Slawyk, see Oesterreich, R. 66, *83*
Sluga, E. 94, 135, 140, *159*
— Seitelberger, F. 94, 135, *159*
— Tomonaga, M. 140, *159*
Smirnova, J. O., see Suetina, J. A. 37, *87*
Smith, A. D., see Azzopardi, J. G. 190, 191, 193, *213*
Smith, G. M., see Gardner, W. U. 19, *75*
Smith, J. M., see O'Leary, J. L. 94, *157*
Smith, Th. C. 17, 23, 24, 27, 57, *86*
— Braverman, L. B. 19, 50, *86*
— Richterich, B. 20, 24, *86*
Smithcors, J. F., Leonard, S. L. 23, 26, 50, *86*
Soemarwoto, J. N., Bern, H. A. 26, *86*
Solcher, H., see Linneweh, F. 145, *155*

Solcher, H., see Peiffer, J. 133, 134, *157*
Sourander, P., Olsson, Y. 129, *159*
Spatz, H., see Lüers, Th. 93, *156*
Speer, F. D., see Ozzello, L. 29, 63, *83*
Speert, H. 21, *86*
— sec Geschickter, C. F. 20, *75*
Spellacy, W. N., Carlson, K. L., Schade, S. L. 66, *86*
Spielmeyer, W. 92, 94, *159*
Spuler, A. 3, 4, *86*
Stadler, H. 133, *159*
Ställberg-Stenhagen, S., Svennerholm, L. 144, *159*
Stampfli, V., see Neimeier, R. 66, *82*
Stancer, H. C., see Sastry, P. S. 129, *158*
Stein, O., Stein, Y. 37, *86*
Stein, Y., see Stein, O. 37, *86*
Steinbeck, H. 2, 57, *86*
Stevenson, L. D., see Alvord, E. C., Jr., 133, 145, *149*
Stewart, F. W. 182, 199, 200, *219*
— see Foote, F. W. 59, 60, 63, *74*, 199, 200, *215*
Stiebitz, R., see Kaufmann, F. 190, *217*
Stillians, A. W. 192, *220*
Stöcker, E. 9, *87*
Stoner, H. B., see Magee, P. N. 136, *156*
Sträussler, E., Koskinas, G. 92, *159*
Strauss, I., see Globus, J. H. 98, *153*
Stricker, P. *87*
— Grueter, F. 40, 41, *87*
Strong, L. C., see Gardner, W. U. 7, 19, *75*
Stuart, D., see Clasen, R. A. 136, 137, *151*

Suchenwirth, R., Bues, F. 66, *87*
Suetina, J. A., Chentsov, S., Chentsov, Y., Smirnova, J. O., Samoilov, W. J. 37, *87*
Surmont, J., see Peyron, A. 187, 190, *219*
Suzuki, K. 123, *159*
— Chen, G. C. 144, *159*
— Kikkawa, Y. 95, 136, 147, *159*
— Poduslo, J. F., Poduslo, S. E. 144, *159*
— Poduslo, S. E., Norton, W. T. 144, *159*
— Suzuki, K., Kamoshita, S. 144, *159*
— see Kamoshita, S. 102, 127, 128, 137, 143, 144, 145, 146, *154*
— see Norton, W. R. 144, *156*
— see Rapin, I. *157*
Suzuki, T., Mostafi, F. K. 141, *159*
Svennerholm, L., see Ställberg-Stenhagen, S. 144, *159*
Swan, J. M., see Vigneaud, P. G. du 45, *88*
Swedlow, M., see Humphrey, L. J. 54, *77*
Sykes, J. F. *87*
— Wrenn, T. R. 21, 26, 40, *87*
Sylven, B. 27, *87*
Symmers, W. St. C., see Nangle, E. J. 192, *218*
Szelozynska, K., see Damska, M. 134, *151*

Takahashi, N. 14, 48, *87*
— see Oota, K. 191, *218*
Talmage, R. V., see Garrett, F. A. 20, *75*
Talwalker, P. K. *87*
— Meites, J. 39, 41, 50, *87*
— Nicoll, C. S., Meites, J. 50, *87*
Tamarin, A. 48, *87*, 165, *220*

Tandler, B. 48, *87*, 164, 166, *220*
Tani, E., Ametani, T., Handa, H. 95, 140, *159*
Tannenbaum, M., Weiss, M., Marx, A. 166, *220*
Tariska, S. 100, *159*
Taylor, H. C. 61, 64, *87*
— Waltman, C. 65, *87*
Taylor, J. M., see Scheinberg, L. C. 94, 140, *158*
Terlecki, S., see Shaw, I. G. 135, *159*
Terry, R. D., see Gonatas, N. K. *94*, 135, 139, *153*
Terry, R. T., see Aleu, F. P. *94*, 135, 136, 140, *149*
Terzakis, I. A. 48, *87*
Thackeray, A. C., Lucas, R. B. 192, *220*
Thölen, H. 3, 4, *87*
Thaenes, W. 34, *87*
Thomas, L. B., see Levine, H. J. 67, *80*
Tidwell, M., see O'Leary, J. L. 94, *157*
Tillingen, K. G., see Diczfalusy, E. 63, *73*
Tindal, J. S., see Benson, G. K. 21, 24, 44, 49, 57, *69*
— see Cowie, A. T. 26, *72*
Tingey, A. H., see Bignami, A. 131, *150*
Toker, C., see Deppisch, L. M. 191, *215*
Tomonaga, M., see Sluga, E. 140, *159*
Torack, R. M. 94, 95, 135, 140, *160*
— Barrnett, R. J. 95, *160*
— Dufty, M. L., Gordon, J. S. 95, *160*
Traurig, H. 9, 10, 11, *88*
Trentin, J. J. *88*
— Turner, C. W. 17, 19, 23, 24, *88*

Treves, N. 64, *88*
Tucker, H. A. *88*
— Reece, R. P. 10, *88*
Tucker, S. M., see Blackwood, W. 92, *150*
Turner, C. W. 2, *88*
— Gomez, E. T. 20, *88*
— Yamamoto, H., Ruppert, H. L. 26, *88*
— see Anderson, R. R. 24, *67*
— see Berswordt-Wallrabe, R. v. 26, 56, *70*
— see Damm, H. C. 40, *72*
— see Djojosoebagio, S. 56, *73*
— see Gardner, W. U. 43, *75*
— see Gomez, E. T. 40, 54, *75*
— see Griffith, D. R. 10, 53, *76*
— see Grosvenor, C. E. 49, *76*
— see Hancock, J. 26, *77*
— see Kirkham, W. R. 7, 10, 24, 27, *78*
— see Lewis, A. A. 17, 20, 40, *80*
— see Meites, J. 43, *81*
— see Mixner, J. P. 20, 21, 23, 24, 27, 40, 54, *81*
— see Moon, R. C. 10, 17, 24, 53, *82*
— see Trentin, J. J. 17, 19, 23, 24, *88*
— see Yamamoto, H. 26, 27, *89*
Tymms, V., see Crome, L. 133, 145, *151*

Ule, G. 94, 95, 97, 102, 126, 136, 137, 148, *160*
— Kolkmann, F. W. 94, 95, *160*
— see Kolkmann, W. 94, 135, *155*
— see Rein, H. 94, 137, *157*

Urban, J. A., Adair, F. E. 59, *88*

Valcke, R., see Hooft, C. *154*
Van Bogaert, L., see Bogaert, L. van 91, 98, 100, 104, 128, *150*
Van der Hoeven, E., see Waugh, D. 165, 208, *220*
Van Wagenen, G., see Duran-Reynals, F. *73*
Verhaart, W. J. C. 100, *160*
Verley, J. M., Hollmann, K. H. 37, *88*
Vernandakis, A., Woodbury, D. M. 95, *160*
Verne, J. 30, *88*
Veronesi, U., Candiani, M. A. 27, *88*
Vial, J. D., see Marin, O. 94, 135, *156*
Victor, M., Adams, R. D., Cole, M. 133, *160*
— see Banker, B. Q. 100, 104, 143, *149*
Vigneaud, P. G. du, Ressler, C., Swan, J. M., Roberts, C. W., Katsoyamis, P. G., Gordon, S. 45, *88*
Vigneaud, V. du, Lawler, H. C., Popenoe, E. A. 45, *88*
Villani, G., Zanella, E. 63, *88*
Visscher, M. B., see Ferguson, D. J., 20, 53, *73*
Vitry, G. 29, 63, *88*
Völzke, E., see Kolkmann, W. 102, 114, 137, *155*
Vogel, St., see Alvord, E. C., Jr. 133, 145, *149*
Vogler, E. *88*, *88*
Volk, B. W., see Adachi, M. 94, 102, 111, 125, 127, 129, 142, 143, 148, *149*

Volk, B. W., see Aronson, S. M. 104, 128, *149*
— see Kanoff, A. 128, *154*
Volkmann, H. 45, *88*
Volpone, S., see Gaburro, D. 102, *152*
Voss, H. E. 44, *88*

Wagenen, G. van, Folley, S. J. 53, *89*
— see Duran-Reynals, F. 29, 63, *73*
Waisman, H. A., see Chou, S. M. 133, *151*
Walberg, F., see Mugnaini, E, 141, *156*
Wald, F., see Zadunaisky, J. A. 95, *160*
Walker, J. M., see Chaudhury, R. R. 46, *71*
Walker, R. J., see Banerjee M. R. 9, *69*
Wallace, B. J., see Adachi, M. 94, 102, 111, 125, 127, 142, 143, *149*
Walter, S. 67
Waltman, C. A., see Taylor, H. C. 65, *87*
Wasan, S. M., see Robertson, D. M. 94, *158*
Wattenwyl, H. v. 17, *89*
Watzka, M. 45, *89*
Waugh, D., Hoeven, E. van der 13, *89*, 165, 208, *220*
Weber, A. T., Kitchell, R. L., Sautter, I. H. 8, *89*
Weber, H. W. 175, *220*
Weber, W. 42, *89*
Wechsler, W., see Schröder, J. M. 94, 95, 96, 139, 143, *158*
Wegener, K., Kolkmann, F. W., Rein, H. 136, *160*
Wehinger, H., see Sander, C. 134, *158*
Weichert, C. K., Boyd, R. W., Cohen, R. S. 16, *89*

Weingarten, K., see Seitelberger, F. *159*
Weinmann, J. P., see Bhaskar, S. N. 190, 194, 197, *214*
Weiss, M., see Gonatas, N. K. 94, 135, 139, *153*
— see Tannenbaum, M. 166, *220*
Weiss, P. 164, 175, 181, *220*
Wellings, S. R., Nandi, S. 37, *89*
— Philp, J. R. 37, *89*
— Roberts, P. 208, *220*
Welsh, R. A., Meyer, A. T. 191, *220*
Wenner, R. *89*
— see Neimeier, R. 66, *82*
Werner, K. H. 17, 24, *89*
Wersäll, J., see Eneroth, C. M. 191, *215*
Westall, R. G., see Dancis, J. 134, *151*
Westman, A., see Diczfalusy, E. 63, *73*
White, A., see Gardner, W. U. 20, *75*
White, W. D., see Browning, H. C. 41, 70, *71*
Whittam, R., Blond, D. 142, *160*
Whyte, H. M., see Calov, W. L. 64, *71*
Wider, J. A., Marshall, J. R., Ross, G. T. 66, *89*
Wiedemann, H.-R., see Henn, R. 102, *153*
Wiegenstein, L., see Goldenberg, V. E. 64, *75*
Wiener, Z., see Wolman, M. 140, *160*
Williams-Ashman, H. G. 38, *89*
— see Price, D. 44, *83*
Willis, R. A. 189, *220*
Wilson, C., see Katzman, R. 136, 140, *154*

Winkelmann, R. K., Wolff, K. 194, 196, *220*
Winkler, C. E., see Shaw, I. G. 135, *159*
Wislocki, B., see Bunting, H. 166, *214*
Wislocki, G. B., see Dempsey, E. W. 27, 30, 46, 73, 164, 165, 166, 167, *214*
Wolf, A., see Newman, W. 166, *218*
Wolff, E., see Girardie, J. 30, *75*
Wolff, K., see Winkelmann, R. K. 194, 196, *220*
Wolman, M. 100, 138, 143, *160*
— Wiener, H. 140, *160*
Womack, N. A., see Hemplemann, L. H. 190, *216*
Woodbury, D. M., see Vernandakis, A. 95, *160*
Woolf, L. I., see Crome, L. 133, 145, *151*
Wrenn, T. R., see Sykes, J. F. 21, 26, 40, *87*
Wyk, J. J. v., Grumbach, M. M. *89*

Yamamoto, H., Turner, C. W. 26, 27, *89*
— see Turner, C. W. 26, *88*
Yanagihara, T., Cumings, J. N. 144, *160*
— see Cumings, J. N. 134, 145, 146, *151*
Yardley, J. H., see Gonzales-Licea, A. 203, *216*
Yasunor, K. T., see Nara, S. 141, *156*
Yokoyama, A., see Cowie, A. T. 26, *72*
Young, F. G., see Folley, S. J. 43, *74*
Young, S., see Hadfield, D, 39, *76*

Zadunaisky, J. A., Wald, F., De Robertis, E. D. P. 95, *160*
Zak, K., see Zarzycki, L. 30, *89*
Zaks, M. G. 46, *89*
Zanella, E., see Villani, G. 63, *88*
Zappella, M., see Bignami, A. 131, *150*
Zarzycki, L., Peryt, A., Klubinska, B., Hjac, T., Zak, K. 30, *89*

Zelman, I. B., Czochanska-Kruk, J., Borowicz, K. 133, *160*
Ziehl-Nielson 170
Ziehrer, L. M., see De Robertis, E. 94, 137, *152*
Zimmerman, H. M., see Gonatas, N. K. 94, *153*
— see Hirano, A. 94, 95, 96, 136, 139, 143, 147, *153*

Zimmermann, H.-D., see Kracht, J. 65, *79*
Zimmermann, K. W. 163, *220*
Zondek, B., Bromberg, Y. M., Rozin, S. *89*
Zuckerman, S., see Folley, S. J. 7, 20, 53, *74*
Zu Rhein, G. M., Eickman, P. L., Puletti, F. 100, 138, 147, *160*

Subject Index

The numbers set in italics refer to those pages on which the respective catch-word is discussed in detail

A-cells   12, 13, 14, 16, 178, 208
acetylcholine   19
— activity in SDI   110
acid mucopolysaccharides in connective tissue of the mammary gland   29
— phosphatase   30
acidophil cells of adenohypophysis   65
acidosis, respiratory   94
acromegaly   64, 66
acrospiroma, eccrine   197
ACTH   20, *39*, 57
active transport of ions   95
adenine   9
adenohypophysis   *40*, 45
—, acidophil cells, in Akumada-del Castillo syndrome   65
adenocarcinoma of the salivary glands   208
adenofibroma   187
adenofibromyoma   187
adenoid cystic carcinoma (cylindroma)   24, 189, *192*, 199
adenoma, glycogen-rich, reticulated (Feyrter)   197, 198
—, intracanalicular   64
—, pleomorphic   190
—, solid (Feyrter)   190, 198
—, tubular-solid (Feyrter)   190, 198
— of mammary gland   188
— of the nipple   187
adenomatous intralobular proliferation of epithelium   60
adenomyoepithelioma   194, 197
adeno-myothelioma   24, 189, 190, *194*
—, malignant   203
adenosintriphosphatase see ATP-ase
adenosis   59, 60, *64*
—, fibrosing   *182*, 211
—, sclerosing   59, *175*, 183
—, papillary, of the lobules   60
—, —, of the tubular system   60
adrenal cortex, hormones   *49*
adrenalectomy   16, 19, 38, 39, 49, 51

Ahumada-del Castillo syndrome   65
β-alaninemia   133
aldolase in SDI   110
Alexander's disease   129
alkaline phosphatase   14, 30, 31, 32, 33, 45, 46, 47, 166, 190
Alper's disease   92, 131, 133
Alzheimer type I cells   117, 133, 136
— type II cells   117, 125, 130, 131, 133, 141, 142, 143
amastia   5
amaurotic idiocy   93
—, Spielmeyer-Vogt variant   130
amenorrhoea   65
amino acid metabolism, inborn errors   132, *133*
androgens   5, 38, 44, 53
—, lack of   5
androgenic effect   5
angiosarcoma of the pituitary   66
anoxic parenchymal necrosis   93
anti-androgens   *6*
Anti-STH-serum   45
argyrophilia of myothelia   164
asphyxia   139
astroglial reactions in SDI   *141*
AT 10 (dihydrotachysterol)   *54*, 56
athelia   5, 6
ATP-ase   30, 190
—, activity   141, 142
—, membrane-bound   95
— in SDI   127
atrophy, cystic   59
—, senile   59
— of the mammary gland   59, 64, 168, 169
atypical papillary proliferation   64
axodendritic synapsis   126
axonal dystrophy   116, 132

B-cells (chief cells)   13, 14, 15, 16, 178, 208
Babinski signs   106

Subject Index

basal cells 166
basement membrane, formation 166
basket cells see myothelia
benign dysplasias of the mammary gland 58
— — — —, etiology *63*
— — — —, pathogenesis *63*
benign lymphoepithelial lesion 181
β-glucuronidase 45
biscyclohexanone oxalyldihydrazone (CUPRIZONE) *136*
bone in mixed tumors of the salivary gland type 193
Border disease of sheep *135*
brain lipids in SDI *127*
— weight in SDI 110
budding stage 4
bud-shaped primordia 4

Calciferol 56
calcification, interstitial 57
—, intra-alveolar 56
— of the mammary gland *56*
calciphylactic reactions of the mammary gland 56
calcium in milk 55, 56
— in serum 56
Canavan's spongy degeneration 91, 92
— sclerosis (disease) 91, 92
carbohydrate catabolism in mammary gland 8
carcinoma, clear-cell 208
—, gelatinous 208
—, lobular 60
—, scirrhous 29, 208
—, solid 29, 205, 213
— of mammary gland 13, 14, 27, 30, 37, 54, *205*, 213
— of the ovary 64
"carcino-chondro-osteoid-sarcoma" 202
carcino-osteoid-sarcoma 203
carcino-sarcoma *208*, 213
cartilage 191, 193, 198, 202, 203, 211
casein synthesis 8, 9, 35
castration 5, 16, 17, 19, 26, 35, 38, 39, 50, 52, 53, 54, 57, 67
ceramine dihexoside in SDI 128
cerebral lipidoses 93
cerebrosides 127, 128
cerebrospinal fluid in SDI 109
ceroid pigment 170, 198, 211
Chiari-Frommel syndrome *65*
chief cells (B-cells) 13

chlorpromazine 66
cholesterol *173*
— in SDI 127
chondroblasts in malignant mixed tumors 200
chondro-carcinoma 211
chondroid syringoma of skin 192
chondroitin-sulphate 190
chondroitin-4-sulphate 190
chondroma, epithelial 211
chondro-osteoid-sarcoma 200, 201
choriogonadotropic hormones 63
chorion epithelioma 66
chorioretinal atrophy 107
Christensen-Krabbe disease 92
chromophobe adenoma of the pituitary 66
chronaxies, neuromuscular 109
—, vestibular 109
"chronic edema disease of the brain" *139*
chronic cystic mastopathy *64*
— mastopathy 174, 178
circumcanalicular fibrosis 23
circumductal mastitis 61
circumlobular connective tissue *60*
circumscribed hyperplasia of myothelia 176
circumtubular connective tissue 23
clasmatodendrosis 93
"clear cells" (Feyrter) 12, 13, 16
clear-cell carcinoma 208
— epithelioma 194
— hidradenoma 198
— myoepithelioma 198, 205
— organ of the mammary gland 190, 208
"clear epithelia" (GRAUMANN) 12
clonic spasms 106
clonus 106
congestion of secretion 14, 56
connective tissue in the mammary gland *60*
— — during hormone action, histochemistry 27
contraceptive hormones 66, 67
— therapy 64, 66, 67
contraction of myothelia 165
convulsions 106, 108
cord-shaped hyperplasia *176*
corpus luteum hormone 23, 37
cortisol 8, 43, 49, 66
cortisone 37, 50, 51, 57

cryptococcus polysaccharide implantation 139
Cuprizone intoxication 95, 133, *136*, 137, 139
Cushing's disease 62, 64, 66
cyanide encephalopathy 94, 97
— poisoning 94, 97
cylindroma (adenoid cystic carcinoma) 189, 190, *192*, 199, 211
cylindroma-like formations 181
cylindromatous transformation 179
cyproterone acetate 6
cystadenoma, papillary 60, *64*
cystadenosis 59
cystic atrophia 59
— hyperplasia 54
cystin-lysinuria 133, 134
cystosarcoma phyllodes 187
cysts, formation in mammary gland 17, 19, 21, 23, 26, 44, 51, 54, 58, 59, 60, 64, 65

decerebrate state 107, 108
decorticate state 107, 108
deformities of the mammary gland, induction by hormones 4
dégénérescence spongieuse familiale 91
desoxycorticosterone acetate (DOCA) 19, 26, 38, 49
development of the duct system, inhibition by progesterone 6
— of the mammary gland, phases *3*
diethylstilboestrol 40
diffuse cerebral sclerosis of the degenerative type (WOLMAN) 138
— hyperplasia of myothelia *178*
diffuse Form der spongiösen Dystrophien des Nervensystems — Typ Canavan 91
digitalis 64
dihydronicotinamide adenine dinucleotide diaphorase in SDI 127
dihydrotachysterol (AT 10) *54*, 56
dimorphism, sexual 4
—, sexual, intrauterine *4*
disgerminoma 64
DNA 45
DNA-synthesis in mammary gland 8, 9, 10, 24, 37
DOCA (desoxycorticosterone acetate) 19, 26, 38, 49
Donnan equilibrium 142

duct system, inhibition of development by progesterone 6
dysplasias, benign, of the mammary gland *58*
—, —, — —, etiology *63*
—, —, — —, pathogenesis *63*
dysregulation, endocrine 59
dystrophies of the cerebral transport structures 93, 97
dystrophy, infantile, and encephalopathy *134*

early infantile cerebral sclerosis 91
— — "diffuse sclerosis" of the brain 91
"early ripening" 63
eccrine acrospiroma 197
— spiradenoma 194
edema, cerebral 93, 94, *95*, 139
—, cytotoxic 96, *139*
—, histotoxic 95
—, perifocal 95, 96
—, vasogenic type 95, 139
—, vasoglial type 139
EEG in SDI 109
elastosis 63
electrolytes in SDI 127
electromyogram in SDI 109
electroretinogram in SDI 109
Emden-Meyerhof cycle 8
encephalopathy in infantile dystrophy *134*
endemic goitre 54
endocrine dysregulation 59
— regulatory mechanisms, classification 2
epimyothelial islands *181*, 211
— proliferation 59
epinephrine 19
epithelial chondroma 211
— myoma 211
— proliferation 26
epitheliosis 59, 60
epitheliotic intralobular proliferation of epithelium 60
eponyms for "Spongy degeneration of the CNS in infancy" *91*
ethionine 56
ethanol phosphatides 128
euthyroidism 54
experimental cyanide encephalopathy 94
— Kuru 94
— spongy encephalopathies *135*
extradural balloon compression 139

familial glycinosis (hyperglycinia) 133, 134
— idiocy with spongy degeneration of the CNS 91
— — — — of the neuraxis 91
— nonpuerperal galactorrhoe 66
— spongy degeneration of the brain 91
fat deposition in myothelia *173*
— tissue, regulating influence on glandular growth 8
fatty acids, unsaturated 171
female primordium 5
fibroadenoma 30, 61, 64, 175, 185, 203
fibroadenomatosis 59
—, simple 64
fibroma 211
fibrocystic mastopathy 13, 19, 27, 59, 60, 61, 63
fibrosing adenosis of the mammary gland *182*, 211
fibrosis, circumcanalicular 23
— of mammary gland 29, 30, 44, 59
fluorocytes 170, 171
follicular hormone 17, 23, 63
Forbes-Albright syndrome 66
funicular myelosis 93
fructose-1-phosphate aldolase in serum 192

galactic band 3
galactin, see prolactin
galactinokinetic effect 45
galactolipids 127
galactopoesis *41*, 44
galactopoetic effect 48
galactorrhoea 65
— accompanied by disorders of thyroid function 66
— after castration 67
—, familial, nonpuerperal 66
— in tumours of the pituitary and brain discorders 66
galactostasis 46, 48, 63
galactosuria 133
gangliosides 128
Gaucher's disease 104
gelatinous carcinoma of the mammary gland 208
gemistocytic astrocytosis 131
gestagenous steroids 6
glandular growth, regulating influence on 8
— primordium 3

glandular structure of the mammary, gland growth 2
glial dystrophies *97*
glio-neuronal dystrophies *97*
glio-vasal dystrophies *97*
glucocorticoids 57
glucose-6-phosphatase 30, 31
glucose-6-phosphate-dehydrogenase 8, 31
glycinosis, familial (hyperglycinia) 133, 134
glycogen 208
— content of myothelia in mixed tumors 191
— -rich reticulated adenoma (Feyrter) 197, 198
— storage of myothelia *168*
glycolipids 128
Gonadectomy 5, 49
gonadotropin 65
granulosa-cell tumour 64
growth hormone (STH) 19, 20, 26, 37, 38, 43, 45, 51, 53, 54, 56, 65, 66
guanine 9
gynaecomastia 11, 12, 13, 15, 17, 21, 61, *64*, 66, 176
—, lobular 64
—, tubular 64
— of puberty 63

haemoblastosis 61
haemopoiesis in the mantle tissue of mammary gland 61
Hallervorden-Spatz disease 132
Held's space 114
hemochromatosis 133
hemoglobin 173
hepatic encephalopathies *133*, 142, 147
hepato-cerebral degeneration 133
— disease 93, 97
hexoestrol 26
hidradenoma, clear cell 198
—, papillary, of the vulva 188
—, solid 194
—, solid-cystic 197
hillock-shaped primordia 4
hirsutism 65
histochemical enzyme model of the mammary gland *30*
histotoxic edema 95
homocystinuria 133, 134
Hurler's disease 144
hyaluronic acid 190

hyalinisation of mantle tissue 27
hyalinosis 63
hydrazine monoamino oxidase inhibitors (Iproniazid) 133, *136*
hydrocortisol acetate 49
hydrocortisone acetate 50
hyperacusis 107
hyperammonemia 133, 134
hyperglycinia (familial glycinosis) 133, 134
hyperoestrogenism and fibrocystic mastopathy 65
hyperplasia, cord-shaped of myothelia 176
—, cystic 54
—, diffuse of myothelia *178*
—, lobular, adenomatous 59
— of the lobules of the mammary gland 59
— mammary gland 17, 63
— of myothelia, intracanalicular 183
— of myothelia, rosette-shaped *176*, 180
hyperplasie myoide 182
hyperthyroidism 53, 66
hypertrophy, lobular 59
—, virginal 61, 64
hypogenitalism 65
hypophysectomy 8, 16, 17, 19, 24, 26, 27, 38, 39, 44, 50, 52, 53, 54
hypoplasia of the genitals 65
— of the mammary gland 64
hypothyroidism 53, 54, 66

Idiotie amaurotique atypique 91
— familiale avec dégénérescence spongieuse du névraxe 91
inborn errors of amino acid metabolism 132, *133*, 146
inclusions, metaplasmatic 15
—, paraplasmatic 14
indirect mammotropic effect 57
individual primordia 3, 4
induction of deformities of the mammary gland by hormones 4
infantile dystrophy and encephalopathy *134*
— Wernicke's syndrome 92
INH-induced encephalopathy 94, 97, 133, *136*, 137, 139, 140, 141, 147, 148
insulin *56*, 57
intercellular substances 213
— — in malignant mixed tumors 199
interstitial calcification 57

intra-alveolar calcification 56
intracanalicular adenoma 64
— hyperplasia of myothelia 183
— papilloma of mammary gland 64, 186
intracystic papilloma 59
intralobular connective tissue *60*
— proliferation of epithelium 60
intrauterine sexual dimorphism *4*
involution 30, 32, 59
iodine deficiency 54
ionic pump 142, 148
ions, active transport 95
Iproniazid-induced encephalopathy 133, *136*
islands, epimyothelial *181*

Jakob-Creuzfeld disease 94, 97, 137, 144
juvenile cerebro-retinal degeneration 130

koilomastia 5
Krabbe's globoid cell leukodystrophy 129
— type of diffuse sclerosis 98
Krebs citric cycle 141
Kuru, experimental 94

lactation 9, 10, 14, 29, 30, 32, 33, 46, 48, 54, 56, 60, 63, 65, 165
—, abnormal 65
— (electron microscopy) 33
— hormone, see prolactin
lactiferous ducts (tubules) 9, 10, 11, 13, 16, 17, 19, 20, 27, 39, 40, 45, 48, 52, 59, 60
— —, ramification 7
lactogen, see prolactin
lactogenesis 35, 37
lactopoesis *41*, 44
lactose 67
lamprocytes 168, 169
late infantile neuroaxonal dystrophy 132
Leigh's disease 138
leiomyoma of the mammary gland 187
leiomyosarcoma 205
"let-down" of milk 165
leukodystrophy 91, 93
—, sudanophilic 131
leukoencephalitis 93
lipidosis 91
—, cerebral 93

lipids in brain in SDI *127*
lipofuscin 198, 208, 211
— in myothelia *170*
lipomatosis of the glandular body 63
lobular adenomatous hyperplasia 59
— carcinoma 60
— gynaecomastia 64
— hypertrophia 59
lobuloalveolar growth factor 24
Lowe's syndrome *133*, 134
luteotropin, see prolactin
lymphoid-myo-epithelial sialadenitis 182

macromastia 60, 61, 62, 63, *64*
—, angiomesenchymal form 63
— due to hormone-active tumours of the ovary 64
— in Cushing's disease 62
— of pregnancy 65
— of puberty 61, 63
maladie oedémateuse progressive cérébrale de la première enfance 91
male primordium 5
malic dehydrogenase activity in SDI 110
malignant adeno-myothelioma 203
— mixed tumors of the salivary gland type 199
malnutrition 65
mamma see mammary gland
mammary cancer 205
mammary gland, action of sex hormones on 2
— —, adenoma 188
— —, atrophy 64, 168
— —, autoradiography *8*
— —, benign dysplasias 58
— —, — —, etiology 63
— —, — —, pathogenesis 63
— —, — tumors, containing myothelia 185
— —, biochemistry *8*
— —, biometry of normal glandular growth *7*
— —, calcification *56*
— —, calciphylactic reactions *56*
— —, carcinoma 205, 213
— —, carcino-sarcoma 208
— —, circumlobular connective tissue 60
— —, connective tissue 60
— —, cysts 17, 19, 21, 23, 26, 44, 51, 54, 58, 59, 60, 64, 65

mammary gland, cytomorphology *7*
— —, deformities, induced by hormones 4, 5
— —, determination of total surface *7*
— —, development *3*
— —, —, dependancy on hormones *4*
— —, — after castration by X-rays 5
— —, — during pregnancy and lactation 32
— —, dimorphous histogenesis 5
— —, dysplasia 2
— —, effect of experimental administration of hormones 16
— —, electron-microscopy *13*
— —, — of hormonally stimulated gland *32*
— —, embryology *3*
— —, endocrinology 2
— —, epithelial cells of A-type 178
— —, epithelial cells of B-type 178
— —, epithelial proliferations 26
— —, fibroadenoma 175, 185
— —, fibrocystic mastopathy 13, 19, 27, 59, 60, 61, 63
— —, fibrosing adenosis *182*
— —, fibrosis 29, 30, 44, 59
— —, formation of cysts 17, 19, 21, 23, 26, 44, 51, 54, 58, 59, 60, 64, 65
— —, galactorrhoea 65
— —, gelatinous carcinoma 208
— —, growth *7*
— —, growth of glandular structure 2
— —, gynaecomastia 11, 12, 13, 15, 17, 21, 61, *64*, 66
— —, gynaecomastia of puberty 63
— —, histochemical enzyme model 30
— —, histochemistry of connective tissue 27
— —, histometry *8*
— —, hormonal regulation of growth 2
— —, hormonal regulation of metabolism 2
— —, hyperplasia 17, 63
— —, hypoplasia 64
— —, intracanalicular papilloma 186
— —, intralobular connective tissue 60
— —, leiomyoma 187
— —, macromastia 60, 61, 62, 63, *64*
— —, — of puberty 61, 63

mammary gland, malignant mixed tumors *199*
— —, mantle tissue *60*
— —, mastopathy 29
— —, micromastia 5
— —, morphology of proliferating epithelium *11*
— —, myoma 200
— —, nucleic acid synthesis *8*
— —, papillary proliferations 21
— —, pathomorphology 2
— —, — of the lobules *58*
— —, phases of development 3
— —, — — (BALINSKY) 4
— —, progressive changes of the lobules *59*
— —, protein synthesis *8*
— —, quantitative morphology 2
— —, regressive changes of the lobules *59*
— —, sarcomas *200*
— —, scirrhous carcinoma 208
— —, secretory function 2
— —, vascularization 26
— —, virginal hypertrophy 61, *64*
"mammogen C" 40
mammotropic effect, indirect 57
— substances *8*
mammotropin, see prolactin
— of the child 63
mantle tissue 27, 29, *60*, *64*
— —, oedematous swelling 60
— —, proliferation 60
Maple syrup urine disease 133, 134
masculinization 5
mast cells 29
mastitis, circumductal (periductal) 61
— in adolescence 63
mastodynia 60, 61, *64*
mastopathy 29
—, chronic, cystic *64*
—, fibrocystic 13, 19, 27, 59, 60, 61, 63
—, proliferating 54, 176, 181, 182
mazoplasia *64*
membrane-bound ATP-ase 95
metachromatic leukodystrophy 129, 144
metamorphosis of lobules, combined 60
metaplasia 58, 59
methionine sulfoximine 94, *137*
micromastia 5
Mikulicz's disease 181
miliary tuberculosis 61

milk, calcium content 55, 56
— ejection reflex 45
"milk let down" 45, 165
"milk let down factor" 45
milk-line 3
—, mineral content 54
— ridge 3, 4
— secretion 41
milk-streak 3
mineral content of milk 55
mitosis index in the primordium 4
mixed tumors, glycogen content of myothelia *191*
— — of the salivary gland type 189, *190*, 211
— — — — —, malignant *199*, 211
monoamine oxydase inhibitors 141
monosialo-gangliosides $g_{4,5,6}$ 128
mucopolysaccharides, acid 29, 63
—, neutral 63
— in connective tissue in mammary gland 27
mucus 190, 191, 193
—, epithelial 190
—, mesenchymal (myxomatous) 190, 191
myelin deficit in other spongy encephalopathies *144*
— destruction in SDI *143*
myoadenoma 188
myoepithelial cells (myoepithelium) 10, 11, 13, 14, 15, 30, 31, 33, 45, 46, 47, 48, 57, 59, *161*
myoepithelioma 194
—, clear-cell 205
myofibrils in myothelia 178, 208, 211
Myoma 211
—, epithelial 211
— of the mammary gland 200
myo-carcinoma 211
myothelia (myoepithelial cells) 10, 11, 13, 14, 15, 30, 31, 33, 45, 46, 47, 48, 57, 59, *161*
—, ability of contraction 165
—, alkaline phosphatase activity 166
—, argyrophily 164
—, benign tumors *184*
—, biochemistry *165*
—, carcino-sarcomas *208*
—, circumscribed proliferation *176*
—, cord-shaped hyperplasia *176*
—, development *164*
—, diffuse hyperplasia *178*
—, electronmicroscopie investigations 48
—, epimyothelial islands *181*

Subject Index

myothella, fat deposition *173*
—, function *165*
—, glycogen content in mixed tumors 191
—, glykogen storage *168*
—, histology *164*
—, hyperplasia *176*
—, intracanalicular hyperplasia *183*
—, malignant tumors *199*
—, myofibrils *178, 208*
—, normal shape *162*
—, occurrence *162*
—, pigment deposition *170*
—, pumping-effect 165
—, regressive changes *167*
—, rosette-shaped hyperplasia *176*
—, transport-function 166
—, uptake of water *167*
— in carcinomas of the mammary gland *205*
— cases of atrophy *175*
— fibrosing adenosis of the mammary gland *182*
— of the excretory ducts 164, 165
— secretory glands 164
myothelioma 211
myotonia congenita 129
myxoedema 54

neuroaxonal dystrophy 93, 132
— —, late infantile 132
neuromuscular chronaxies in SDI 109
Niemann-Pick's disease 93, 104, 144
nipple, adenoma 187
Nissl's acute cell disease 97
nodular hidradenoma 194
nucleic acid synthesis in mammary gland 8
5-nucleotidase 31
nystagmus 107

Oasthouse urine disease 133
Ödemkrankheit des ZNS im frühen Kindesalter 91
Oedema lakes 27
Oestradiol 5, 6, 9, 40, 49
— benzoate 17, 24, 26, 40
— dipropionate 17
— propionate 17, 19
Oestrogen 5, 7, 9, 10, 11, 12, 13, 15, *16, 24*, 29, 31, 34, 35, 37, 38, 39, 44, 51, 53, 54, 56, 57, 61, 63, 64
— actions, biochemical mechanisms *37*
— -progesteron ratio in experiments 27
— -progesterone-treatment combined 41

oestrone 40, 53, 54
oncogenic transformation 174
opisthotonus 107
optic atrophy 107
oral contraceptive therapy 64, 66, 67
osteoblasts in malignant mixed tumors 200
osteoid sarcoma 202
osteoid-osteo-sarcoma 203, 211
Ouabain intoxication 94, 97, 133, *136*
ovarian insufficiency 65
ovarectomy 7, 27, 56
Oxytocin *45*, 165
Oxytocinase 46

pallidonigral neuro-axonal dystrophy 108
papillary adenosis of the lobules 60
— — of the tubular system 60
— cystadenoma 60, *64*
— hidradenoma of the vulva 188
— proliferations 21
— syringadenoma 188
padilloma, intracanalicular, of mammary gland 64, 186
—, intracystic 59
papillomas of the lactiferous ducts 60, 187
papillomatosis 59
parathyroid hormone *54*
parathyreoidectomy 26, 55, 56
Parkinsonism, post-encephalitic, and galactorrhoea 66
Pelizaeus-Merzbacher disease 129
pentose-phosphate cycle 9, 31
periductal mastitis 61
perifocal edema 95
Periston infusion 8
phases of development of the mammary gland 3
phenylketonuria 133
phosphatase in SDI 110
phosphatides in SDI 127, 128
phospholipids 127
Pick's disease 93, 104, 144
pidgeon crop test *41*
pigment 211
— deposition in myothelia *170*
— in adenomas of the salivary glands 198
pinocytosis 30
pituitary, angiosarcoma 66
—, anterior lobe, extract 20, *40*
—, — —, transplants *40*

pituitary, tumors, and galactorrhoea 66
— hormones 38
— tumours, transplanted 41
pivot nipple 5
placenta 9, 63
plasma cell mastitis 61
pleomorphic adenoma 189
porto-caval encephalopathies 133
post-encephalitic Parkinsonism and galactorrhoea 66
post-partum abnormal lactation 65
— amenorrhoea 65
prednisolone 19
pregnancy 9, 10, 30, 32, 39, 40, 46, 57, 59, 60, 165
pregnandiol 64, 64
pregneninolone 23
presenile spongioform encephalopathy 135
primordia, bud-shaped 4
—, globular individual 4
—, hillock-shaped 4
—, individual 3, 4
—, supernumerary 3
primordium, female 5
—, glandular 3
—, male 5
progesterone 6, 9, 10, 19, 20, 21, 22, 23, 24, 29, 31, 35, 36, 37, 39, 40, 44, 53, 54, 56, 57, 64
progressive cerebral poliodystrophy 131
— degenerative subcortical encephalopathy 91, 98
— infantile poliodystrophy (CHRISTENSEN-KRABBE) 92, 97
— poliodystrophy 130
Progynon 17, 18, 21, 22, 25, 29, 55
Prolactin 8, 19, 20, 22, 23, 26, 31, 32, 37, 38, 39, 41, 45, 53, 54, 57, 65, 66
proliferating glandular epithelium, morphology 11
— mastopathy 176, 181, 182
proliferation circumscribed, of myothelia 176
Proluton 22, 29, 55
propylthiouracil 54
protamine-zinc-insulin 19
protein synthesis in mammary gland 8, 10, 12, 13, 37, 38
pseudobulbar palsy 108
pseudocartilage 191
"pseudoextracellular spaces" 96
psychoses 65

ptosis 107
pumping-effect of myothelia 165

ratio of oestrogen-progesteron in experiments 27
Refsum's disease 133
regressive changes of lobules of the mammary gland 59
relaxin 57
reparative gliosis 93
reserpine 66
respiratory acidosis 94, 137
rigidity 106
RNA-synthesis 38
Rosenthal fibers 129
rosettes 24
rosette-shaped hyperplasia of myothelia 176, 180

Sarcoma phyllodes 185
sarcomas of the mammary gland 200
Schilder's disease 98
Schimmelbusch's adenosis 60, 64
Scirrhous carcinoma 29, 208
sclerosing adenosis 59, 175, 183
SDI = spongy degeneration of CNS in infancy 90
—, atypical cases 130
—, biochemical aspects 127
—, clinical aspects 105
—, clinical laboratory findings 109
—, clinical symptomatology 106
—, differential diagnosis 128
—, Eponyma 91
—, etiological problems 147
—, genetic and geographic aspects 99
—, histological findings 112
—, historical aspects 98
—, infantile form 105
—, juvenile form 105, 130
—, late infantile form 105
—, localization problems 146
—, nosological aspects 130
—, pathogenesis of myelin destruction 143
—, pathogenetic aspects 138
—, pathological aspects 110
—, peripheral nerves and muscle 123
—, relationship to other spongy encephalopathies 132
—, topography of the lesions 119
—, transition to progressive poliodystrophy 130

SDI, transition to sudanophilic
    leukodystrophies *131*
—, ultrastructural findings *124*
secretory function of the mammary
    gland 2
seizures 107
selective parenchymal necrosis 95
— partial necrosis 93
senile atrophy 59
serous imbibition of cerebral tissue
    92, 93
sex hormones, action on the mammary
    gland 2, 7, 8
— —, synthesis 2
sexual dimorphism 4
— —, intrauterine *4*
sialadenitis, lymphoid-myoepithelial
    182
Sialuronic acid 190
silver nitrate implantation 139
simple fibroadenomatosis 64
Sjögren's syndrome 181
skin, benign tumors, containing
    myothelia *188*
sodium pump 142
solid adenoma 190, 198
— carcinoma 29, 205, 213
— hidradenoma 197
— cystic hidradenoma 197
somatotropin (STH) 19, 20, 26, 37, *38*,
    43, 45, 51, 53, 54, 56, 65, 66
spasms, clonic 106
—, tonic 106
spastic amaurotic axonal idiocy 132
Spasticity 106
Spiegler tumor 193
Spielmeyer-Vogt variant of
    amaurotic idiocy 130
spiradenoma, eccrine 194
spongy dystrophics, classification 97
spongy encephalopathies, experimental
    135
— degeneration of the cerebral white
    matter 91
— — of the CNS (van Bogaert-
    Bertrand type) 91
— — — in infancy, see SDI
— — of the nervous system 91
— neurodystrophies 93
— state, gliogenic type *93*
— —, neurogenic type *93*
— transformation resulting from
    loss of nervous tissue components
    94

spongy transformation without primary
    loss of neural elements 94
— type of diffuse sclerosis 91
status prespongiosus 93
— spongiosus *92*
— —, gliogenic type *93*
— —, neurogenic type *93*
STH (somatotropin) 19, 20, 26, 37, 38,
    43, 45, 51, 53, 54, 56, 65, 66
steroids 66
stilboestrol 8, 21
strabismus 107
subacute combined degeneration of
    the spinal cord 94
— necrotizing encephalomyelopathy
    92, 97
— necrotizing encephalopathy 97
succinic dehydrogenase in SDI 127
succinodehydrogenase 31, 45
sucking pressure 45
sudanophilic leukodystrophies 129,
    131, 133, 134
superficial cells 15
supernumerary primordia 3
supporting connective tissue in the
    mammary gland *60, 62*
syntocinon 47
syringadenoma, papillary 188
syringoma 188
—, chondroid, of skin 192

tapetoretinal degeneration 107
Tay-Sachs disease 104, 128
testosterone 21, *50*, 54
testosteron-propionate 5
TET-edema 96, 97
— intoxication 95, 133, *135*, 136, 137,
    139, 140, 141, 147, 148
thiamine deficiency 94
thyroidectomy 19, 24, 26, 53, 54, 56
thyroid function, disorders, and
    galactorrhoea 66
thyrotoxicosis 54
thyroxin 19, 20, *53*, 57
tonic attacks 108
— extensor spasms 107
— reflex movements 107
— spasms 106
— tendon reflexes 107
toxic encephalopathies 132
transitional types of cells 191
transformation, cylindromatous 179
transport, active, of ions 95
— -function of myothelia 166

transport structures, dystrophies 93
triethylin (TET) 95, 133
triple operation 16, 37, 38, 39, 43
trisialo-ganglioside G_1 128
tuberculosis, miliary 61
tubular gynaecomastia 64
— -solid adenoma (FEYRTER) 190, 198
turban tumor 194
tyrosinemia 133

unsaturated fatty acidys 172
uridine 9

Van Wyk-Grumbach syndrome 66
vascularization of the mammary gland 26

vasogenic edema 95, 96
vestibular chronaxies in SDI 109
virginal hypertrophy 61, 64

wallerian degeneration 123
water content of brain tissue in SDI 127
Wilson's disease 93
Werdnig-Hoffmann's disease 129
Wernicke's syndrome, infantile 92
— tissue syndrome 97
"witch's milk" 60, 62, 63
Wolff's duct 4

Zondeck-Bromberg-Rozin syndrome 66

Index to Volumes 37—53
Ergebnisse der allgemeinen Pathologie und pathologischen Anatomie

Volume 37

L. H. Kettler, Parenchymschädigungen der Leber 1
G. Axhausen, Die Ernährungsunterbrechungen am Knochen 207
G. Kahlau, Der Lungenkrebs 258

Volume 38

P. Gedigk, Die funktionelle Bedeutung des Eisenpigmentes 1
E. Lindner, Der elektronenmikroskopische Nachweis von Eisen im Gewebe . . . 46
R. Gieseking, Aufnahme und Ablagerung von Fremdstoffen in der Lunge nach elektronenoptischen Untersuchungen 92
L. J. Rather, The significance of nuclear size in physiological and pathological processes 127

Volume 39

Dominos de Paola und J. Rodrigues Da Silva, Histopathologie der Kala-Azar . 1
J. Schoenmackers, Technik der postmortalen Angiographie mit Berücksichtigung verwandter Methoden postmortaler Gefäßdarstellung 53
W. Florange, Anatomie und Pathologie der Arteria bronchialis 152
G. Zbinden, Biochemische, funktionelle und morphologische Organveränderungen durch Beeinflussung des 5-Hydroxytryptamin-Stoffwechsels 225

Volume 40

H. A. Hienz, Die Pfaundler-Hurlersche Krankheit 1
E. W. Chick, H. J. Peters, J. F. Denton und W. D. Boring, Die Nordamerikanische Blastomykose 34
A. Fialho, Die pathologische Anatomie der Südamerikanischen Blastomykose (Lutzsche Krankheit) 99
O. Fresen, Orthologie und Pathologie der heterotopen Hämopoese 139

Volume 41

G. Hieronymi, Über den durch das Alter bedingten Formwandel menschlicher Lungen 1
F. Gloor, Die doppelseitige chronische nicht-obstruktive interstitielle Nephritis . . 63
H. Selye, Nonspecific Resistance 208

Volume 42

H.-D. Bergeder, Grundlagen der biologischen Strahlenwirkung und Strahlenschäden 1
N. Schümmelfder, Die experimentelle Strahlenschädigung des Zentralnervensystems 34

A. Georgii, Die Virusätiologie der Mäuseleukämien 93
C. A. Salvatore, The Significance of the Myometrial Cell Hypertrophy during Pregnancy (Critical Review) 148

Volume 43

A. Studer und K. Reber, Der Tierversuch in der Arterioskleroseforschung . . . 1
A.-M. Novi, Die subvalvuläre Aortenstenose 88
W. Hartung, Untersuchungsmethoden an Lungen und Thorax zur postmortalen Analyse der Atmungsfunktion 121

Volume 44

G. Schneider, Über die Pathogenese der Amyloidose. Immunologische, histochemische und morphologische Untersuchungen 1
G. Seifert, Die Sekretionsstörungen (Dyschylien) der Speicheldrüsen 103
Volume 45
A. Engström, Der Einfluß strahlender Energie auf das Knochengewebe 1
G. Liebaldt, Das „Kleeblatt"-Schädel-Syndrom, als Beitrag zur formalen Genese der Entwicklungsstörungen des Schädeldaches 23
R. Böhmig, Mastopathia fibrosa cystica, ihre Epithelproliferationen und deren Beziehungen zum Carcinom 39

Volume 46

F. J. Lang und J. Thurner, Arthropathia deformans coxae (Coxarthrose, Malum coxae) 1
K. A. Rosenbauer, Die granulierten Zellen am Gefäßpol der Nierenkörperchen . . 81
H. Görsch, Über die Gastritis hypertrophica gigantea (Ménétriersche Erkrankung) 156
Nachtrag zur Literatur des Beitrages „Lang und Thurner, Arthropathia deformans coxae (Coxarthrose, Malum coxae) 206

Volume 47

N. Koppang, Familiäre Glykosphingolipoidose des Hundes (Juvenile Amaurotische Idiotie) 1
H. Ch. Löliger, Ergebnisse der experimentellen Leukoseforschung beim Huhn vom Standpunkt der vergleichenden und speziellen Pathologie 44
H. J. Zschoch, Die Herz- und Gefäßkrankheiten in der Sektionsstatistik 58
H.-A. Müller, Die Chromozentren in den Leberzellkernen der Maus unter normalen und pathologischen Bedingungen 144

Volume 48

K. Hübner, Kompensatorische Hypertrophie, Wachstum und Regeneration der Rattenniere 1
H. Görsch, Die Neuroblastome des Olfactorius 81
W. Wöckel, Die Infektion mit Pseudomonas aeruginosa (Bacterium pyocyaneum) 102
Volume 49
G. E. Schubert, Die pathologische Anatomie des akuten Nierenversagens 1
W. D. Walther, Tierexperimentelle intravitale und postmortale Untersuchungen der normalen Niere, der postischämischen Nephrose und der Crushniere 113

W. REMMELE, Die Osteopoikilie: Klinik, pathologische Anatomie, Differentialdiagnose 182
G. W. DOMINOK, Der alternsbedingte Wandel des feingeweblichen Bildes menschlicher Knochen 229

Volume 50

R. POCHE und H. ALTENKÄMPER, Vergleichende Untersuchungen über die Altersverteilung der Sterbefälle der allgemeinen Bevölkerung und der Obduktionsfälle des Pathologischen Institutes in Düsseldorf von 1908—1963 1
R. POCHE und U. HOFFMANN, Über die allgemeine Krebshäufigkeit und die Altersverteilung einzelner Organkrebse in Düsseldorf von 1908—1964 26
H. MÜNTEFERING und G. KAISER, Die Mißbildungen im Obduktionsgut des Pathologischen Instituts der Universität Düsseldorf in den Jahren 1929—1939 und 1952—1965 63
W. GUSEK, Neue Befunde zur Morphologie und Funktion der Epiphysis cerebri . . 104

Current Topics in Pathology

Volume 51

K. BENIRSCHKE, Spontaneous Chimerism in Mammals: A Critical Review 1
P. J. FITZGERALD, B. CAROL, Quantitative Autoradiography: Statistical Study of the Variance, Error and Sensitivity of the Labeling Index (Thymidine-H^3 and DNA Synthesis) 62
W. REMMELE, A. HINRICHS, Renal Siderosis. Morphology, Etiology, Pathogenesis and Differential Diagnosis. With Special Reference to Traumatic Hemolytic Anemia 97
M. MARIN-PADILLA, Morphogenesis of Anencephaly and Related Malformations . . 145
G. A. PADGETT, J. M. HOLLAND, W. C. DAVIS, J. B. HENSON, The Chediak-Higashi Syndrome: A Comparative Review 175

Volume 52

Z. LOJDA, P. FRIČ, J. JODL, V. CHEMELÍK, Cytochemistry of the Human Jejunal Mucosa in the Norm and in Malabsorption Syndrome 1
M. WANKE, Experimental Acute Pancreatitis 64
J. WIENER, Ultrastructural Aspects of Delayed Hypersensitivity 143

Volume 53

R. BÄSSLER, The Morphology of Hormone Induced Structural Changes in the Female Breast 1
K. JELLINGER, F. SEITELBERGER, Spongy Degeneration of the Central Nervous System in Infancy 90
H. HAMPERL, The Myothelia (Myoepithelial Cells). Normal State; Regressive Changes; Hyperplasia; Tumors) 161

Current Topics in Pathology

Ergebnisse der Pathologie

Reprint from   Vol. 53

The Morphology of Hormone Induced Structural Changes in the Female Breast

R. Bässler

With 26 Figures

Springer-Verlag Berlin · Heidelberg · New York 1970

Current Topics in Pathology

Ergebnisse der Pathologie

Reprint from **Vol. 53**

Spongy Degeneration of the Central Nervous System in Infancy

K. Jellinger, F. Seitelberger

With 15 Figures

Springer-Verlag Berlin · Heidelberg · New York 1970

Current Topics in Pathology

Ergebnisse der Pathologie

Reprint from **Vol. 53**

The Myothelia (Myoepithelial Cells)

Normal State; Regressive Changes; Hyperplasia; Tumors

H. Hamperl

With 29 Figures

Springer-Verlag Berlin · Heidelberg · New York 1970

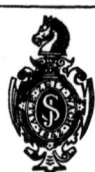

SPRINGER-VERLAG
BERLIN · HEIDELBERG · NEW YORK

J. Gershon–Cohen
Atlas of Mammography

By Jacob Gershon-Cohen, M. D., D. Sc. (Med.), Professor of Radiologic Research, Temple University Medical School, Philadelphia, PA; Director Emeritus, Division of Radiology, Albert Einstein Medical Center, Philadelphia, PA; Assistant Professor of Radiology, University of Pennsylvania School of Medecine, Division of Graduate Medicine; Consultant radiologist to various hospitals in the Philadelphia area

With 300 figures
Approx. 280 pages
Due September 1970
Cloth DM 96,—
US $ 26.00

This Atlas of Mammography acquaints the reader with roentgenography of all phases of breast development, from normalcy to the many forms of disease. It is illustrated with 300 roentgenograms gleaned meticulously from some 50,000 collected by the author during 30 years of mammographic study. The preferred technique is described, and the proper training of radiologic technicians emphasized. When cancers are discussed, it is noteworthy that every one was verified by histologic examination. It is felt that no other mammographic atlas has the foundation upon which this book has been built.

The dysplasias, singly and in various combinations — the so-called mastopathies — are categorized and illustrated with special clarity. All cases were confirmed by biopsy.

■ **Prospectus on request**

Contents: Introduction. — Some Pertinent Remarks on Histology of the Breast. — Technique. — The Normal Breast. — The Dysplasias. — Differential X-ray Diagnosis of Benign Breast Lesions. — Cancer of the Breast. — Miscellaneous. — Medico-Legal Implications. — Suggested Reading. — Subject Index.

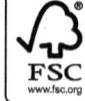
MIX
Papier aus verantwortungsvollen Quellen
Paper from responsible sources
FSC® C105338

If you have any concerns about our products,
you can contact us on
ProductSafety@springernature.com

In case Publisher is established outside the EU,
the EU authorized representative is:
**Springer Nature Customer Service Center GmbH
Europaplatz 3, 69115 Heidelberg, Germany**

Printed by Libri Plureos GmbH
in Hamburg, Germany